Before the Storm

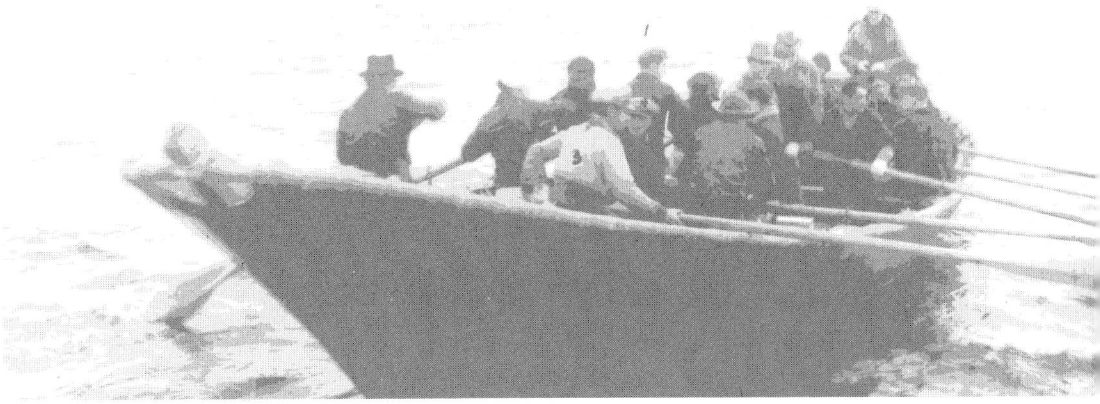

Before the Storm

A Year in the Pribilof Islands, 1941 – 1942

Fredericka Martin

Edited with supplemental material by

Raymond Hudson

UNIVERSITY OF ALASKA PRESS
FAIRBANKS

UNIVERSITY OF ALASKA PRESS
P.O. Box 756240
Fairbanks, AK 99775-6240

Library of Congress Cataloging-in-Publication Data

Martin, Fredericka I.
Before the storm broke : a year in the Pribilof Islands, 1941–1942 / Fredericka Martin ; edited with supplemental material by Raymond Hudson.
p. cm.
Originally an unpublished manuscript written in 1942 entitled The wind is no river.
Includes bibliographical references and index.
ISBN 978-1-60223-076-7 (pbk. : alk. paper)
1. Pribilof Islands (Alaska)—Description and travel. 2. Pribilof Islands (Alaska)—Social life and customs—20th century. 3. Aleuts—Alaska—Pribilof Islands—Social life and customs—20th century. 4. Pribilof Islands (Alaska)—History—20th century. 5. Natural history—Alaska—Pribilof Islands. 6. Seals (Animals)—Pribilof Islands—History—20th century. 7. Medical care—Pribilof Islands—History—20th century. 8. Martin, Fredericka I. 9. Berenberg, Samuel R. 10. Saint Paul Island (Alaska)—Biography. I. Hudson, Ray, 1943- II. Title.
F912.P9M37 2010
969'.9—dc22
2009035377

This publication was printed on acid-free paper that meets the minimum requirements for ANSI / NISO Z39.48–1992 (R2002) (Permanence of Paper for Printed Library Materials).

Publication of this book was made possible in part by a generous donation from the Aleut Corporation.

Interior layout and composition by Alcorn Publication Design.

Contents

Introduction

Raymond Hudson

The year Fredericka Martin and her husband, Samuel Berenberg, lived on St. Paul Island was a pivotal year in the history of the Pribilof Islands. It was the last year of continuous occupation of St. Paul and St. George since permanent communities had been established in the early nineteenth century under the Russian-American Company. For over a century, life had been rigidly controlled by that company and by companies and agencies the United States had designated to harvest fur seals. For the Unangan residents, conditions were those reflected in the titles of two books about the islands, *Slaves of the Harvest* and *A Century of Servitude.*[1] Less than a year after the Berenbergs arrived on June 24, 1941, Japanese forces attacked Alaska. The St. Paul and St. George people were summarily removed to evacuation camps in southeastern Alaska. As Martin foreshadowed at the conclusion of her work, although three decades of struggle remained, the evacuation irrevocably altered the lives of the Pribilof people. What they learned and saw during the years away propelled them to intensify efforts that eventually won their emancipation from the federal government.

In 1940 the Bureau of Fisheries and the Bureau of Biological Survey consolidated to form the U.S. Fish and Wildlife Service.[2] A year later the service hired Samuel Berenberg as the physician for St. Paul. The F&WS had never seen a partnership quite like that of the Berenbergs. Highly trained, experienced in public health, and uncompromising in their views on social justice, they found themselves in a corner of America where serfdom had become institutionalized. Martin's sympathies were wholly with Aleut families.

Fredericka Martin began the manuscript she titled *The Wind Is No River* in mid-February 1942, although she had started drafts as early as the autumn of 1941.[3] On May 18, 1942, she wrote John P. Harrington of the Smithsonian Institution that her decision to write the book had been prompted by a possible Japanese invasion of Alaska. Sixteen days later, the war began in Alaska. "So I have a manuscript of over four hundred pages," she wrote, "which I think is very readable and quite a skillful admixture of personal experiences with the history, the details of seal life, botany, social life of the Aleuts, etc., every aspect imaginable.

Not an easy combination. I have some gaps to fill in and some cutting to do but I was determined to have the fun of writing it no matter what happened."[4] The final manuscript totaled over five hundred pages.

Although it follows a rough chronological progression, Martin's work is not a diary. She used daily events to reflect on the social and natural history of the island. She recorded life as she observed it in her home, the hospital, and across the landscape of the island. Disturbed by what she found, she attempted to uncover the historical causes. Her investigations ranged across disciplines as she perused books and reports, interviewed residents, queried visiting experts, and initiated a vast correspondence. The task she set for herself was daunting. "I want to be ten people up here as usual," she wrote on July 9, 1941, "to encompass everything."[5] While writing, she had in mind specific people with whom she shared a professional background as a trained nurse and a political activist. Early in her manuscript, she described her methods and purpose:

> Armed with notebook and pencil I began to spend more of each day poring over the pertinent books in the island library, winning the confidence of the Aleuts I knew best, and recording the facts they chose to disclose. Simultaneously with my detective work I prepared mail for all my friends and acquaintances for the last outgoing boat of the autumn to carry south. . . . Instead of distributing random bits of the story to my friends, I ought to be writing that story for a wider public, for Americans such as I had been a few months before, to whom the name *Pribilof Islands* was strange and alien. I vowed to record the story of one small island mothered by Alaska, a realm of birds and flowers, a refuge for sea animals, and a cruel prison to the dreams and aspirations of a people whose past was forgotten and whose present was a sea-bound secret.

The F&WS library on St. Paul had a remarkable collection of original documents and early publications. There were books by Henry W. Elliott and David Starr Jordan, over a dozen volumes of the 1891 fur seal arbitration hearings, and various published reports on the fur seal industry. Most important were the daily logs kept by the government representatives from the early 1870s through the 1930s, with only a few missing years. She borrowed H. H. Bancroft's *History of Alaska* and Clarence Andrew's *The Story of Alaska*. Father Makary Baranoff, the Orthodox priest on St. Paul, allowed her access to his extensive files, and the two of them had frequent discussions on the history and conditions of the islands. Martin rummaged in the attic of the hospital and the doctor's residence as well as in dusty corners of the Company House. Among other finds, she uncovered two original letters from Elliott to the vituperative agent George Tingle.[6] Back in Washington, D.C., she consulted material in both the National Archives and the Library of Congress. Unfortunately, Martin's manuscript lacks citations for her sources. I have identified many, but some remain to be unearthed. Martin's notes herein are indicated by *F.M.* The translations from Veniaminov's *Notes on the Islands of the Unalashka District* are the unpublished ones made by Richard Henry Geoghegan that he shared with Martin. I have footnoted references to corresponding passages in the 1984 published edition.

Fredericka Imogene Martin was born June 2, 1905, in Cooperstown, New York.[7] After high school, she lived and worked with the St. Margaret Episcopalian Order of Nuns in Jersey City, New Jersey, graduating with honors from the affiliated nursing school of Christ Hospital in 1925. She then worked in hospitals in New York City. After marriage to Alexander Cohen in 1929, she began a study of Russian and Yiddish. In 1935 she visited England, Russia, and Germany and became aware of the growing threat of Fascism. Following her return to the States, she became an active member of the Medical Bureau to Aid Spanish Democracy. Initially organized to provide medical supplies, food, and clothing to the beleaguered Spanish Republic, by late 1936 the bureau was recruiting personnel to send directly to Spain. Martin volunteered in January 1937 and became part of the first American medical unit there. She was the head nurse in one hospital and later served as an administrator for six hospitals.[8] She returned to the United States at the beginning of February 1938 as part of a national speaking tour that included a representative of the Catalan government and the writer Dorothy Parker.[9] In 1939 she was invited to establish and direct a hospital in Greenbelt, Maryland, under a federally funded housing initiative created by the Resettlement Administration. During this period, her marriage to Cohen ended, and in 1940 she married Dr. Samuel Berenberg. Following their year in the Pribilof Islands, they settled in New York City. In 1944 her edited edition of Geoghegan's *Aleut Language: The Elements of Aleut Grammar* (based on Veniaminov) was published by the Department of the Interior. In 1946 she published *The Hunting of the Silver Fleece: Epic of the Fur Seal.* This was followed in 1960 by *Sea Bears: The Story of the Fur Seal.* When the marriage to Berenberg dissolved in 1950, she moved to Cuernavaca, Mexico, with nine-year-old Tobyanne. For the next forty years she made her living as a translator, a travel book writer, and an instructor at a Spanish language institute. Because of her long support for the Aleut people, she was awarded an honorary doctorate by the University of Alaska in 1986. That same year she was made an honorary lifetime citizen of St. Paul Island. She died on October 4, 1992, in Cuernavaca. In 2007, with the cooperation of the people of St. Paul Island, her daughter Tobyanne Berenberg was able to bring her ashes to the island for burial.

This book must be taken for what it is: a sensitive and critical first-person account of a significant year in the history of the Pribilof Islands by an intelligent, inquisitive, and determined writer. It is published over fifty years after it was written. During the intervening decades, the literature on Alaska during the Russian and early American periods has significantly increased, with the publication of studies and translated primary sources. Martin used what was available to her at the time, works by Henry W. Elliott, William Healy Dall, and Ivan Petroff. She accepted them as eyewitnesses and experts. Dall, for example, was one whose "testimony is unimpeachable." Elliott was "a human volcano whose brimstone and sulphur would scorch many a reputation [and] . . . shake the very foundations of government bureaus and topple bureaucrats." Her extensive use of Elliott is enhanced by personal recollections of him from Pribilof residents. Occasionally, historical and biological material she excerpted from earlier writers overwhelmed her narrative. A great deal of this has been cut for the present edition. Nevertheless, I have retained much of what she wrote about the fur seal and its centrality to life on St. Paul. Her extensive descriptions of conditions and practices surrounding the harvest of the seal document a way of life now gone. This material is historically important. Her reactions to what she saw in 1941–1942 were colored by what she understood to be the history of the islands that she was gradually unearthing. To correct her misunderstandings (and there are certainly instances where she got the history wrong) would be to undermine the basis for her outrage and lessen our appreciation for her conclusions and subsequent actions.

The greatest value in Martin's book is found in her own observations and reflections, focused primarily on conditions relative to the Native population but also on the community of government workers. She found the self-imposed isolation of the "Service families" from the larger Native community inherently unhealthy. The subservience shown by government employees toward superiors struck her as intolerable. Although her comments are frequently harsh and uncompromising, they provide insight into the workings of a bureaucratic system that dominated Native life. As with any account of a very closed society by an "outsider," insurmountable problems exist with her perceptions regarding the Aleut community. Whether supplying patients with cigarettes or suggesting measures to improve the required inspections of Aleut homes, Martin was clearly a woman from the Washington Beltway in 1941, an emissary of "civilization" to an Alaska village, an activist for social rights. Her voice was always clear and unequivocal. For example, in discussing the sanitation inspections made by the doctor and the government manager, she wrote, "But to ensure actual sanitation and cleanliness, inspection should include bedrooms to see if beds were made and the slop jars emptied and should be made at unannounced intervals." Today, of course, such intrusions into private homes would be considered outrageous if not actually criminal. Nevertheless, Martin provided illuminating contrasts between Aleut homes and those of the "white" management families:

> Despite Sam's descriptions, the first time I accompanied him I was amazed. Some kitchens looked like magazine advertisements except for the bulky coal range. They contained glass-doored dish closets, enameled modernistic cupboards, gay dishes posed ornamentally on the shelves, frilly curtains, shining oilcloth on the floor, and flowering plants on the

> windowsills. Some contained beautiful sinks, very different from the worn old ones in the homes of the officials. The gleaming enamel and chrome trimmings were ironical. Our old faucets poured out water copiously, sometimes rusty, sometimes a bit muddy, but water. Their shining spigots were only ornaments. The drain pipes were serviceable, and the soiled used water drained out into the earth under the house.

She continued this passage by describing how Aleut had tried to secure running water and how government officials had persistently raised excuses to frustrate their attempts. Martin was not a dispassionate social scientist but an ardent participant in the unique and troubling society into which the Pribilofs had evolved. When she discussed the role radio and motion pictures might play in improving English vocabulary, she pointed out a pervasive paradox. The films were paid for by proceeds from purchases made by Aleut at the Native store or canteen, but when it came to seeing the films there was a clear racial demarcation:

> [A]s long as the "whites" of the Island sit in the small gallery without paying admission, leaning back against plush seats, enjoying the movies paid for by the Aleuts who sit below on hard, backless benches, how can English become their own beloved natural language? Not until their American associates open the gates and admit the Aleuts to mingle in their society and converse with them can English be the natural speech of the Pribilofs.

Martin's portrayals of St. Paul residents and visitors bring to life the events of 1941–1942. We meet a host of local residents including Gabriel Stepetin, Metrofan Krukoff, Elary Gromoff, Anna Stepetin, Peter Kochergin, Paul Merculieff, Heretina Kochergin, and the siblings Alexandra and Ishmael Gromoff. We are given glimpses of the government workers: L. C. McMillin, Carl and Geneva Hoverson, Edward Johnston, and Doc Moore. We meet the obsessive visiting linguist John P. Harrington, and we are introduced to the aged eccentric linguist Richard Henry Geoghegan. Among those whom the Berenbergs came to most appreciate were the devoted Orthodox priest Makary Baranoff and the talented John Yatchmenev, son of the great chief Alexei Yatchmenev of Unalaska.

To heighten the immediacy of Martin's narrative, I have incorporated sidebars from her typed journal and from a few other sources. More personal and intimate than the text she produced, these excerpts bring us nearer to the village as war inexorably closed around the island. Like her narrative, the sidebars are generally but not always in chronological order. Martin addressed her book to her daughter Tobyanne, who was born during the year her parents were on the island. Martin's original introduction is found in appendix 1. Excerpts from Samuel Berenberg's remarkable 1941–1942 annual medical report are in appendix 2. An afterword summarizes events in the Pribilof Islands following World War II, with emphasis on Martin's contributions.

Whenever possible, the spelling of Aleut words has been standardized with Bergsland's *Aleut Dictionary.* I wish to thank the Alaska and Polar Regions Collection, Elmer E. Rasmuson Library, University of Alaska, Fairbanks, for permission to use the Martin texts and photographs in their collection. Bruce Parham and Diana Kodiak at the National Archives and Records Administration, Pacific Alaska Region, in Anchorage retrieved Samuel Berenberg's annual report from material in the process of being cataloged. Staff members at the Middlebury College Libraries were very helpful in providing early government documents. The book has benefited from careful readings by Betty A. Lindsay, John A. Lindsay, and Patricia Partnow. I am indebted to Marvin Collins for discussions about the early history of the Alaska Commercial Company. Special thanks to the exemplary folks at the University of Alaska Press for bringing this work to fruition: Elisabeth Dabney, Sue Mitchell, Kathy Cummins, and David Alcorn. David Hales encouraged the editing of this book and has had a tenacious belief in its historical value. Tobyanne Berenberg has been supportive of the project from the very beginning. I hope she finds the final publication a fitting tribute to her remarkable mother.

Before the Storm

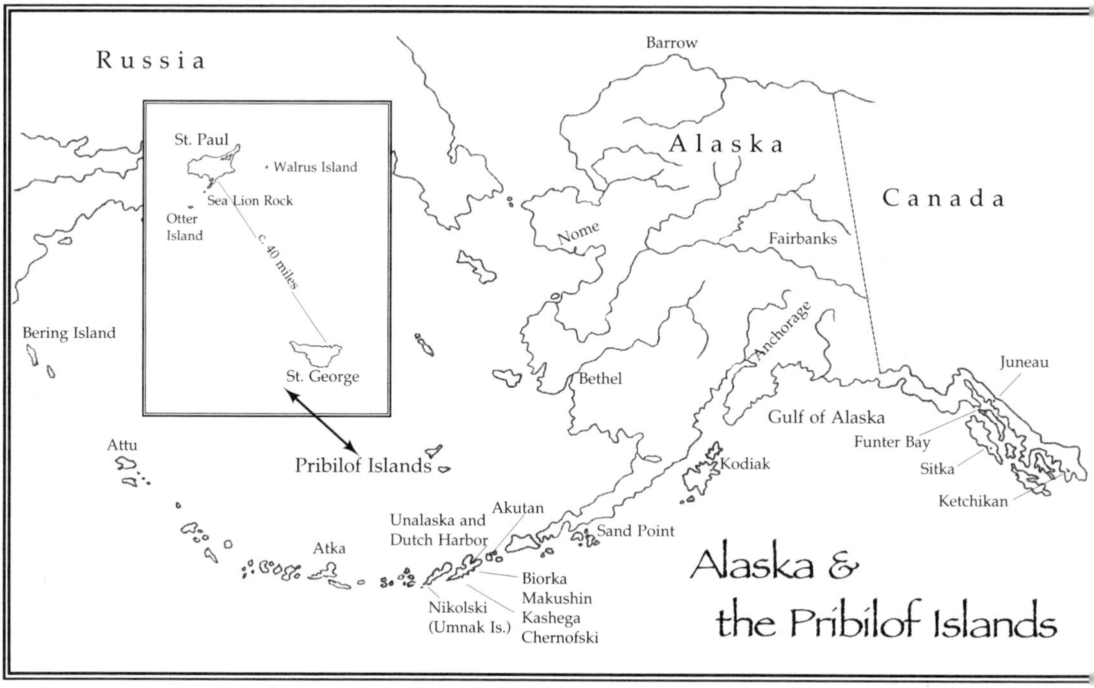

The Bering Sea and the Pribilof Islands

Chapter 1

We came to the Pribilof Islands with the last snow and the first flowers.[1] For days the sea had been stretching endlessly, alive with tiny tinsel-tipped waves. Then to our north my husband and I saw a thin shadow that grew darker and larger. Standing at the rail of the U.S. Fish and Wildlife Service motor ship *Penguin* in late June 1941, we watched the staunch lava sea-walls of St. George Island stand clear against the blue horizon, growing taller and taller in the luminous air. Beyond the high rim of the land, a plateau streaked with browns and reds, stained with black shadows, a rough sloping plain castellated with high outcroppings of tumbled rocks and tumulus hills of burned volcanic cinder, drowsed in the sun. St. Paul and St. George, the two inhabited Pribilof Islands, arrogant upstarts in the Bering Sea's smoke-grey emptiness, bear no identifying family resemblances. Unlike St. Paul, St. George was no timid nestling of earth cradled anxiously in the sea but a braggart of an island, indifferent to the pull of the tides, the endless pawing waves seeking greedily to draw it down into the depths again.

St. George lies about forty miles southeast of St. Paul. It extends for nearly twelve miles and is almost five miles across at its widest part. Its shape has been compared to a stone battle-ax. The approximately thirty-six miles of area are bound by nearly thirty miles of formidable coastline, the sheer perpendicular cliffs being broken only occasionally by sloping rocky beaches and one or two small sandy coves. The average altitude of St. George is three times that of St. Paul. Among the many volcanic cones that stud its surface is the peak of Ulakaia, over eight hundred feet in height. Although the few accessible beaches have offered little living space to the fur seals, the rocky uplands have been friendly to the little Pribilof fox. Hundreds of them lurk among the boulders, alert to seize an unwary seabird from the millions that occupy the cliff walls. Sated by kittiwake, puffin, or murre, the foxes can retire easily to natural burrows in the rumbled rocks. Instead of regular roads, the seal rookeries are connected by plank tracks laid across the rocky terrain.

Just a month before we saw St. George rise out of the sea, the name *Pribilof Islands* had sounded strange and unfamiliar to my ears, not even awakening echoes of childhood delight in Kipling's story "The White Seal."[2] The two tiny brown flecks on the blue-paper Bering Sea of our globe, initialed *P.I.*, were as unreadable to us as the dots and dashes of a strange code. As the cliffs lifted the broad tableland of the heart of St. George into view, I thought back to that afternoon when I had been loafing in a lawn chair in the scanty shade of pine trees in our Greenbelt, Maryland, garden, trying to endure patiently the hottest May afternoon I had ever known.

My husband was in the house answering the telephone. He called from the window, "How would you like to live on an island in the Bering Sea?"

His query was as refreshing as a plunge into a cold mountain stream. A vision of snow-covered islands and glistening bluish icebergs thronged with enormous polar bears floated for an instant in the shimmering sunlight.

"I would love it," was my immediate response. "When do we start?"

Two weeks later we were in Seattle on the motor ship *Penguin*. Sam was to be the resident physician for the Fish and Wildlife Service of the Department of the Interior on St. Paul, largest of the Bering Sea island group. Some household effects had been safely stored. Others had been hastily entrusted to friends. We had little baggage besides three hundred favorite books and a layette for the baby we expected in August. Officials had assured us we needed nothing but personal articles and clothing for weather no colder than the average Washington, D.C., winters. Limited shopping time forced us to rely on their assurances. A helpful hint in Seattle sent us scurrying to buy raincoats.

Our friends had bid us good-bye with faces that displayed contradictory emotions of incredulity, disapproval, and envy. Even at Pennsylvania Station in New York they had difficulty in realizing that we were actually climbing out of a placid, happy, secure rut for an adventure. They were shocked that I, a registered nurse, dared forsake the comforts of modern hospitalization and the service of an obstetrical specialist for my first baby.

It was easy to understand how they could feel slightly horrified and wistfully envious at the same time. In 1941 the shadows of war had crept so near the United States that most people were trying to close their eyes to the danger and were clinging resolutely to every outward symbol of security. That we, however, actually presumed to act as if the world were peaceful and safe to go traveling in was disturbing. We had faced the specter of war, aware of the probability that Japan might attack America. Nevertheless, we decided to try to obtain a year of close companionship in a lonely place that promised a degree of leisure unattainable by a busy physician in the States. We had balanced the emotional strain of a father serving as accoucheur against his privilege of sharing intimately the child's first year of life, a joy beyond the reach of a father occupied with the pediatric care of hundreds of Greenbelt babies. The year ahead promised new interests and

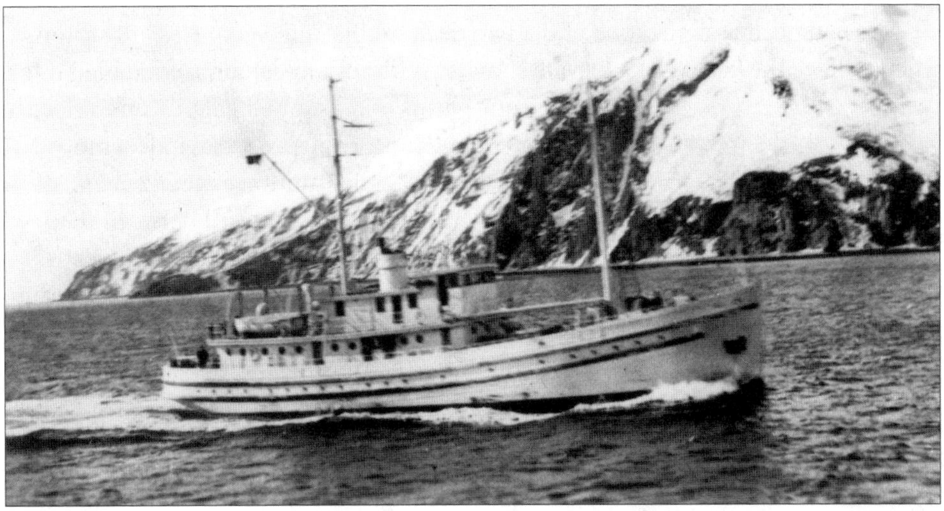

The U.S. Fish and Wildlife Service vessel *Penguin* (from the Martin Collection, USUAF210, Archives, Alaska and Polar Regions, Rasmuson Library, University of Alaska Fairbanks).

hours for study. We hoped for experiences to rest our minds and bodies from the stresses of modern life and to strengthen us for the tests Americans must face in—we dared not guess how many months.

Our first glimpse of the *Penguin* was disquieting. The pier at the end of Stoneway on Lake Union lay in dense shadow. A few dim lights outlined the ship. Pictures of toylike arctic vessels against a background of towering ice or wallowing in tumbling seas enliven travel books. Confronting the small vessel that must carry you thousands of miles north and west, across the wide stretch of the tumultuous Gulf of Alaska into the shifting windy wastes of the Bering Sea, your respect for explorers increases. In the darkness the outlines of the *Penguin,* built in 1930 especially for the Pribilof run, belied the claim of a four-hundred-ton displacement. Even the mountains of crates and boxes hiding the deck failed to add bulk to its size.[3]

As the *Penguin* pulled lazily away from the dock one minute after midnight on the fourteenth to appease marine superstition about setting out on Friday the thirteenth, we stood at the railing watching the twinkling lights of Seattle's hills, wondering about the year ahead of us. We felt like explorers setting out to open up an unknown portion of the globe. Inquiries to museums and individuals possessing reputations as authorities on Alaska had given us scant information about the Pribilofs. We knew only that the herd of two million Alaskan fur seals was bred there and that the native inhabitants were called Aleuts, were considered government wards, and attended the Russian Greek Orthodox Church. The vague answers of Washington officials of the Fish and Wildlife Service to our questions about our future home had been puzzling. Whatever life on St. Paul might be, we hoped to have the satisfaction of exploration and investigation.

We had been assigned one of the two deck cabins and were pleasantly astonished to have the luxury of a private shower. Without unpacking we tumbled into our berths and dropped happily off to sleep.

> June 14, 1941
> Sam's dismay when he saw the *Penguin* was comical. Such a small boat to be going through the perilous waters the Navy *Coastal Pilot* has been describing. I liked the boat and am hoping that its size is not going to make me lose my record as one of the blessed who is never seasick. . . .
>
> Sam asked a couple of officers who were chatting on the dock if they could assign someone to help him. They told him to ask the sailors who were busy tying on freight on the deck. All deck space seems to be covered with boxes and barrels. . . . Finally deciding he had to be a rugged individual whether he felt like it or not, Sammie began to lug the bags aboard. I managed a few parcels myself after he had made a few tries and finally saw our quarters. . . .
>
> On board it was more evident that there would be no deck space to tramp for fresh air and escape from seasickness. Every inch except for a tiny strip between the galley door and the dining salon door was crowded with supplies. I wonder how such a toy can carry so much and stay afloat. I begin to share Sam's discomfiture.

In the morning we woke to feel the pleasant rocking motion as the *Penguin* steamed steadily northward between the islands of the Inland Passage. Anxieties aroused by our nocturnal glimpse of the ship were forgotten. We surrendered to the charm of one of the most beautiful waterways in the world. For several days we spent most of our waking hours perched on sacks of potatoes or crates of oranges watching the endless variations of the shoreline. The mountainous islands that we left in our wake never palled. Out of rock and coniferous trees and silvery waterfalls nature had wrought a series of designs devoid of monotonous duplication. The sky was always dramatic with swirling, shifting masses of clouds, assuming myriads of shapes to tantalize the imagination.

The *Penguin* was alive with people.[4] Some twenty young college students were aboard, employed to blubber seal skins for the Fouke Fur Company. They swarmed noisily over the freight, wandering restlessly from one bumpy nook to another or sprawled out uncomfortably for sun baths. A group of regular employees of the fur company were more sedate and delighted mainly in painting the terrors of seasick days to come. Despite the crowding, the confines of the deck tended to separate the passengers so that many faces were nameless until we had been on St. Paul for some days. Everyone sought out a crevice in the freight and maintained squatter's rights determinedly. Aside from the frolicking of the college lads there was little social life in the daytime beyond brief conversations at mealtimes. Most of the old-timers stayed up until dawn playing cards for small stakes and retired to their berths after breakfast to sleep the day away.

Pleasant table companions were the superintendent of the islands, Edward C. Johnston; Ralph Baker, a minor official from the Washington office; and Doctor

Moore, a chemist employed by the fur company.[5] Other employees of the company and ship's officers were less interesting messmates.

Late Monday afternoon we idled up Revillagigedo Island Channel and docked at Ketchikan, the second-largest town in Alaska, to fill our water tanks.[6] Captain Knudsen, a Napoleonic blue-clad and brass-buttoned martinet, could be heard for several blocks from the pier when he learned the ship's tanks were nearly dry. "Them college boys and their baths," he bellowed in his Norwegian-flavored speech. "There'll be no more baths on this trip." As far as I know there were none except a skimpy shower I stole in desperation one miserable afternoon.

Ketchikan, derived from the Indian name *Kach Khanna,* meaning the "outstretched wings of a pinioned eagle,"[7] is located on the western side of Revillagigedo Island, named in 1793 by the English explorer George Vancouver in honor of the Viceroy of Mexico. The town clings to a long, narrow strip of shore at the base of Deer Mountain, a stern guardian peak of three thousand feet. Canneries and boats, the latter sprouting a forest of bare masts, shut the town away from the water's edge. Houses zigzag erratically up and down the slopes. Sidewalks of silvery worn planks cut the landscape with bright crisscrossing lines. The heart of the business section backs away from the main pier with fur stores and curio shops crowding numerous saloons and liquor stores. We stepped ashore to confront the blackened skeletons of buildings, where fire, that evil genie of Alaska, had wreaked great havoc in the spring.

June 14, 1941
The cook was a joy to meet. Andy, the jovial Swede. He had just come back to the ship after an absence of several years while he was securing citizenship papers. Everyone seemed glad to see him. He was bustling around the galley, preparing sandwiches at a terrific rate of speed. Morton brought in a paper that he asked Andy to sign. Andy tried to ignore the request and brandished his knife in midair as he sliced liverwurst. "I'm too busy. Have to get a nice lunch. What kind of paper anyway?" he parried.

"To prove you are not a Communist," explained Morton.

"Oh, man, I'm no Communist but why should I sign a paper to prove it," claimed Andy with a sideswiping gesture of his knife that looked really dangerous. About an hour later, just before we were to sail, poor Andy, looking very glum, was ushered into the dining salon by the captain who stood over him threateningly till poor Andy had laboriously drawn his signature. Poor Andy, all his ferocity to hide his inability to write well.

Anxious to send mail to our friends we hurried first to the post office. Too late we learned the shops had closed promptly at six. We stood longingly in front of the music store, looking at stacks of records. We had brought a portable Victrola, expecting to buy records along the way. And now we had missed that last opportunity to stock up with musical entertainment. Regretfully we thought of our many record albums left behind with friends.

Many passengers had run ashore for a last highball before being marooned on the government reservation of the islands where liquor was illegal. I had a different thirst. Very reverently I sat in the drugstore sipping, as I thought, my last chocolate soda for a year.

[Undated]
Plans for our route were changed from time to time as the weather shifted. We had expected to cut out into the open sea soon after Port Walter, and the old-timers were busy extolling the horrors of being tossed about for so many extra days. So the bad weather was a mild blessing and we continued inside until we reached Icy Straights. We passed the glacial fields at night and missed the views we had been looking forward to.

So many ports we passed that called to us. I felt extremely bad to think how close we were to Sitka when we passed Baranof Island. But Sitka, the important center of Russian settlement, is on the ocean side of the island.

The doors of the "Alaska Sportsman" were still open. Disregarding the tourist bait of garish totem poles, leather articles, poorly carved animals, many of them stamped "Made in Japan," we examined the few shelves of books. When the *Penguin*'s whistle blew warningly we staggered under our burden of volumes that included *Alaska Wild Flowers* by Ada Sharples, *Hunters of the Great North* and *Ultima Thule* by Stefansson, *Western Bird Guide* by Reed, a handsome edition of Rockwell Kent's *Wilderness,* and the *Alaska Guide* edited by Morle Colby.

I shall always remember Ketchikan because of the Indian youngster crowned with an Indian headband blazing with lurid feathers, obviously new and obviously the product of a trinket factory in the States. Decked in the imitation war bonnet, he lived his dreams striding down the quiet street, shooting off his cap pistol at imaginary foes.

For several days we loafed on up the Inland Passage. We watched legions of giant jellyfish floating past and uprooted fields of kelp smearing the water with tobacco-colored stains. Occasionally we roused from our somnolence to catch the sleek gleam of a whale as he broke slightly above the surface of the water. Our eyes followed the flight of kittiwake, albatross, and murre.

At Little Port Walter we lingered for a brief half hour to drop off freight. The nearer we approached the Gulf, the more intensive was the campaign of the old-timers to dishearten us. When we answered questions about our welfare cheerfully, the doleful prophets would mutter, "Just you wait until you get out on the Gulf."

True to the forecasts, Sam succumbed to the *Penguin*'s sportive antics soon after we passed Cape Spencer and encountered the impact of ocean waves. My immunity still withstood attack. But I felt better on deck, even at the risk of freezing to death. Of course the trunk that held warm clothes had accidentally been buried deep in the hold. Sam found the courage to join me on deck while we traveled through Kupreanoff Strait between Kodiak and Afognak islands. I kept my eyes glued to the shores of Kodiak, hoping some extrovert among the famous bears would exhibit himself on shore. Of course, one never did.

I shall never be certain whether I was the victim of the stormy seas or the combination of lukewarm, greasy food, tepid, revolting drinking water, and the constant sounds and sight of other people's illness. At any rate, feeling tired and disgusted with the increasing filth of the dining room and unable to remain on the storm-lashed decks, I retired to my bunk with *Pride and Prejudice* and finished the book I had been trying to read to the end for years.

Late Saturday afternoon we arrived at Sand Point on Popoff Island and stopped to fill the ship's tanks again. The cold dank rain seemed to fall in large masses, but everyone was eager to step ashore. The boys had crowded into the store run by the owner of the salmon cannery and carried off every scrap of candy before we could even get inside the building. Two cans of grapefruit caught my eye. The price was terrifying. As I consumed them later I felt as if every mouthful were encrusted with gold. I should hate to be poor in Alaska.

By dusk we were off on the last portion of our journey, cutting through Unimak Pass to cross the barrier of the Aleutian archipelago. In a gracious mood the reputedly termagant Bering Sea welcomed us. Less than twenty-four hours later we were off St. George.

When the *Penguin* dropped anchor in the shallow roadstead opposite the sole village, which bears the island's name, an awkward squarish boat was already being rowed rapidly toward us. The few employees of the Fish and Wildlife Service and the permanent Aleut residents were anxious to open the bulging mail sacks the seamen were heaping on the deck. For almost another twenty-four hours we swung at anchor. When the tide ran smoothly the freight was unloaded into the picturesque boats, the *baidars,* fashioned after the ancient Aleut pattern but covered with canvas instead of animal hide. The stocky, muscular Aleuts sped the heavily loaded boats easily through the waves. When the tide changed and the current pulled too strongly against the oarsmen, unloading was halted. Most of our fellow passengers went ashore to explore. Sam and I stayed aboard, contenting ourselves with reading the face of the island, watching the circling flight of curious and hungry seabirds, and keeping a lookout for the dark brown shadows in the water that were fur seals. I was so weary of the sea I wanted no brief visit to land. I wanted to stay ashore for a long, long while.

At last the final baidar was loaded and we weighed anchor for St. Paul, forty miles to the north.

St. Paul lay dark and low upon the sea wrapped in veils of twilight. The rolling lowland ran in waves beyond our range of vision. The skyline was embossed with the cones of red- and brown-tipped volcanoes. The little red hills wore the dignity and majesty of rugged mountains. The landscape was strong, serene, aloof from the clamor of the waves lashed by a wind loosed suddenly in the quiet of evening. Here was the island I was looking for, that I had dreamed of for weeks.[8]

I heard someone shout, "There's a seal drive from Reef." On our left I saw a cloud of dust and dark figures moving slowly within the haze. Shadowy men with shepherd's crooks surrounded a phantom flock.

Everyone else was eager to land. I was still cautious. The physician my husband was replacing would still be resident in our new home. I dreaded the possibility of sleeping on someone's narrow couch or staying up half the night entertaining the news-starved islanders. Sam sympathized with my fears. He sought out Mr. McMillin, the agent and caretaker in charge, who had come aboard.

"Will there be any place for us to sleep tonight if we go on shore?" Sam asked pleasantly.

"You won't be sleeping in a tent," retorted McMillin rudely and turned his back.

I excused his churlishness that night because I thought him overburdened with unloading details and supposed that he reacted to Sam's query with the thought, "Fine time to think about a bed after you've arrived." Had I known that the remark was his normal manner of speech I might have turned back with the *Penguin.*

We stayed aboard, creating a precedent. We were the first victims of the *Penguin*'s bucking bronco tactics who did not desert her at the first opportunity, even if they had to be taken over the side in the unloading net. We had an enjoyable evening listening to the yarns of the ship's officers. Andy, the cook, who had worked around the clock throughout the voyage, joined in the jollity and told the most uproarious tales about his experiences as a vaudeville comedian. As he talked he played solitaire. He finished dozens of games because at every possible opportunity he cheated. "It rests me to play quick" was his excuse.

Chapter 2

We rose early June 25. Just a month had passed between the hot afternoon when we had first heard of the Pribilofs and our first glimpse of the islands. After a relaxing sleep we were pulsing with excitement at the prospect of setting foot on St. Paul. Captain Knudsen snorted when he saw us on deck, "They won't send a boat out until after ten o'clock. They've been sitting up all night talking and are sleeping late this morning. The lights at Government House were on all night."

```
June 25, 1941
[Government House] is a fine,
large, rather nicely furnished
building that sits next to the
highest terrace of the vil-
lage and has a view over the
houses below of sea and sky.
Equipment includes such luxu-
ries as a gas refrigerator.
Unfortunately, all this com-
fort is locked up for the
greater portion of the year.
The superintendent, visiting
officials from the Washington
office, the chief employees
of the Fouke Fur Company, and
visiting heads of the same
outfit and important visitors
are taken care of during the
few weeks of the summer when
such people are here. Usually,
then, the building is open
only six weeks of the year.
We were most fortunate to be
introduced to life on St. Paul
from this comfortable station.
```

The *Penguin*'s engines came to life. Slowly we steamed about the tip of the island to Village Cove and West Landing, where the seas were calmer.

The captain's forecast was correct. Mr. McMillin was cheery enough when he arrived in a small motor dory that towed a large, flat freight barge. Soon it was loaded with freight. Carefully I climbed down the short rope ladder, waited for the barge to ride the top of the wave, jumped, and landed safely. Perched precariously on a sack of onions, clutching my typewriter, I watched the shore emerge from a blur of browns and greys and separate into low, boulder-strewn beaches and jagged cliffs. Under the latter, patches of unmelted snow gleamed whitely.

Mr. Johnston guided us across the large cement wharf to his car. Temporarily we were to stay at Government House, the official name of the summer quarters of the superintendent and other ranking officials. Crowded in a small Ford

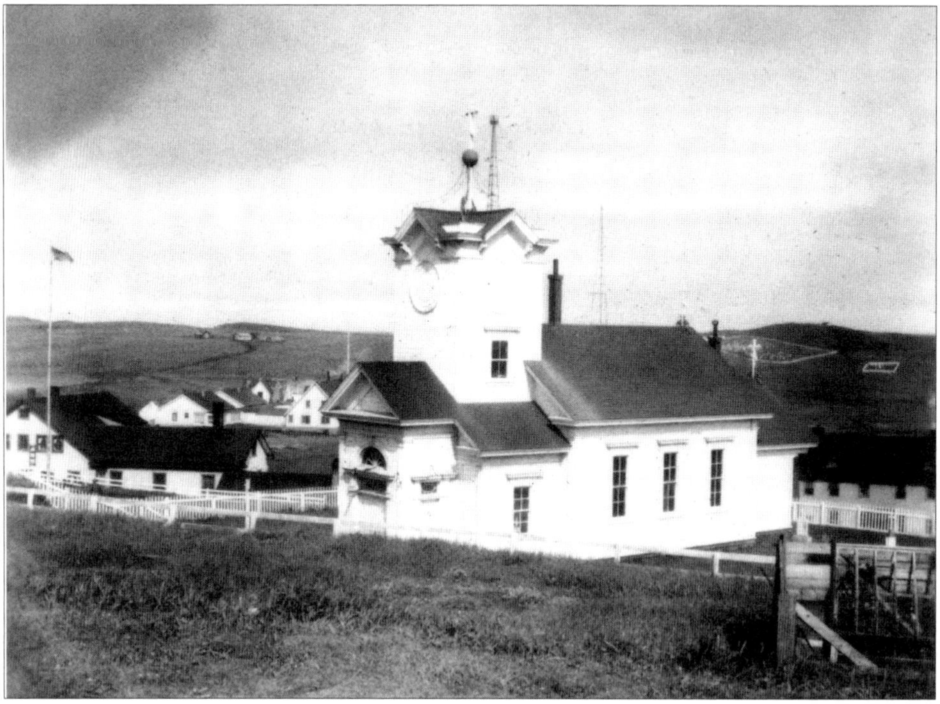

The Church of Saints Peter and Paul, St. Paul Island (from the Martin Collection, USUAF210, Archives, Alaska and Polar Regions, Rasmuson Library, University of Alaska Fairbanks).

we drove so quickly along the lowest street of the village that I had only a blurred impression of dingy grey buildings, which Johnston identified as the office, the Company House, "your new home," and the hospital. A flash of white as we circled up a hill was the Russian Orthodox church. Just beyond it the car stopped. On a broad terrace stood Government House, trim, adorned with peaked gables. In the yard were two small cannons, the only relics of Russian days. Our trunks were waiting in our large, bright bedroom.

Two reborn individuals bathed and wearing clean clothes went down to lunch to join our shipboard mess companions and meet Harry May, jocose manager of Fouke Fur activities on the Pribilofs.[1] After lunch we met Elary Gromoff and Paul Merculieff, the two Aleuts who served the Government House mess. Had I met them in the States, I would have taken for granted that they were of Russian descent. Elary was thin, pale, and nervous. He burst immediately into a long history of the sickness in his family. Paul was short, plump, and exceedingly shy. Sam misunderstood Elary's name, perhaps subconsciously affected by the detective yarns he had read on the boat. As a result *Ellery* became a fairly permanent name for poor Elary, who worried about it but was finally comforted by the thought that Ellery was an American name. He wanted people to call him Larry, but no one did. *Ellery* was at least a step toward the fulfillment of his dreams.

After lunch we called upon Dr. Migliori. Our spirits sank as we surveyed our new home. The exterior was dispiriting enough in the greyish daylight. Having seen the delicate pastel walls of rooms in Government House and been charmed by the spacious, bright rooms, the interior of the doctor's cottage was extremely depressing. I looked at Sam and his face betrayed the same dismay that I felt. The windows were closed. Steam heat engulfed us as we entered the living room. Long ecru curtains pinned together in the center and half-drawn blinds shut out the light of day. Ugly tan walls frowned at us. The woodwork was funereally dark. The furniture, battered by many previous residents, was a collection of the largest, most uncomfortable, unwieldy specimens of the worst era of Mission furniture. I caught a glimpse of the kitchen beyond, where the same darkness reigned. Had the curtains been drawn back, the outlook from the front windows would have been ugly and gloomy. Directly across the muddy street stood a huge barnlike structure, the bunkhouse where seasonal workmen from the Aleutian chain were housed. The bunkhouse, itself a dull grey eyesore, shut off all view of land or sea and most of the sky. We seemed to be in the squalid section of an industrial city or opposite the grim coal breakers of a mining town.

Depressed by the atmosphere, made listless by the extreme heat, we sat listening to Dr. Migliori's account of St. Paul medical practice and island social life. The Aleuts, he claimed, were the world's worst patients, who delighted in disobeying doctor's orders. Having inherited an appetite for fishy flavors, adults guzzled in a day the supply of cod liver oil prescribed for the children of the household for a week. They were, he excoriated, without a single exception, filthy and germ ridden. As for the government officials and their families! And then we listened to

[Undated]
Mrs. Migliori seemed very sweet. She and the doctor began talking very carefully about their experiences but gradually warmed toward us and poured out a host of troubles. They had trouble with the Natives, who demanded enormous amounts of cod liver oil, which the whole family drank because they liked the flavor. They were always noncooperative in carrying out medical directions. They were all dirty and would not comply with sanitary regulations. All of them. No exceptions. As for the white people. Be careful of them. One family asked for supplies in large quantities in order to report the physician for squandering supplies. Hence Dr. Migliori had requested and received a signed order from Mr. Johnston that the white employees were to get only necessary medications. Some information about bureau people Migliori spilled freely with details. But he and his wife employed a great deal of circumlocution in advising us that happiness would be ours if we shunned social contact as they had for the greater part of their life here and that by holding ourselves aloof from all bureau employees we could obtain a minimum of the respect due a physician. A great deal of this confession sounded pretty cockeyed . . . Their kindliness was most apparent. I began to feel sorry that they had not been able to enjoy their stay here more.

interminable tales of petty feuds and disagreeable incidents. For the past year of their stay the Migliori family had refused all social invitations and kept away from other government employees. Finally we were warned that the small official community had little respect for physicians because its members believed only incompetent doctors would bury themselves, even temporarily, at such a post.

The Miglioris were very sweet and charming people. It was discouraging to listen to their experiences. But as I listened I was confident that Sam and I were equipped to avoid most of the pitfalls they described. The perils of insularity could be overcome by a sense of humor, sympathetic understanding of human foibles, and enough studies and hobbies to fill leisure hours. Their accounts had been tinged with the apprehensions of sensitive people caught in a net of bureaucracy. They shared the dread that paralyzes so many government employees and turns them into bureaucratic automatons, the fear that freely voiced opinions and independent action may displease a superior and cost them their economic security. No such cautious considerations would hamper our actions or disturb our peace of mind.

June 25, 1941
The village looks twice as drab as it need, because of the ugly paint. The houses of the Natives are plastered one against another as if there were a tremendous need to conserve space. Because of their proximity, the yard space is beaten earth with no green stuff growing. Yet every window we passed was filled with flowering plants, which proved the Natives do care for growing things.
As far as coping with social relations, the doctor's warnings fell on deaf ears. We have no qualms about being disliked or not having the proper respect shown us. We are accustomed to being ourselves wherever we are and do not curry favor.

It was late afternoon before we could excuse ourselves on the plea of exploring the village. We made a hasty survey of the house before we left. All the rooms were drab, dark, shut away from light and air, and cluttered with heavy, clumsy furniture. Outside we gulped in lungfuls of air in relief. "That ugliness is a real challenge to our ingenuity," I told Sam. "I can stand everything but the lack of a view. Of course we shall be spending as much time as possible out of doors. Imagine putting up that huge barrack directly across the road. They had hundreds of empty acres on which to build but they just plopped it there and gave no thought to the mental health of the occupants of the doctor's cottage."

Our walk through the village, interrupted by constant greetings from friendly children, failed to cheer us. The dun cottages sat in yards that were filthy with trash and littered with cans and rubbish. The hospital overwhelmed us with its ancient dirt and dark atmosphere. It was merely a roof over some very rickety beds and not a house of healing.

Until Dr. Migliori left a few days later we had little to do but write letters, explore, and ask questions. Brief excursions to the shore refreshed us and gave us courage to recover from our first impressions, to plan to make our residence livable, to create a real hospital, and to extract all the knowledge and joy that out-of-doors life on the island could afford. We were attentive listeners to all who would tell us about the Pribilofs. In a few days we had absorbed the equivalent of volumes of information, misinformation, and opinions that had to be tested by our own observations and studies. We were soon as well equipped as older inhabitants to act as guides to newcomers. From our first to our last day on St. Paul we were insatiable students. It was inevitable, having been lured so far from home by the phrase *volcanic islands,* that our first serious studies were about the geography and most conspicuous geological features of St. Paul.

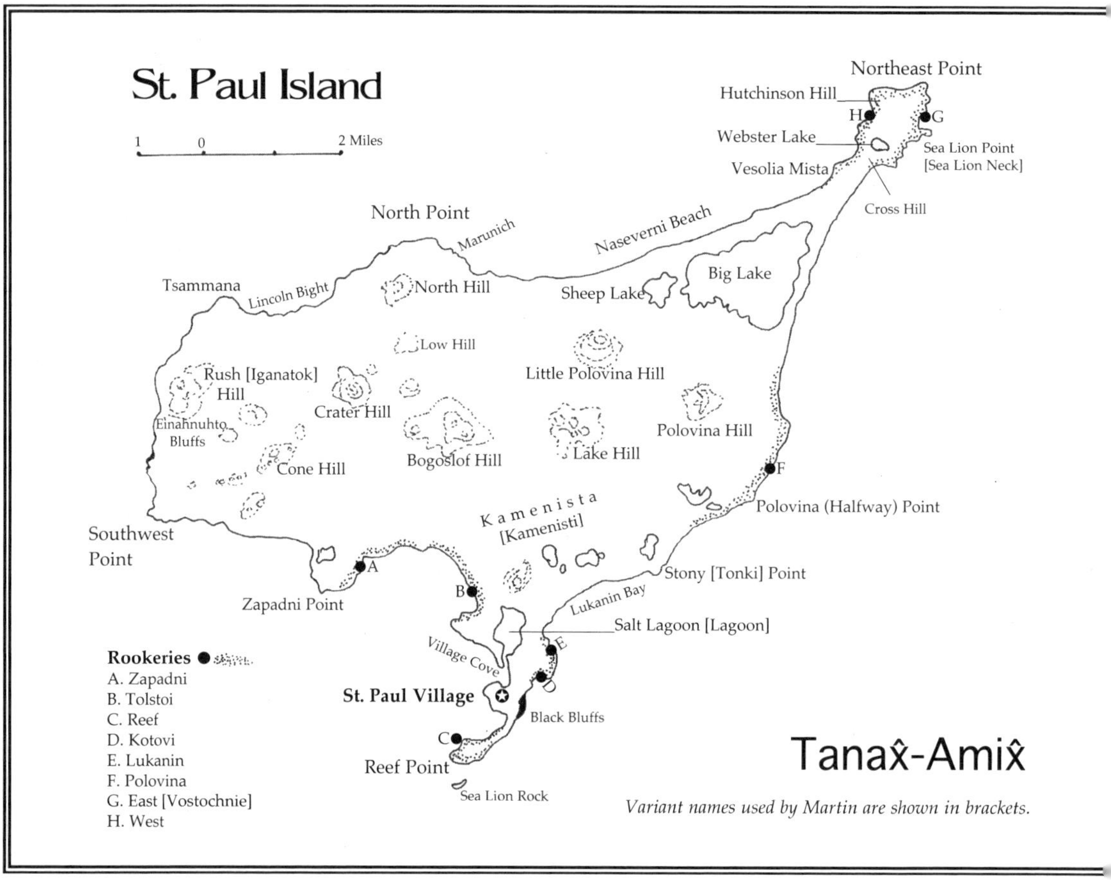

St. Paul Island.

Chapter 3

There are five islands in the Pribilof group, although only the two large islands of St. George and St. Paul are commercially valuable as the land habitation of the Alaskan fur seal.

Sivuchii Kamen or Sea Lion Rock, a calf of St. Paul, is a rough crescent of barren tumbled rocks a few feet above the sea, a scant third of a mile from the southeastern tip of its mother island. At its highest point, wedged firmly into the rocks, is an old wooden Russian cross, placed there when the Aleuts braved the swift current of the channel to kill sea lions. Only an occasional sea lion has been seen there for many years. After the sea lions deserted the isle, the Aleuts still sought and secured their first fresh meat since autumn there when the earliest returning seals hauled ashore each spring to loaf before going on to St. Paul. Regulations against killing seals for food put an end to annual trips. Unmolested, a bull seal or two generally sets up harems or a party of bachelors takes up residence on this rocky suburb each season.

Bobrovyi or Otter Island, about six miles to the southwest of St. Paul, has a total area of about a hundred and fifteen acres. While *Sivuchii* crouches low in the waves, Otter Island breasts the seas like a proud vessel, its westernmost volcanic peak broken into an abrupt cliff suggesting the sweep of the prow of the ship. The shimmering air, the motile sea, and the restless mists constantly evoke the illusion of motion. The cone at its eastern promontory bears traces of the most recent volcanic activity in the whole group although so long ago that no human eye witnessed the upheaval. A subterranean passage, perhaps a genuine lava tunnel, leads from the crater to the beach below and is accessible at low tide.

The heart of the island was built up by the debris from the volcanoes. Its southern coast is a steep unbroken cliff where seabirds throng. Toward St. Paul the land slopes gently down to the shoreline. During the summer young male seals often sojourn temporarily on the low accessible beach. Occasional summer human visitors have encountered a few arctic foxes, stranded by floating ice, lean and emaciated from the poor, uncertain fare of birds. Gone forever is the sleek gentle sea otter for which the early Russian hunters named the island, *bobrovyi.*

Actually, the Russian word meant *beaver* but had been applied to the sea otter by the Russian fur seekers who first observed them on Pacific shores. It has been unoccupied except for a few summers during the latter years of the past century when the United States maintained guards there to ward off poaching sealers and to discourage the seals themselves from staying ashore. The guards had to bring even their drinking water from St. Paul, for Otter has no water supply except the pools of brackish rainwater in rocky hollows, too often tainted by the overflow of high seas.

Otter Island awakened the spirit of animism in my heart. The theatrical structure, the sensation of motion, the elusive appearance and disappearance into veils of mist, were too exciting to result from a mass of inert land and atmospheric action. When the sun beat down on the grassy heart of the island, turning it into a bowl of fire scintillating with luminous gold-tipped flame, it seemed dull to credit the dark storm cloud with dropping a heavy curtain over the scene or quenching the flame with rain. Surely the island had capriciously shut itself off from the glances of mere mortals. In autumn the sun kindled the harsh brown vegetation into flowing gold, creating a fleece the Argonauts might well have risked death to win. When snow spread a soft white mat over its unbroken slope, the island was transformed into a strange mythical swan brooding upon the smoke-grey sea.

Six miles from the northeastern coast of St. Paul, *Morzhovyi* or Walrus Island was generally a thin dark line on the horizon. In storms the waves dashed across the flat table of irregular lava blocks, only a quarter of a mile long and a hundred yards across at its widest. On clear days watching from St. Paul, we saw gigantic waves break against the island, great spouts of frothy spume spurting high in the air as if an immense herd of whales sported there. Only a few clumps of hard grasses maintain their rootholds in rocky interstices against the frequent washings of the sea.

Morzhovyi belongs now to the birds who return each spring to breed and no longer to the hundreds of walrus that rested there on their journeys north and south. Until a few years ago, St. Paul Aleuts made several trips each spring to gather eggs or kill birds for food. As other foodstuffs became more easily available, the dangerous trips grew less until it is as much tradition as desire for fresh eggs that inspires an annual spring outing on a day when the Bering lolls in a placid mood. Egg gathering is so simple, once the dangers of the sea are eluded and a landing has been safely made from the swaying boat to the abruptly squared face of the shore. The eggs lie scattered in profusion on the level surface, retained on their smooth platelike nest by their natural contours. The extreme tapering form of the murre egg and the blunter stubbiness of one tip of the kittiwake egg enable the eggs to swing circularly back to safety as if on a pivot when disturbed by wind or other contact. Dangerous as the trip to Walrus Island may be because of the threat of a storm off the Bering, the venture is less risky than dangling over the high cliffs where the bird rookeries on St. Paul are located. The Natives of St. George have no choice on their bluffy coast but to seek eggs while dangling from ropes.

St. Paul is the most important of the Pribilof Islands and was the pivot of our studies of the entire group. In the latitude of 57 degrees north and longitude 170 degrees west, it lies across a map like a lazy swimming turtle with the peninsular Northeast Point forming the outstretched neck and head. The ultimate southern point of the island, Reef Point, frequently referred to as simply "Reef," is a hind leg trailing lazily in the sea. Between the two the distance is a bird's straight flight of thirteen miles. Between Polovina Point on the east coast and Marunich, where the island shore swerves from west to north, seven miles of level tundra stretch across the widest part of the island.

The twenty thousand acres of St. Paul present the most diversified landscape of the Pribilofs. Everywhere the earth betrays the violence of its volcanic birth. Doubtless when St. Paul first emerged from the sea's depths, it was no single island but a bevy of peaked islets. Undoubtedly the stately two-crowned peak of Bogoslof first pushed aside the waves. Hot tongues of vesicular lava rich in olivine coiled out of its multiple mouths and solidified into the island fundament. A second mighty flow of spongier lava overspread the first sheet. The mother peak and vents and cracks in the lava field continued to erupt. The little red-topped hills are genuine craters choked with the fractured segments of lava during successive explosive upheavals. The seething blocks and chips of lava hardened during their brief upward flight in the cold air and fell backward solidified. The descending shower of fragments packed one piece firmly upon another, erecting the inverted funnel-shaped peaks. Between the elevations thousands of tons of basaltic blocks tumbled, linking the bases of the hills together. The finer bits, scoria cinders and tuff, settled down between and over the large rough chunks. The terrain became more level and hard packed. The basaltic boulders must quickly have bridged the areas where the cones are closest together. Centuries may have elapsed before some of the more isolated ones were joined to the main body of the expanding island by sand drifts. Throughout the lowlands the grey, unkempt toppled boulders litter the landscape, picturesque monuments of the volcanism that created the island.

By word of mouth the story has been handed down among Aleut families that when the first Aleuts accompanied Russian hunters to St. Paul, Northeast Point was still a separate island to which the seal hunters traveled by boat and where they camped during their hunt. Now a broad isthmus has linked the Point to the mainland, joined the neck to the carapace of the turtle. The largest dunes are long-lived because the frost has solidified the heart so that no exuberant wind can shatter the mound. Stubborn-rooted grasses and flowers have settled on the sites and summits and hold the elusive grains of sand firmly within a matted network of rootlets. As if in revenge the wind covers the vegetation in winter but each spring the plants push up above the extra covering and proclaim their hardiness with triumphant spears of grass and blazing banners of flowers.

The ice of the southward-advancing arctic ice pack almost annually hacks at the shore boulders. The ice pushes at the land and breaks against the unyielding stone. The broken blocks, impelled by the pressure of the ice field, are pushed up and over the rocks, filing and grinding the softer basalt surfaces. The dust sifts into the crevices. The stone surfaces are rounded, polished smooth, and shiny by the ice burrs.

Unlike St. George and the three small isles, St. Paul has long sweeps of sandy beach that curve in sickles here and there along the forty-two miles of coastline. Between the sand beaches lie the rocky shingles that delight the fur seals. The occasional line of bluff affords the seabirds nesting space. Along the shore there are flowing glassy black terraces where a lava flood fled backward to the sea. Most beaches are composed of basalt blocks scattered helter-skelter or laid out with the precision of a human builder.

The brooding cones of the quiet volcanoes, actually attaining but a few hundred feet of elevation above sea level, tower above the flat plateau areas with the majesty and insolence of real mountain peaks. In all weather they expose their outworn craters or rubble-tipped peaks indifferently to the sky. Snow or rain or fog or brief benediction of the sun all serve to adorn and beautify the hills. A band of scoria, reddish, brown, or black, girdles their summits. The alpine vegetation that climbed up the hills ends abruptly and forms an undulating boundary of summer green or winter amber to the colored stone ring.

Small lakes lie snugly in the shallow depressions of the flatlands, fed mainly by the rain and melting snow. Antone Lake is the most picturesque and Big Lake is the largest. Big Lake once possessed a more pleasing name, spelled by its first American recorder as *Mee-sulk-mah-mee.* Oral legend still calls it *Mishelki.* Neither the old spelling nor the modern pronunciation gives a single clue to the meaning of the old name.[1]

The term *tundra,* while not actually correct, has been most often applied to the terrain of the lowland. The unbroken appearance of the broad fields and the summer vegetation mislead the newcomer into expecting pleasant meadow rambles. Under the thick growth of flower and grass lurk basaltic blocks of varying sizes and the sharp corners and spines of cinder clumps. "Eyes down" was the first law of hiking we learned on the island. If I wanted to savor sky or landscape I halted and walked on only when my eyes were ready to watch out for the traps underfoot.

Always the air was sibilant. Birds swept eternally through the skies. The lively chatter of the waves carried far from shore. The wind whispered to the grasses in summer or rattled the dry stalks after seedtime. And in summer, like the faint blurred melodies of distant breakers, the clamor from seal beaches reached far across into the very heart of St. Paul, where it rose to the red lips of the old volcano craters.

Chapter 4

My first night's sleep on St. Paul had been broken at dawn by the raucous clamor of roosters. I lay feeling faintly irritated that my slumbers should be interrupted by any noise. Faintly the mooing of a cow floated in through the window. Suddenly my sleepy brain exploded.

"Sam," I demanded, for I could hear him stirring, "what kind of noises are these to wake us up in the center of the Bering Sea? Roosters crowing and cows mooing! Where is that uproar of the seal rookeries we feared might deafen us? I feel cheated."

Faintly from far away a thrumming surflike sound reached us when the domestic animals were still. The nearest rookery was at least a mile away. The sound that welled through the air was a soughing lullaby with no hint of animal origin. Had we not known the truth we might have thought it sea sound entirely. But the harmonious ululation was not wave sung. It was a composition of tens of thousands of seal voices. Discordant and strident, piercing the seal chant from the reef, the cries of the village domestic animals burst against our ears.

"Adventure," I grumbled as I buried my head in the pillow, since the clock hands pointed only to three thirty. "I expected to have to force my way among throngs of seals to get into the house but so far except for that glimpse from the ship and another across Zolotoi Bay, I have seen no animals but chickens, cows, and cats. This village is too civilized. We might as well be on a farm in Maryland as on the Seal Islands."

The village of St. Paul lacked every aspect of a wilderness or frontier town. The drab buildings, the unpaved streets, the exterior aspects of the town could be duplicated in hundreds of poor little towns in the States. Forty-nine cottages for Aleut families, three large hilltop bungalows for government employees, the school, the Russian church and priest's residence; Government House, the Community Hall, the office, the Company House, and an additional dormitory for Fouke Fur workers, the Aleut bunkhouse, the tiny jail, warehouses, garage and repair shop, the carpenter shop, the barn, the hospital, and close by the doctor's home; the coal sheds; the salt houses, the blubbering shed, the packing rooms—all

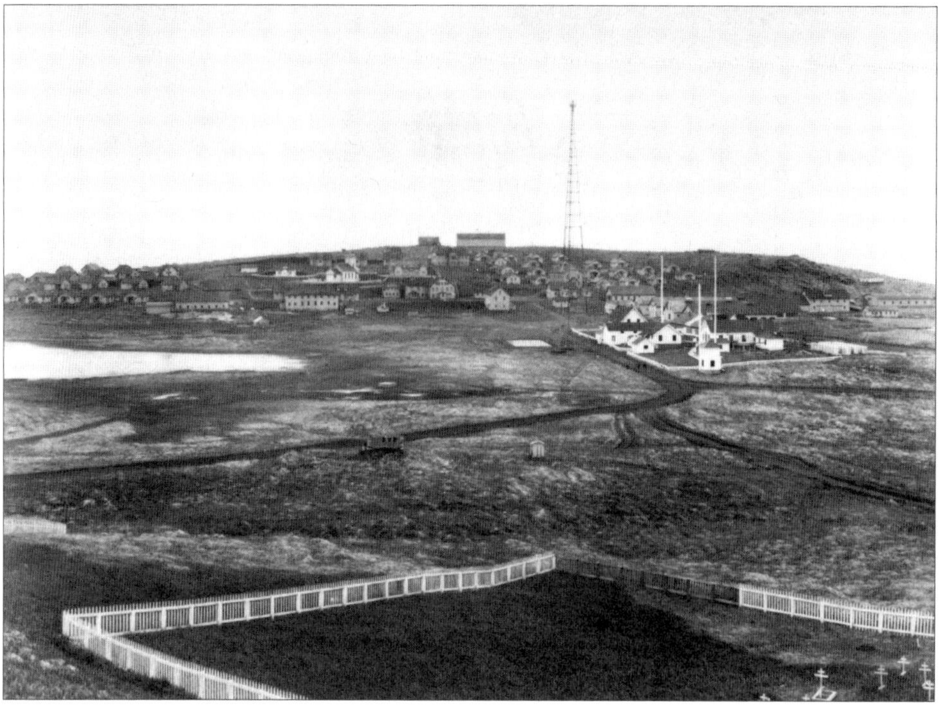

A view of St. Paul Village.

for the seal skins; the power house and refrigerating plant: all these buildings composed a nicely functioning community.

Accommodated to the natural terraces of the slopes of the bulging promontory of Village Hill, the horizontal streets seemed amazingly straight. Only the roads that climbed the hills were curved. The houses fitted snugly back against the hillside on broad shelves of earth until one lonely Aleut home and the big schoolhouse stood exposed on the level hilltop. A few hundred feet behind them, the land dropped abruptly to broad coiled lava platforms on the shore.

In the flats below the village stood the group of buildings that the Navy had erected and used for a radio station (discontinued a decade before).[1] Some Fish and Wildlife Service employees were housed there in 1941 and a smaller radio unit that was in daily service was established in one of the buildings. On the flats between the barn and Village Lake, which one day deserved the designation and at a later date had dwindled to the status of a mere pond, a small glass-roofed and windowed greenhouse for government employees only stood inside a rough, high-fenced outside garden.

The by-products plant, where the bodies of skinned seals were converted into commercial products, was built three-quarters of a mile away on the bank of the lagoon, to keep the village atmosphere free from disagreeable odors. It was clearly visible, however, and sometimes faintly malodorous.

St. Paul Village had just grown. As buildings were required and as appropriations for them were included in the budget, the agent in charge at the time, with more or less supervision from the Washington office, chose the site and superintended the construction. The pattern on Village Hill owed its normal appearance more to natural appropriateness of the more level and most easily cleared space for building than deliberate harmonious planning to create a pleasant village. Consequently there had been clumsy additions, such as the erection of the ugly barrack across from the hospital and doctor's residence on the village main street. Another example was the unnecessary proximity of barn and hospital, the former possessing a score of manure tumuli that mounted faster than the wind-built sand dunes.

Village Hill was one of the many heights composed of scoria bedded down upon a base of large basaltic blocks. Once digging almost to sea level for a well, diggers found deep deposits of blue marl, a soft lime clay that may have been scooped up from the sea bottom and retained between the igneous rocks when the island was born. The village today bears the English name of the island. The Aleuts term it simply "the village" in their tongue or as *tannak,* a living place [*tanax̂,* a dwelling place]. They often allude to the hill itself as "the rocky place" and have designated an out-jutting rock arrangement of the cliff back of the village as "the place that has a nose."

Across the flats, so low that occasional tidal inundations caused the early settlers to fear the sea might transform Village Hill into an island once more, two cemeteries occupy the grassy inland slope of Black Bluffs. Inevitably the hill is called Cemetery Hill in both languages. The larger, enclosed by a white picket fence, bristles with the slanting arms of Russian crosses. Here the Aleut dead lie. No inscriptions identify the graves. The unmarked white crosses denote only a grave site. Family memories must retain the knowledge of the location of their forebears' graves. A few yards away a small fenced plot is set aside for the "whites," exclusive and superior to the Aleuts even in death. Since the first Protestants who died on the island were buried in the churchyard alongside Aleut dead, the separate plots are not due to religious differences. The small yard contains eight graves. Three pathetic little mounds are headed by bronze plates that describe infants of naval men at the radio station, who never left their island birthplaces. Three long barrows stretch horizontally in front of a large wooden shield. Weather and a coating of white paint have worn the raised cutout inscription. I climbed the fence one day for there was no gate and traced the outlines of the lettering. Three sailors home from the sea. The inscription read, "Three seamen of the U.S.S. *Lincoln,* Drowned, October 9, 1869." According to Henry W. Elliott the three were victims of vanity,[2] for the sailors of the ship that gave its name to a beautiful bight on the west coast of the island were deceived by the ease with which the Aleut boatmen rowed their big baidars through the rolling waves. They launched a boat when strong tides were running. Unfamiliar with the currents they were also probably not watchful enough in observing the oncoming waves. The boat capsized and the three sailors lost their lives.

The still more worn inscriptions on two other shield-shaped wooden headboards would have been indecipherable had I not known the names of the deceased. I could make out the *D* and *V* of Dr. Voss and a letter or two of the name Edward Hughes, the famous Ned who for nearly a quarter of a century was the Company House cook. The latter was the reputed grandfather of a number of sealers. Dr. Voss at first practiced his medical profession. Then he took a more remunerative post on the company staff. One day he was supervising the loading of a cart drawn by a team of frisky mules. The lines dropped between the animals and startled them into flight. He leaped upon the wagon tongue and leaned forward to catch the dragging reins. Losing his balance he fell between the mules and was dragged for several yards before the runaways were stopped. He died almost immediately.

The graves of the Aleuts possess the solemnity of any burial ground close to a community. On certain dates, particularly the name days of the dead Aleuts, villagers took flowers and religious ornaments to their dead. The smaller graveyard was more poignant. Within it lay those adults who died far from their homes and tiny babies, whose parents could probably never revisit their graves. I never glimpsed those tiny mounds without a pang of grief. No one on the island tended the plot or brought flowers. But both cemeteries were unkempt with shaggy grasses, looking forgotten and forsaken.

Cemetery Hill deprives the village of a complete view of the Bering. Opposite the center of the village is *Navastok* or East Landing, a low shingle from which extends a long cement pier. Between this and Black Bluffs lie rusty iron rails, partially embedded in cement, great rugged chunks of cement, and other rubbish, the remains of an earlier wharf that had been connected with the fur storage bins by a small-gauge railway. It was predicted that winter frosts and beating surf would destroy man's work with such ease that dock building would be a waste of time. The first dock wore away and crumbled under the attack of the elements. The larger, stronger pier that could support a dozen large trucks was man's defiant answer to natural forces. It has resisted decay for a long time and can last a good many more seasons.

Once the slopes of Cemetery Hill housed the quick instead of the dead. The exact site of the first settlement there is obscure. Elliott recorded the calamity that made the spot most suitable for a graveyard.[3] In the early fall of 1835 the ice came sweeping down from the north, hemmed in the island behind high ramparts that remained around the islands until late the next summer. The dwellers in the semi-underground homes (*barabaras*) of Black Bluffs had no stores of driftwood and blubber with which to warm their dank huts for so long. Many died from the cold, others from malnutrition and disease.

It will never be known how many and where all the earliest communities or camps were. Around 1787 Gavriil Pribylov stationed Aleuts from the islands of Atka and Unalaska somewhere on the north shore to hunt for his company.[4] Separate, rival colonies existed later from Marunich to Northeast Point. Rapacious killing spurred on by competing companies would wipe out the animals at one point. Then the group of hunters would move to another spot. Polovina on the east became one of the largest and more stable settlements. By 1796 the ruthless killing had depleted the herd so badly that hunting became unprofitable. Some traders withdrew their men. Three years later, the Russian-American Company gained the sole right to the island as part of the whole vast Russian American territory. They expelled the agents of their former competitors and ordered the remaining hunters to move to the one village at Polovina.[5] In 1806 sealing was halted to permit the herd to recuperate and the islanders were removed. In 1809 hunters returned to St. George and commenced sealing. In 1810 sealing was resumed on St. Paul and it is likely that the hunters settled down again at Polovina and Northeast Point. Toward the close of the second decade the company managers ordered the population to move to the environs of East Landing, Zolotoi, and the Lagoon, because the area was adjacent to the two best roadsteads at East Landing and off Village Cove. Furthermore, the small Russian vessels could sail directly into the quiet waters of the Lagoon at certain tides. Records of happenings in the new village contain allusions to dates between 1821 and 1824 and the exact time of consolidation is obscure.

In "Early History of the Pribylov Islands" Veniaminov wrote, "Aleuts who have migrated thither, Creole and Russians, to the number of 137 souls, dwell in two villages. The first and principal village is situated at the southwest end of the island along a bay; the other at the southeastern extremity. In the principal village, named the Harbor, there are the following buildings: (1) a wooden oratory, named after the Apostles Peter and Paul, constructed in 1821 and embellished within with very passable ikonostases and figures, furnished at the expense of the natives living there, (2) a house for the [Russian-American Company's] manager, and (3) a store or warehouse for merchandise; both of these buildings being of wood, very well and commodiously set up. Besides these, there are: a barrack, constructed after the customary style of Aleut yurts, and some other like buildings belonging to the company and thirteen barabaras belonging to the natives. A small windmill has lately been erected.

"In the second village, known as 'Stochnoye,' that is Vostochnoe (eastern), buildings are extremely few, principally two barabaras."[6]

It seems so peculiar to consider the few buildings behind Black Bluffs, so close to the Harbor, a separate community. However, the distance that takes five minutes to cover by foot on the road today probably was a half hour of hopping from hummock to hummock in his day. The Americans had been on the island several years before they began to build a road halfway across the swampy terrain toward

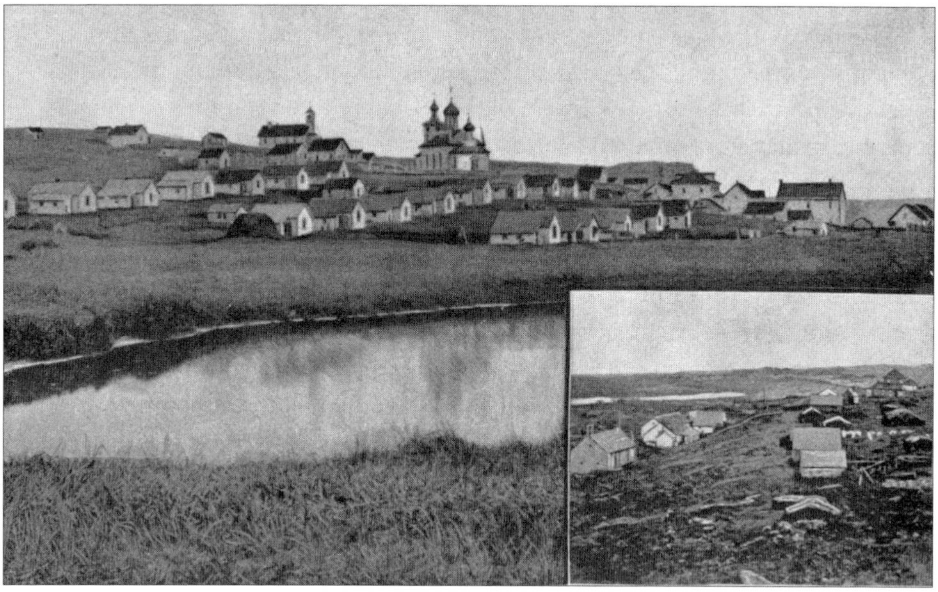

The village of St. Paul in 1891 with an insert showing the village in 1870 (*Fur Seal Arbitration. Proceedings of the Tribunal of Arbitration,* Vol. 3, 1895, facing p. 95).

the landing. There is no doubt that the Harbor is the vicinity of Village Hill because Veniaminov alludes to the possibility of a tidal wave sweeping in from the Golden Bight to cut the village off from the rest of the island.

The impermanence of barabaras (the Russians introduced the Siberian term and blotted out of daily usage the Aleut word *ulak* [*ulax̂*]) gave a nomadic character to the communities so that dates and locations became blurred in oral history. It is very likely that the actual Harbor straggled backward and forward in the area between East Landing and Village Hill. John Hanson, chief foreman of the work gang, informed Father Baranoff and me that as a lad he played in old barabara ruins just where the radio station was erected.[7] He remembered vividly the deep depressions, half-choked with whalebone timbering. A very old lady placed the earliest chapel that Veniaminov praised so lavishly just where the greenhouse and gardens are now. Some habitation was there. Father Baranoff sifting soil for his garden found a delicate smoky brown ivory spoon about the size of an incense ladle. Dimitri Tetoff insisted that either another settlement had been among the sand dunes off toward Lukannon or that part of the early village had extended sprawlingly to that point.

Eventually the main body of the village became settled on the dry, well-drained scoria slope of Village Hill, where its modern successor was erected.

The Alaska Commercial Company erected frame dwellings for the sealers in the first fifteen years of the American occupation and earned a fine reputation for caring for their workmen. Actually the company fought the desire of the sealers to erect their own homes on plots of land set aside for their indefinite use, even if they bought their own lumber and supplies. A government agent accused the company of preventing the Native residents' getting a vested interest in the island.[8] After the First World War the Bureau of Fisheries, predecessor of the present government agency, erected the cement bungalows that line the streets today.

Only two traces of the past are conspicuous today, the three [*sic*] small Russian cannons in the yard at Government House and a tiny broken-windowed, frame hovel across from the dispensary window, the last of the American frame dwellings. I tried to picture an average-sized sealer's family wedged into that frame hut. It was easier to imagine when I learned how few articles of furniture they possessed and that they frequently slept in rows on the floor. To eyes accustomed to the houses of less windy climates the small dwellings must have represented a step toward civilization. I have no doubt the Aleut was far warmer and comfortable in the stale atmosphere of his sod-covered barabara. Even some of the latest cement houses had cracks through which the wind penetrated.

The cannons painted in coats of aluminum paint appeared as toys to modern eyes. Until quite recently they had been fired on New Year's, Fourth of July, and the most important church holidays, usually just after midnight ushered in the holiday. Their racket had delighted the Aleuts and irritated the more sedate and less holiday-minded officials. When the Alaska Commercial Company was packing its gear to remove from the island [around 1890], its employees claimed the right to take the cannons. The exasperated sealers insisted that the cannons belonged to the village and its inhabitants. They won their case, the only known instance of a victory over the grasping tendencies of the first lessee.

Once the seals neighbored with the human beings. Elliott's map of 1872 shows the site of Nah Speel rookery in a curve of the spiked sea cliffs of the hill behind the settlement.[9] The seals lingered near the village for a long time. In 1889 no official could recall the last date seals had been seen there. Since no bachelors hauled out, island officials paid slight attention to the harems almost under their noses. The proximity of man could hardly be blamed for their desertion. They were shut away from the noise and odors of the village by the backdrop of cliff. Elliott testified to their indifference to an audience hanging over them, even when small boys pelted them with bits of wood and pebbles. He gave the seals credit for knowing that, because they were the breeding animals, the humans would not deliberately harm them. Probably when the seal herd was in danger of extermination in the late 1880s, the seals found sufficient landing places on the southeastern side of the island and did not bother to return to their old hangout.

Over twenty thousand seals lived in harems opposite the village landing place on the boulder barrier that almost transformed the Lagoon into a lake. They were just opposite the killing field that the Russians had used for over fifty years, located on the sandy plain that might aptly have been the village common. Elliott computed that by the time of his visit over twenty-three million seals had been slaughtered there. Digging a well close to the first cliffs of Village Hill in 1868, [workers found that] the deposit of sea lion and seal bone was twelve feet thick.[10] Farther the shovelers did not investigate. The water was fit only for laundry purposes because of the bone debris. Since hundreds of thousands more animals were slaughtered farther from the slope the layer of decaying animal matter must be much thicker. Neither the protests of the victims, the noisy clamor of the killer, nor the stench of rotting bodies disturbed the inhabitants of Lagoon Reef, for the site was only deserted a couple of decades ago.

On our first evening we leaned over the brim of Nah Speel and looked down upon the untenanted coves. That twilight excursion, from the most southerly tip of the headland to the dock at West Landing and back through the village to the comfortable bed at Government House, cast a spell over me from which I shall never be free. It drove away all but a faint exasperation over the defects of our house. Before I went to sleep I wrote to an artist friend who had pitied us for coming to a land where no trees grew. I thought of him as I watched the melting changes of greys and whites of clouds close to the dark horizon and the subtle blending of purples and reds of the faces of the cliffs and the nearest volcanic cones. Not lush enough for his brush in most moods but I wondered if he would mind as much as he thought a land that does not support trees. For this beauty has a charm, a compelling quality that seizes the heart immediately. There is an independence in the starkness that wins respect at once and repels melancholy, a sense of majestic age wrought by great violence, now serene, strong, and inflexible. This is the mood the landscape evoked in us that night. The wind, fog, and other elemental forces would soon be inspiring new impressions.

Trees! But we have trees. If willows cannot spring up toward the sun and drop toward fresh flowing waters, they can sling lovingly to the earth that is still being formed slowly over the cold volcanic rocks. They can spread widely over that earth in a protecting mantle and provide a furry carpet of pussy willows for careless feet to crush. Life is so awesome. It insists upon growing, if not upward and skyward, then outward from the center to some periphery. And the mosses and the lichens everywhere! Colors to tempt an artist's brush. The boulders and pebbles are adorned with gay orange and green snoods. At a distance many a rock looks like a fairy-tale animal mottled in fantastic designs, crouching in the grass. The sky, the sea, the land, if we find no congenial friends here, we shall have these three to companion us.

Chapter 5

The most terrible indictment of Bering Sea weather I have read occurs in Henry Elliott's description of sea otter hunting during the closing years of the past century. "It is a region so gloomy, so pitilessly beaten by wind and waves, by sleet, rain and persistent fog," he wrote, "that the good Bishop Veniaminov, when he first came among the natives of the Aleutian Islands, ordered the curriculum of hell to be omitted from the church breviary, saying as he did so that these people had enough of it here on earth!"[1] Elliott was describing the immediate vicinity of the Aleutian archipelago but melancholy pictures of similar conditions around the Pribilof Islands are a continuous monotonous repetition in writings of people who have known the Seal Islands.

Fog is the principal victim of Pribilof complaint. I once spent a year in London during which loyal Londoners assured me that the pleasant weather we experienced was exceptional, that on subsequent visits I should live like a wraith in the mist. My doubt that London was always perpetually enveloped in a dense fog seemed to hurt the national pride of my friends. On the other hand, Parisian friends ignored the miserable weather I encountered there, while my clothes curled miserably around the hems from the damp drizzle that seeped constantly from the mist. Taxi driving, perilous at best in that city, became a real test of courage as buildings loomed up in the thick haze. My French friends lifted their eyebrows at my complaints. "Fog?" they would murmur skeptically, "You think it is foggy?" Residents and ex-residents of the Pribilofs belong to a clan of fog devotees similar to my London acquaintances. I found myself, almost at once, becoming a follower of the Parisian school.

Fog, the majority insists, blankets the islands day and night. The sun seldom vouchsafes light or warmth. Ships find their way to the coast through dense fogs only by harkening to the tumult of seal voices crying like lost souls in the mist. The fog! The fog! It pursues the seal even into the realms of advertising where fertile pens concoct paeans dripping moisture to enhance milady's garment with magical mystery. Long before the advertising copywriters wrote of the Pribilofs, the Misty Islands, the Isles of Mist, the Land of White Fog were familiar nicknames for the islands. I heard about the fog in Washington. I read more about it on my way north. Imagine my disillusionment when we approached St. Paul late in the evening and saw the low coastline of the southern shore clearly thirty miles away. The next morning I ran to the porthole wondering whether I could still see the shore. The land and the buildings were clear-cut in a fine grey rain. Where was that fog, that ever-constant, ever-enveloping fog that perpetually curtained off the home of the fur seal?

Of course I eventually discovered the fog, a lot of fog, but never the fog in which I had expected to dwell for a whole year. Not trusting my own impressions, in case my stay should actually be limited to a period of exceptional weather, I turned to the weather reports of the years and became busy questioning the Aleuts to determine the truth.

The winters, which may be said to begin in October, have few foggy days or hours. The usual season of fog is summer, which blooms abruptly in June or occasionally in late May. But not the fog that romantic writers have conjured nor doleful mariners have spun into their weird yarns. Extremely rare is the fog dense enough to shroud St. Paul from approaching ships or to cause a hiker to pass a fellow stroller a few feet away.

Generally, Pribilof fog is a soft white or light-grey mist that rolls up from the sea and spreads with amoeboid motions and grace until it diffuses thinly through the atmosphere. The fog may lie easily in the air around the village while a mile away the scoria road winds over Telegraph Hill glinting in the sunlight and the flowers glow with soft radiance. A trip from the village to the other end of the island, to Northeast Point, may be a game of playing hide-and-seek with drifting patches of fog or the entire journey may be made in a soft grey haze that softens the landscape. The fog is usually friendly, cottony tissue, at its most beautiful delicately lacy, at its grimmest a grey somber shadowy web.

The terror of old mariners in uncharted seas, in crude boats, lacking modern instruments, inspired the first dread of the fog but did not deter the Russian fur seekers. The legend began shortly after Vladimir Atlasov and a band of Cossacks and Tartars in search of furs trekked across Siberia in the seventeenth century and reach Kamchatka. There they found the beautiful shy sea otter whose skins brought golden wealth. Unrestrained hunting soon drove the animals away.

In 1742 before completing his second voyage of exploration in northern waters, Vitus Bering died of scurvy on an island that still bears his name. Bering Island and neighboring Copper Island form the Commander Islands, situated about 110 miles from Kamchatka and about 240 miles from the western tip of the Aleutians. Bering died without reaping fame or wealth for his journeying and without himself realizing the value of his wanderings and the changes the discoveries should make in history. Perhaps the animals that thronged the coastline of Bering Island, sea otter, seal, sea lion, and the little foxes that boldly invaded the damp cave in which he lay, half buried in sand for warmth, prophesied to his failing mind that he had opened the sea routes to a rich commerce for his foster country.

In his wake followed hundreds of tiny boats, thousands of fur seekers, hungry for wealth. The clumsy *shitkas,* the wooden craft whose planking was sewn together, often came to grief on beaches of the Commander and Aleutian islands. But numerous shipwrecks did not deter others from the hunt. Eventually the Russians extended their search as far south as the Spanish settlements of California and maintained hunting camps on the Farallones Islands. The Chinese fur market was never sated with peltry. That the rich merchant might walk adorned in sea otter fur, men died quickly in the cold seas or slowly and painfully succumbed to scurvy. But there were always other adventurers fired by dreams of gold and ease, undeterred by fog, to replace the dead.

Gradually the supply of furs from the Aleutians diminished. The wary sea otter fled to safer kelp beds. The insatiable hunters sought out new haunts of marine animals. If the vanishing sea otter could not be captured, the pelt of the fur seal, though less valuable, became more desirable. Yet the seal had almost disappeared from the shores of the Commander Islands. Only, not all the seals spent their summers on this group of islands. The Russians had noted what the Aleuts had known for centuries, that the fur seal passed northward between the islands of the archipelago in the spring and returned southward accompanied by young seals in the autumn without pausing to come ashore on the islands. Where did these seals, so elusive to spear in the water, haul out upon dry land? Through a tribal legend, the Aleuts of Unalaska knew of *Amix* [*Amix̂*], islands that lay to the north, but they were none too anxious to help their conquerors find new wealth. And if the seals had a summer habitat north of the Aleutians, the Aleuts reasoned, they must have warmer islands somewhere in the Pacific for a winter home. The Russian hunters either accepted or formed the same theory. Southern islands were more alluring to seek, so many ships sought blindly back and forth across the reaches of the Pacific, trying to pursue the swift swimming seal to his winter residence. An occasional vessel turned north but was soon discouraged by storms and winds and shifting currents.

For nearly two decades men searched the seas but the retreat of the fur seal remained a secret. Then Gavriil Pribylov, navigator in command of the *St. George,* owned by Lebedev-Lastochkin Company, set out northward. He is supposed to have heard of the guarded song of the Aleut that told of Igadik, son of an Unimak chief, who was lost north of the archipelago in a great storm.[2] The winds drove his kayak to the shores of St. Paul. Hostile winds prevented him from turning homeward that season. So he wintered on the island, killing many animals. In the spring on a clear day he looked southward and saw the peaks of his own fair island. Loading his kayak with otter tails and pelts as proof of good hunting, he set out for Unimak and reached there after four days of travel.[3]

When Bishop Veniaminov wrote his history of the Pribilof Islands nearly fifty years after their discovery, he believed the testimony of Pribilof hunters that Unimak mountains could be seen from St. Paul. The Aleuts showed him the campsite where Igadik wintered. Igadik must have been fired with homesickness to be so tricked by his imagination. And the Aleut informants of the bishop were either victims of mirages or possessors, too, of powerful imaginations. For even St. George, only forty miles away, is none too clear on the finest day from the highest vantages of St. Paul. To glimpse Unimak was and is an impossible feat for human eyes.[4]

Perhaps Pribylov had really listened to and believed the song of an Aleut shaman. More likely, being a practical mariner, he figured that since many years of voyaging south had revealed no trace of seal islands, it were best to seek them to the north where few had sailed before him.

Secretly, hiding his purpose from masters of other Russian vessels in the harbor on Unalaska Island, he started north. Three weeks of sailing brought him to the high cliffs of an island on June 25, 1786.[5] He observed that where the shores were low, the beach was thronged with thousands of animals. Bringing his ship close to the steep face of Tolstoi Mys, his men went ashore. They climbed the stout seawall in order to avoid disturbing the animals sequestered on better landing places. The island was named St. George, for the patron saint of the discoverer's boat.

Elliott imagined the discovery in the following terms: "And though the fog was so thick he could see scarce the length of his vessel, his ears were regaled by the sweet music of seal-rookeries wafted out to him on the heavy air. He knew then that he had found the object of his search, and he at once took possession of the island in the Russian name and that of his craft."[6]

Elliott was merely carrying on the tradition of the fog recorded by Bishop Veniaminov: "Despite the pre-eminence of Pribylov over all navigators of the time in that region, it did not fall to him quickly to chance on a landfall. While near to one of the islands that later were to bear his name, he noticed unmistakable signs denoting the existence of land, and these were continuously encountered, yet during a period of three weeks, the land itself could not be perceived due to fog conditions. Finally fortune either taking pity on him or abandoning the struggle against the importunity of man, lifted the curtain of fog and the eastern part of the island nearest the Aleutian archipelago showed itself to their indescribable joy, before the eyes of our mariners."[7]

Perhaps Pribylov boasted in his cups, a habit that overcame him fatally on Kodiak Island,[8] that a great mariner like him could only have been delayed by extraordinary fog conditions or he merely enlarged on his experiences in good sailor fashion. The legend was born and it was fostered by the two earliest historians of the islands.

Pribylov left a party of Aleut and Russian hunters on St. George, under the leadership of Peredovshchik [foreman] Efim Popov, to collect a shipload of furs while he returned to Unalaska to winter in a safer harbor and collect supplies. His smaller crew, the stores of fresh furs aboard the *St. George,* and his refusal to tell where he had been aroused much speculation among the crews of other vessels that lay wintering in the harbor. When Pribylov set sail, late the next spring, for St. George, other ships followed and came safely through the fog of ignorance and of the seas to the Seal Islands of the Bering.

Pribylov's party had taken many skins during the winter. But other supplies ran low. When Pribylov failed to return in early spring, the small party became anxious. Perhaps he had forgotten his sea course. Perhaps the *St. George* had fallen prey to Bering winds. Anxiously, on clear days, the men climbed to high points along the shore and scanned the sea in all directions for the sail of the *St. George.* On such a bright forenoon a pair of sharp eyes picked out a dark line on the horizon to the north, undoubtedly land. Immediately Efim Popov manned a baidar, the large skin boat of Aleut make, and set off toward that distant smudge. They came ashore on the new island on the twenty-ninth of June, according to the old Russian calendar or July 10 by today's reckoning, the day of the Apostles Peter and Paul, and dedicated the land to them. The cumbersome title was soon abbreviated to St. Paul. Over the long accessible coastal reaches of the new island crowded millions of the animals the Russians had hunted down the seaways for over a century. The density of the fog that obscured the land was of no avail to the fur seal. Where he could travel, man could follow and finally overtake his last northern retreat.

July 8, 1941

A little before nine this grey morning and I am ready to bang away on this machine. Sam has just satisfied our curiosity about the washing machine and reports that it is definitely on the blink so that now I can sit back with a clear conscience and wait for it to be repaired later today I hope.

I was down in the cellar after lunch (which had broken off my scribbling of yesterday) concluding that the machine needed assistance when Sam came running to tell me to get dressed to go exploring. I flew upstairs and into warm slacks and boots despite the bright shining sun before I learned whether we were going with the Obergs or Harry May. It was the former. McMillin had suggested that he take the afternoon off to go out to Northeast Point because Sunday when he had wanted to go there, M. said it would interfere with the drive [of fur seals to the killing grounds].

What a different world we were driving through as we followed the same road to Big Lake that we had traveled the afternoon before. For now the world was alive with sunlight and the lupine and yellow poppy gleamed like new flowers. Both the silvery beauty of a rainy day and the radiance of a sunny afternoon are enchanting and I do not know which to prefer.

Had I chanced to discover the Seal Islands I might have had cause to cavil at the fog. Arriving a hundred and fifty years later with a mind filled with shipboard yarns and notions acquired from books, I was sorely disillusioned. The early morning fogs were not as dense as the morning mists of late summer in the Catskill region of my childhood. I reveled in the few bright warm days, regular interludes in every summer season according to the weather records. I liked no less the days when the mist rolled playfully in from one coast, was pushed playfully about by the breezes, and finally blown to sea again. Gossamer wisps fluttered in the air like dainty kerchiefs kidnapped by the wind. Little puffs rose from damp hollows like ghostly balloons. The shortest walk was an adventure because of the changing temperament of the weather. If the sun shone, it was well to have a kerchief for the head in the pocket. Suddenly the brilliance would fade and gentle rain fall. Before the kerchief was knotted under the chin, the sun was smiling again. Not often was the fog, the little light fog of the Pribilofs, clammy, cold, and miserable to the bared face. The constant variation as if some errant musician played on the organ of the weather, his fingers lazily, thoughtlessly improvising endless arrangements of his fog theme, provided the charm, the small adventure, the romance of life on the Misty Islands.

Ungrateful is the American who curses Bering Sea fog, be it flimsy or thick, for the cool atmosphere is the chief cause of the fur seal's choice of breeding ground. Were there not enough fine spray in the air to keep the animals comfortable they would have sought other shores. The well-drained beaches of lava boulders, the light rainfalls that do not turn the soil between the rocks into sticky plaster to adhere to furry flanks, are other conditions that fur seals require for comfortable existence during the periods when procreative instinct drives them in from their broad pastures of the sea.

Chapter 6

Since there were no seals to greet us at West Landing our immediate burning desire was to rush out to the beaches where the seals congregated. It proved not to be a simple matter of donning hiking clothes and inquiring the direction toward which to travel. There were other barriers than mere distance. Our first questions brought answers that put us in the humble station befitting amateurs.

The seals must not be unnecessarily disturbed during the breeding season from June to August. Visits to rocks overlooking rookeries were permitted provided a roundup of young males was not scheduled for a few days. Since beaches within walking distance from the village were soon to be culled we were advised to be patient.

We began to sort out the terminology that made so many sentences of general island conversation mystifying. Although a baby seal was a pup, its mother was a cow and its father a bull. They all lived together on a division of beach known as a rookery. Considering the bovine names of the family heads it seemed strange that their resort was not called a pasture. A young male under five years of age, unfettered by matrimony, was known as a bachelor. A herd of bachelors formed a pod and a section of the beach that they occupied was a hauling ground. During the breeding season there is such a strict demarcation between the rookery and the hauling ground, policed by vigilant bulls, that only an occasional bachelor is lucky enough to stray across the invisible boundary and escape unscathed.

Most unexpected was the information that a seal is not a seal any more than the performing seal we have thrown tidbits to in zoos or watched balancing balls on his nose in a circus is a seal. The latter is a California sea lion. The Alaskan fur seal is a very, very distant relative of real seals, who cannot use their hind flippers on land but merely drag the rear portions of their bodies jerkily over the ground and never go far from the water's edge when ashore. The Alaskan fur seal is much more closely related to, of all animals, a bear. But the misnomer is certain to endure indefinitely since years of custom have made the English term fixed and inviolable no matter how strenuously scientists may deprecate the name.

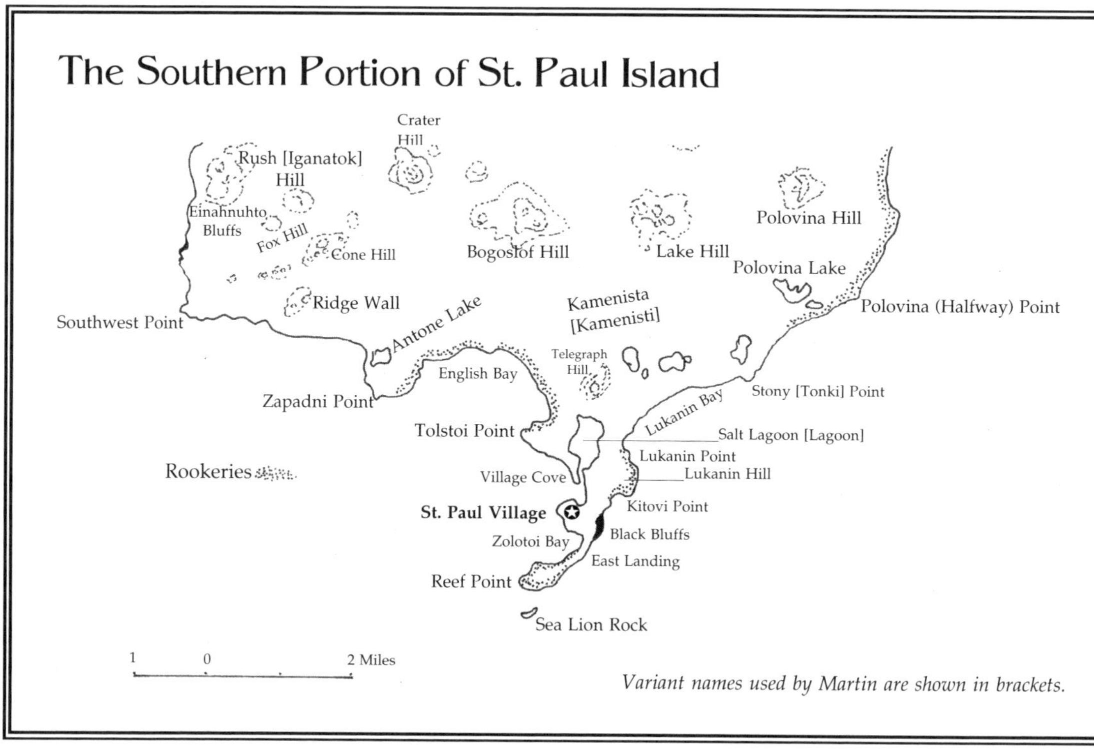

The southern portion of St. Paul Island.

However, scientists dare not criticize the layman's error too severely since the scientific cognomens have not been satisfactorily settled for the three species of fur seal that inhabit the northern Pacific area. One species breeds on the Japanese-owned Kurile Islands. The second spends it summers on the Russian Commander Islands. The third species belongs to the largest herd, which resorts to our own Pribilof Islands.

If we except the shipwrecked hunter from Unimak, probably no man was familiar with the land habits of any of the three species until a more famous shipwreck brought Bering to the island in the Commander group that bears his name. A member of Bering's party was a German naturalist, George William Steller, whose efforts to gather green plants on various shores for anti-scorbutic purposes, were frustrated by Bering's impatience and refusal to linger even a few hours near unknown and possibly dangerous shores. Perhaps Steller's weeds might have saved the lives of Bering and nineteen of his crew. As Stefansson has proven, these men died close to certain remedies for the scourge of mariners of that era, surrounded by millions of animals whose fresh flesh would have restored them all to health in a short time. Steller wasted no moment of his enforced stay on Bering Island. He studied the animal and floral life there and kept lengthy detailed notes of his observations. His keen eyes studied the fur seal well as the scientific name he picked out, *Ursinus marinus* or sea bear, reveals. Today this species is known as *Callorhinus ursinus*, the pretty nosed bear. But the American variety is usually known vaguely as *Callorhinus alascansus*—pretty nosed Alaskan.

The Russian hunters called the fur seals by a more homey phrase, *morskie koticki,* or sea cats. The Russian terms for the various classes of seals are still sometimes found in quite recent fur seal literature but such usage grows more and more infrequent. Even the Pribilof Aleuts employ them rarely although their fathers were still keeping personal records in Russian of their daily seal kill. Only in literature and history will the young fur seal continue to be known as *kotik,* the kitten; the female as *matka* [*maatkax̂*], a Russian endearment for mother; the young bachelor from two to five as *holostiak* [*x̂ulustaakax̂*], or bachelor; the mature male from five until the time that he obtains a mate as *polosikach* [*polusikaachax̂*]; and finally when he becomes a beachmaster as *sikach* [*sekách*]. Only old Aleuts will be able to recall in a few years that *atach* [*aataax*]in their ancient tongue meant the old harem sultan, *ennathact* was the female and that a pup was called *lakuthak* [*laaqudax̂* or *laaq(u)daadax̂*]. Even when David Starr Jordan was conducting an investigation of seal life in 1896 he found only the children calling a pup *lakuthak.*

In accordance with the regulations we curbed our desires and waited patiently until we could join a regular party going out to drive bachelors from their hauling grounds to the killing field to be despoiled of their fur coats and their lives. The opportunity came unexpectedly a night about a week after we had become citizens of St. Paul. Mr. Johnston casually asked us if we should care to accompany him on the drive at Reef Point, which was due to start in a few minutes. We responded with joy. Though the baby's arrival was only two months away, I could maintain a steady walking pace for many miles but I did not enjoy rushing over rough ground. I decided to start ahead of the villagers. Since there was little time I neglected to change to heavier clothes. The day had been warm. The sunlight was still brilliant at seven thirty in the evening. We crossed Zolotoi Sands at a leisurely pace and climbed up some steep bluffs to the level of the long southerly peninsula of Reef. Already the seal drivers who had left the village half an hour after our departure were at our heels, some climbing the cliff, others racing across the soft sands. The first comers settled down by a jutting tower of breccia. From that point to the end of Reef the scoria road lay on open land. The respite gave me time to catch my breath and look about the landscape. Otter Island made me lose my breath again. It sailed across a golden horizon, ethereal and dreamlike. The grassy field sloping toward St. Paul burned like a huge exotic emerald that surpassed any Sinbad found.

As soon as the drivers, armed with long slender poles, were assembled, we tramped rapidly down the road to the great parade ground of Reef. My immediate personal christening of the wide bare central plateau was not original, for a few days later I found the words *Parade Ground,* capitalized, on a map. I sensed rather than saw the movement of masses of life that bordered each side of the Parade Ground for over a mile ahead of us.

The sealers divided into two groups. We followed those who went left to the seaward coast of Reef while the other gang went off at a fast pace toward the Zolotoi Bay side, opposite Village Hill.

July 5, 1941
We have made some sort of beginning for routinizing our lives so that we may have leisure to study and explore and relax. . . .

Sam went on his rounds of the jail and stopped off at the office. He came back with fifty folders, and two packages of paper. U.S. government paper but very sleazy stuff. But at least it will hold lots of words. I want some of the folders in order to start letters to different people and keep them tidily. Others we will be using around the office for records, I guess. Sam also asked McMillin to ask the doctor on St. George's if he had a Bard Parker handle which he could send over when the *Penguin* came by in a couple of days.

Sam also put in a request for bread and meat. The cook at the Company House is in charge of both. He came over in a few minutes with a loaf of old bread and said I would have fresh bread this afternoon. In a few minutes he was back with beef steaks for tonight and a chicken. Both frozen stiff as ice. And the chicken has to be cleaned. So what. I'll manage somehow. He said the bread was dependent completely on his good will. Seems very kindly and jolly. Gave Sam a word of advice-not to baby the St. Louis bunch. Evidently the lads are a trial to him. And he doesn't want to have to send lunches to the hospital. . . .

cont.

As soon as the drive was under way, the sealers acted with clocklike precision going full speed ahead. With extraordinary agility the drivers pranced over the boulder-littered shore. Every few minutes a few men would break away toward the shore rim, racing to get between a pod of bachelors and their one sea passage to escape. Then the sealers began to pound the rocks with their poles and the excited bachelors, choosing the only open way, rushed madly from their foes straight inland. Since the hauling grounds were adjacent to rookeries the old bulls nipped them and roared at them if they sought safety by crossing a harem. If a space happened to be clear, a sealer rushed into the breach, brandishing his club, tapping rocks and shouting. Relentlessly the men drove the seals toward the Parade Ground.

As one pod responded to goading, another bunch of sealers had broken off from the main gang and were busy cutting out the next group of bachelors. The main gang kept going steadily ahead, diminishing after each stop as two or three men were left to herd each captured pod toward slaughter. The air vibrated with the snorting breathing of the bachelors, the cacophony of the disturbed bulls, the cries of the sealers, and the ominous chilling drumbeats of their clubs. Sounds of similar tumult drifted across from the Zolotoi side.

Rushing after the sealers, trying to keep my footing as I jumped from one rock to another in order to keep just behind the main body of sealers, I found the role of spectator difficult. I ran as rapidly as I could for a short space, with my eyes on the ground. But as soon as I felt a reliably steady rock under my feet and knew I was not in the way of the drive, I stopped to observe the roundup.

Fourth of July had been a gala day, not only because of the festive activities, under the blessing of the Fouke Fur Company, but also because of the weather. We were not up until late but went out about eleven to watch some of the races. Mrs. [Geneva] Hoverson came over and brought us a beautiful coconut cake on her way to watch. Most of the white people were chatting together at the head of the steps when ice cream cones were being dished out. Harry May came along with cones for us all. And it was really delicious pineapple ice cream. I could have eaten a quart. After lunch Sam fell asleep. I watched races and the start of the ballgame from the window and finally went into the bedroom and had a nap myself. . . .

Last night was probably the greatest thrill we shall have here. For we went with Baker and Johnston on the Reef [Point] drive and were taken where no other personnel are taken. We didn't realize that but on the way home Johnston asked us not to mention to the other people that we had been out on the tripods.

Nature seems to have had man's tastes for furs in mind when she taught the sea bear its living and mating rites, for the gregarious bachelors make themselves easy prey. Were they of more solitary habits, scattered in twos or threes, hunting them would require caution and skill. But their sociable natures make them as accessible as domestic cattle. The young males have been misled by some ancient propaganda that in unity there is strength. The exception to that rule renders them almost helpless victims of the hunters.

The confusion in the harems constantly diverted my eyes from the bachelors. The timid cows rushed about crazily trying to get to the sea. A fleeing cow gave no heed to the pup it was deserting. The bulls reared up, bellowing and snorting, lunging at frantic bachelors who tried to flee across their territories, yet never losing sight of their nervous panic-stricken wives. Bulls grabbed at cows and slung them back into the harem, often bleeding from deep gashes. The ponderous males moved with such speed that often I got the impression several bulls were in the place of one as almost simultaneously an agile harem ruler routed several bachelors and recaptured three or four wives.

A mile down the Reef when the peninsula was narrowing, Mr. Johnston called us to halt and led Baker and ourselves up to the top of a high heap of basaltic blocks from which we could survey both shores and the Parade Ground. By this time more than a dozen pods had reached the road and were moving slowly toward the Village flats. For the pods nearest us it meant a trip of over a mile, an exhausting journey for flippered animals.

The sunlight that had delighted us all day had dried out the light scoria surface of the Parade Ground. The flippers of the seals beat up a thick red haze of volcanic dust. The pods in the vanguard traveled fantastically within a dull copper cloud. From our gallery seat they appeared as smartly marching military platoons. Only close at hand the struggling, squirming masses of greyish brown bodies were pathetic caricatures of soldiers. I felt my throat grow dry and constricted as I watched them gasp and snort.

When a pod of seals was first driven from its hauling ground, the animals all rushed together into a mad squirming heap, tremulous and agitated as a pile of slithering fish. As some struggled to the top of the heap, others pushed them over and under and mounted on their bodies in turn. The drivers stood beside the furry maelstrom watching the sleek bodies spurt upward as from a fountain and then fall back and be submerged among their fellows. Any animal who got clear of the melee and started back to sea was immediately headed off and driven back with the others. When the panic subsided, the bachelors, disciplined by a few judicious prods of the sealing clubs, stopped their insane jostling and became quiescent from fatigue. Responding to the rock-tapping signals of the herders they flip-flopped over the rough stony ground, trying to avoid the makers of the harsh sounds. They scrambled untidily, nudging and pushing each other. A few resented being driven so much that they missed no opportunity to snap at the hovering seal clubs or a driver who came too close. As the seals moved off, the drivers kept up an intermittent tattoo on the rocks and gracefully manipulated their long poles to prod a laggard or push a recalcitrant back into line.

A fur seal has no sweat glands and consequently no relief from overheating exertions. Frequently the pods rested to let the exhausted animals sink down for a brief respite. The best drivers, as Mr. Johnston pointed out, let the seals chose their own pace and their own rest interludes. When a seal in the lead dropped down panting, his tongue hanging out like a weary dog, good drivers did not interfere. As the leaders halted, the ones behind piled up on top of them in great confusion once more. In a few moments, almost before the rear seals had dropped to their bellies, the vanguard began to move of its own accord and soon the whole furry mass was forging ahead again with its curious abrupt choppy rhythm. If a group lingered too long to please its drivers the men began to whistle and tap the rocks. Some men picked up bits of wood, which they used as clappers. Others slapped their hands together. Slightly macabre to me was the sight of two scapulae of seals being played like cymbals.

As the pods passed our reviewing stand, the clouds of dust swirled higher and grew darker. Proportionately Johnston's anxiety increased.

"There will be many road skins tonight," he predicted ruefully and then paused to translate the term for us. Drivers were supposed to maintain such watchful guardianship over their pods that seals that were tiring too quickly could be cut out of the pod and chased off toward the sea. The exhausted beast usually hated to forsake his fellows and scrambled frantically back to them. When the drivers had successfully beaten him off, he would seek the sea for consolation. If the seal had the strength to reach the water, his chances of survival were good. But if he was overlooked until his strength had ebbed too much, he would die quickly. We watched laggards being chased from pods. Staggering off a few feet they would sink in exhaustion. In a few minutes they would struggle erect on their flippers, drag along a few more yards and then drop down again. Always their instinct led them to the sea and its recuperative coolness.

The fur of animals that died from overheating spoils within a couple of hours. The pelt becomes slimy. The guard hairs become loose. As soon as a drive is finished, the route and the neighboring ground is combed thoroughly to pick up all the dying or dead beasts and skin them. Mr. Johnston always headed the search for road skins. A searcher had to miss no clump of grass, no projection of rock that might shelter a fugitive. Johnston seemed to feel the search was his personal responsibility and that a high number of road skins would be a blot on his own reputation. That seemed a very oversensitive reaction to me, particularly on an abnormally dry evening.

Flip. Flop. Flip. Flop. The army from the sea went shuffling wearily on its wobbly way below us. My eyes were enchanted by them. I tingled with an excitement, half interest, half impersonal pity and revulsion. I was barely aware of the cold breeze against which my light clothing was absolutely no protection. So it was with reluctance that I heard Mr. Johnston say, "Let's go."

But to my amazement and joy he turned away from the departing seal pods as the final group was passing us and led the way down the shore, in the direction of the very end of the Reef. We were going to have an intimate view of life in a Pribilof harem.

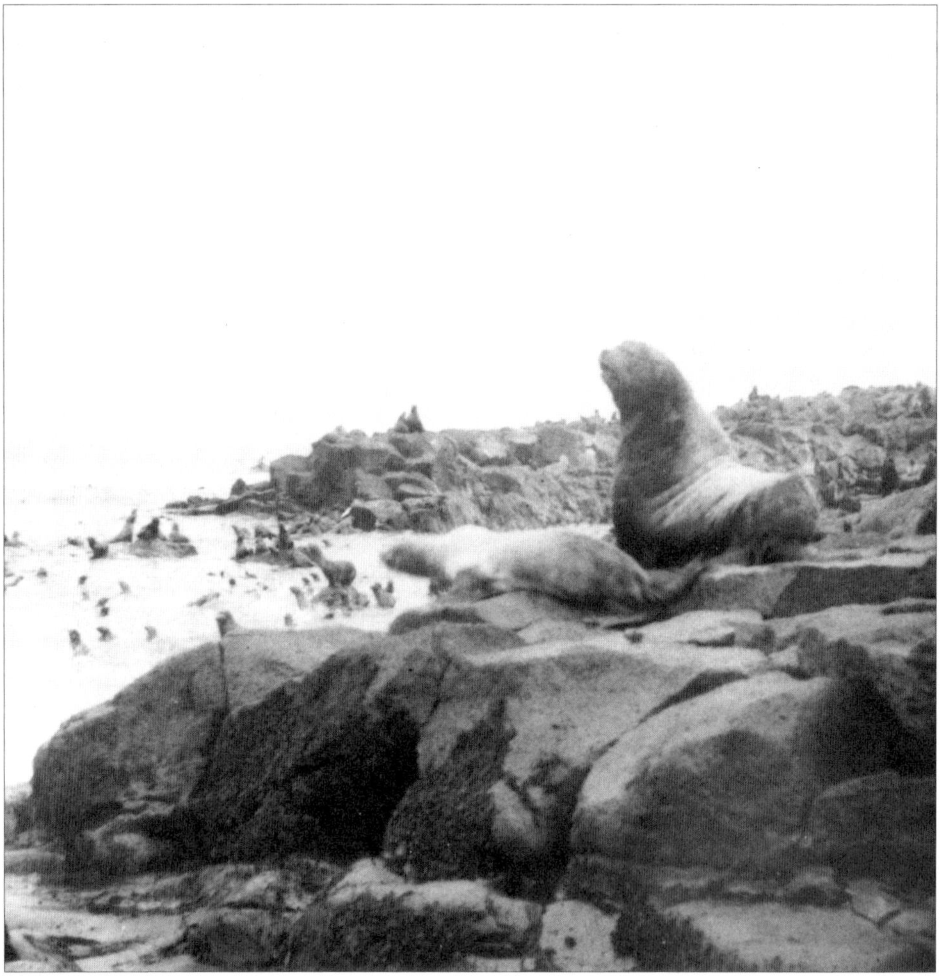

A fur seal rookery.

Chapter 7

As soon as we stepped down from our lava-buttressed reviewing stand and threaded our way a few yards among scattered boulders, we began to encroach upon bulls jealously guarding harem sites, but there were no furry odalisques for several hundred yards. Only at intervals a huge bull seal swaggered back and forth menacingly within narrow confines, lunging about fiercely either in our direction, as we passed near, toward a fellow bull held captive in his realm by similar invisible boundary markers, or just lashing out at imaginary foes. Not even a lion in a rage could look more dangerous to approach, but Mr. Johnston zigzagged as leisurely through the midst of ferocious ravening beasts as if he were strolling in a flower garden. We followed with quaking hearts not completely reassured by Johnston's placid demeanor. As we went along he explained the immutable laws that govern the behavior of the fully mature male seal.

Early in the spring the bulls are the first to arrive from southern seas. Each selects, by what manner of judgment no scientist has been able to discover, a particular portion of the beach for his own domain. The first bulls may just take up squatter's sites near the shore that is unoccupied by rivals. As later bulls arrive they have to fight their way past the original settlers and stake out claims farther and farther from the sea. As soon as his harem site is chosen, the bull begins his sentry duty, warding off all daring *sikachi* [beachmasters] who attempt to oust him and, even when there is no danger, carrying on a playful campaign against imaginary foes exactly like a soldier training for battle. By the time a few hundred bulls are settled, the rookery becomes a field of bellicose, furry fiends, blasting the air with defiant thunderous bellows, challenging the universe. The semblance of fearless independence is a sham. There is no more skilled bluffer, not even among human beings, than a bull seal. The bonds of instinct and habit chain each bull to a wall-less, bar-less prison, once his choice is made, unless he is ousted by a stronger male. Across these enchanted borders he will not or cannot cross. Only on its margins will his belligerence find an outlet in a bloody match when his watchful eye marks out a neighbor as a trespasser.

In June the cows begin straggling ashore. As they emerge from the sea, waiting bulls appropriate them for their harems. Conflicts over an arriving cow rage up and down the length and breadth of the rookery. All the activity that the bull has engaged in since his arrival is a rest cure compared to his exertions now. He must watch his restless cows, flighty, feckless females ready to flee at the slightest disturbance or to succumb to the come-hither glances of neighboring gallants. He must keep off thieving Lotharios who want to snatch his bride away. From the moment the first female enters his harem, he dare not close an eye until the breeding season breaks up in late July. In the early weeks he must also maintain a watch for additional wives as cows continue to arrive. The fortunate beachmasters are those stationed at the shoreline who can easily bar the way of a landing female and add her to his flock. Until late in the season many bulls in the rear of the rookeries are still waiting for females. Some may fail to win one bride. Others may woo and win the young virgin females who arrive in midsummer. Among such patient luckless bulls we were walking.

As I ventured within the network of nebulous borders natural law seemed flimsy and insubstantial. I longed for stout recognizable walls and less spiritual, less gossamer terminative markers. The bull seal might know his rights but would he pity my ignorance if I innocently trespassed upon private property, put one foot within the angle of his plot? Only experience could impart complete smug security. How was it possible that the eight hundred pounds of ferocity rushing directly at me with an open mouth glittering with nasty pointed seaweed-stained yellow teeth, blowing out a cloud of murky steam, roaring awesome threats as he poised to leap at me, was going to sit down abruptly a couple of feet away as meekly as a kitten sated on cream?

Johnston laughed at our doubts. "He won't come any closer," he kept saying. "All this noise is bluff. And a bull seal is a coward, except when you actually invade his harem during breeding times. Just throw a pebble at his chest and he'll run away." Over and over he repeated the guarantee, "No one has ever been killed by a seal."

Over large stretches of the rookeries, six or seven feet above the ground, aerial walks supported on tripod posts ran in irregular designs. From these tripods toward the end of July Johnston and an assistant would estimate the number of seals present. From far off, those walls were fragile tracery on the horizon. Close at hand they looked scarcely more substantial. But I was willing to walk on the air itself to get within the heart of the great throbbing mass of life that tossed up and down in rusty, silver-streaked billows just beyond us. I forgot my skepticism as we came to more densely occupied areas. I walked in a dream animal world. On our planet there could be no such multitude of creatures. The dark earth heaved and swayed, twisted and writhed. The rocks had taken on a covering of soft fur. They had become mobile and sentient, baying at the dome of the sky.

The runway we neared ran in a straight line almost to the water's edge and curved to extend across the forefront of the beach almost to Reef Point where it cut sharply back almost to the limit of the rookery. Johnston warned against more than one person on a plank section of the runway at this time. Mounting the crude ladder I thought his advice was superfluous. The silvery weather-beaten boards looked like strips of paper strung through the air. I followed Johnston across the first single narrow planks, paying deep and silent respect to the entire clan of acrobat and tightrope performers. Thankfully I reached the next segment of the walk, a mighty avenue two planks wide. With a foot on each plank the playful bouncing of the boards was more bearable. There was a low wire rail, which I had to stoop to grasp. Its cold metal strands imparted a confidence that had scant basis in its actual helpfulness. I had the courage to gaze away from my feet and drink in the frenzied scene beneath us as we walked along.

The air was alive with sound, a medley of snorts, whistles, puffings, gruntings, roars, and bleating calls. The heavy bodies slapped rhapsodically on the basalt terraces. The endless beating of flippers was a clapping accompaniment to the cacophony. The sounds were harsh and ugly, each one distinct. There was no unison, no cadence, no blending into a harmonious sonority. Bulls beneath and near the runway leaped up toward us with bared teeth and ear-shattering roars. Their immense bodies springing upward just missed ramming against the planks. The air was full of flying monsters. They stormed and raged and failing to capture us, turned to snarl obscene thunderous profanities against their mates.

The timid cows, so sleekly clad in silvery fur, darted like startled trout amidst the heaving brown billows. The omnipresent beachmaster, poised to leap upward to destroy us, would detour into a swift well-calculated swoop, sinking his teeth into the soft flanks of a fugitive. Callously he would drop or hurl her into the center of the harem and be thrusting his huge bulk up toward us in a twinkling.

Every harem was dotted with slippery black pups indifferent to the furor about them. Delivered into a world of confusion and clamor, they were not disturbed by the heightened pandemonium occasioned by our presence. I gasped when a huge bull sat back heavily on a very small pup. An errant wife brought him to his flipper immediately. Up bounced the pup undamaged to squirm about as lively as before.

Johnston stopped and waited for me. I advanced to the end of my plank to talk to him. Below us lay the flattened body of a dead pup like a black paper pattern for a toy. I concluded his careless foster father had been the steam roller that destroyed him. Johnston assured me pups are rarely killed by such accidents. No matter how clumsily their elders trample them, as soon as the pressure is removed, the pups bounce up buoyantly, unaffected by temporary suffocation. I noticed again and again pups wriggling out from under the massive beachmasters who sat unaware of the frantic squirmings beneath them. Fortunately for the continuation of the species the pups are pliant balls of fat, possessing astounding resilience.

Only by an accident is the pup a member of the harem presided over by his own father. Rare indeed must be the bulls who claim the same females for two seasons in succession. The young exist by mere sufferance of the harem ruler, who pays them little heed unless they chance to annoy him. Then he bites or cuffs the offender with no trace of parental fondness.

> July 5, 1941
> I was amazed to see how the cows fought together, biting each other viciously. The pups squirmed underneath all other activity. I saw one dead pup so flattened out that I thought he had been squashed by some bull or cow sitting too long on him. J[ohnston] said that rarely happens. Something else must have been the cause of death and the flattening process had taken place after death. And then he pointed out a very large bull who was grabbing some of his cows and just bouncing up and down with his immense body on some half-dozen pups. But the pups were completely uninjured. J. said they are practically balls of fat and very resilient. And as I watched, as we loitered along, I saw how the pups were trodden on, rolled over, sat upon. And a few seconds later they were squirming around gaily.

It requires nearly a year for a sea pup embryo to mature. The urge that brings the female upon land in the early summer is probably the intuitional forewarning of impending labor pains. Hardy indeed is the female who must run the rough gamut of wooing bulls before being made captive. Within two or three days of landing her baby is born. Although there have been tales of twin seals no actual proof of twin birth has been established. Considering the ceaseless careful observation of seal life carried on season after season on the Pribilofs, it is extremely unlikely that multiple births could have gone unnoticed, be they ever so rare. So it is accepted as an established truth that the female gives birth to but one pup.

A few hours after delivery the female is ready for impregnation. This accomplished, the beachmaster permits the female to go and come freely. Hers is no comfortable postnatal convalescence. Her life becomes a series of sea journeys, traveling back and forth between the island and regions a hundred and fifty to two hundred miles away where squid abound and returning to nurse her offspring. At first the pup nurses at frequent intervals. As he grows larger he becomes capable of imbibing enough milk to nourish him for several days and at a later period probably as long as a week. The longer intervals between feedings give the mother leisure to rest and travel the long route to the feeding grounds without haste.

Since the pups that sport about a single harem have probably had different fathers it seemed to this sentimental observer that nature might have compensated for this separation from the actual fathers by endowing the females with a capacity for intense maternal affection. To my indignant amazement, I saw the hundreds of seal mothers underneath me behaving with nonchalant indifference to their young. Not a tremor betrayed the slightest sign of love for the pups. Johnston assured me my observation was accurate. I noticed that whenever the cows were frightened and attempting to leave the harem, they scrambled as roughly over the pups as if they were but inanimate lava stones. While still shocked and irritated by the selfish abandonment of pups at the threat of danger, I observed several pups flip-flopping about with their placentas still attached at the navel. That the mother seals do not even gnaw through the umbilical cord seemed the epitome of laziness. In a few days, as the pup wriggles about the stony area, the withering cord is severed by the sawing friction of the sharper rocks.

Johnston halted again and pointed downward. Beneath us a cow was giving birth. The little black body was partially encased in its grey membrane. I still expected the cows to display a motherly trait. But the mother did not lick and clean her baby as a dog or cow would. In the midst of the delirium, due to our proximity, the cow lay quietly, seemingly unaware of the excited clamor and the excessive movement about her and disinterested in her newborn infant. When several panicky cows crowded against her, she roused from her haughty frigid state and snapped savagely at them. They retaliated. Despite the uncompleted birth she snarled and bit and hit out with her flipper, without rising from her supine position. In the fray the little newcomer was frequently trampled on or received a glancing blow. When the fight subsided, some pups began to gambol close to the parturient mother. In their play they backed into her or even scampered across her. Expertly she nipped them and drove them off. When they tumbled over her pup she gave no heed.

I waited as long as I could, hoping to see her drop that mask of disdain or apathy. I might have frozen there before such a miracle would happen. Stupid lethargic female. How I hated her.

I had been hardly aware of my shivers and chattering teeth as the icy wind buffeted us. The fascinating pageant of animal activities blotted out all other feelings. Occasionally I spotted a dead bull who had paid with his life for attempted kidnapping or for trying to protect one of his own wives from a neighboring ravisher. Villain and hero met the same end on the seal beaches, where there was no justice and brute strength ruled. In shallow spaces in and between the rocks pools of bright blood were clotting. Neither the corpses nor the scarlet stains amazed me. Were these the only results of all the furry conflict, this constant battle of rutting males, the casualties were minor indeed.

At the end of the runway we found our way off barred by a huge scarred veteran, guarding a harem of half a dozen cows. He had no intention of letting us pass. When he lunged toward us his body just brushed the end timbers. Johnston clapped his hands at the monster. I could not help laughing aloud. It seemed pathetic and futile to employ against a fiend gestures helpful to divert a child. Something more than a game of pat-a-cake was needed. Perhaps the bridge keeper shared my opinion. He refused to retreat before either gesture or shouts.

He darted backward when Johnston made a short rush in his direction but his rebound was so swift that Johnston had no chance to jump past him. On all sides other excited beachmasters applauded the veteran and waited their turn to block whomever escaped the first beast. To dodge one meant to fall into the maws of another. Since we had no weapons, such as sticks or pebbles, it began to look as if we must retreat the whole way back along the windswept runway.

Mr. Johnston was not going to let a mere bull seal get the better of him. As the monster cast an anxious backward glance at his wives, Johnston jumped and raced between several charging beasts. The air filled with huge lashing brown bodies in his wake. He sprang toward the top of a clump of rocks. He missed and started to fall backward. I felt myself poising to jump in instinctive helpfulness just as he regained his balance by a skillful twist of his body and gained the top of the rocks. I breathed again. I was the next in line to run the gauntlet. Johnston searched busily for pebbles and loose stones beyond his rock of safety. Meanwhile, the foiled guardian of the runway fumed more angrily than ever as he bashed his body against the planks. Although there was always a loose pebble to turn one's ankle in the spaces between the rocks, now, when one was virtually necessary, Johnston searched over a large area and came back toward us with two tiny stones. As he threw them at our dragon, he reached one hand to me. I swung down and raced to the safety of the rock pile. Never had I moved more swiftly. I seemed to feel the hot musky breath of the bulls I passed, but perhaps my imagination was too intense. I began to hunt for rocks. I managed to pull loose a few fragments of crumbling breccia. While I continued to gather ammunition Johnston made two return trips and held off the enemy with a rock barrage that enabled first Sam and then Baker to escape.

July 5, 1941
Mainly because the weather is nice, the seals are late coming ashore. J. says that later they will come in such large numbers that it will be almost impossible to handle them even with the larger crew of workers this year.

And this is the year that extra people were sent in to take a much larger catch than usual in case the Japanese begin pelagic sealing this year and wreck damages upon the herds. When I read even the little I have of the evils of the pelagic sealing, I hope from the bottom of my heart that it is not to start over again. I remember the heart-rending accounts of the pups dying by hundreds on the beach because their mothers have been killed at sea while they are out seeking for food, and I remember that this whole process of animal destruction goes on to get furs for coats . . . I hope no interminable warfare is going to start in over killing rights.

In just a few seconds we were past the remaining bulls. All of us were slightly short of breath except Johnston, who was twinkling-eyed and unruffled as usual, ready to utilize our experience as proof that man has nothing to fear from seals.

Midway along the runway we had stopped for my first close view of Sea Lion Rock. The channel between the islands was dotted with the dark bodies of seals sporting in the water. Bachelors and cows and yearlings splashed and swam and performed dolphin jumps in full view of the poor bulls harnessed by natural law from their favorite and more natural habitat. The rocks were covered with seals and the old Russian cross leaned wearily over them.

So magnetic had been the scenes of seal life during the hours we spent on the runway I had missed the capricious drama of the restless weather. Sun had been replaced by dainty drizzles that would have been pleasant had not the cold wind from the sea whipped the drops into our faces too harshly. While the rain was pattering upon us we had only to glance over our shoulders to see the bright yellow moon painted on the sky's deep blue canvas. One moment a hill to the west glowed as if the sunlight were imprisoned within it and emanated from its heart. The hill was a volcano of glass within which the flames leaped and scintillated. A little later I noticed that the radiance had died away. Dull purple clouds were draped in dignified rippling folds over the hill's multiple cones. When we turned homeward puffs of grey mist like demure old-lady caps rested lightly on the peaks.

As we came back through purple dusk, Johnston pointed out the man-determined division of the Reef. The immense rookery on the Bering side where we had followed the sealer borrowed its name from the peninsula, Reef rookery. On the Zolotoi side a small rookery near the tip of the Point had been christened Ardiguen. From the next cliff, extending nearly to Zolotoi sands, the shore still retained the name Gorbotch, the Russian word for "humpback." There were many crags above the shingle that could have suggested that appellation to the Russians.

The only site nearest Reef that was grass-grown enough to furnish a killing field where little dust and sand could adhere to skins was the flat across from the village, beyond Village Lake. Because of the distance, Reef bachelors were driven in the evening and permitted to rest through the night until three o'clock in the morning. I was in no mood to get up early to watch the butchery of the first seals with which I had established an intimate contact. We fell asleep with the soft sounds of the captured seals streaming through our window. Staccato beats of the guards' sealing clubs rang out infrequently. No wily bachelor could break through the ring of sealers to escape the dawn and the fatal descent of those inevitable clubs. Into my dreams went a procession of clumsy, straining bright-eyed seals enveloped by swirls of red dust that grew more crimson as the animals advanced toward the silver tips of huge knives blooming like spiked grasses in the field by the lake.

Chapter 8

The very next afternoon we went driving with the Obergs. Earl was the island mechanic, an old Alaskan resident who had come to St. Paul just a month ahead of us. He had three topics of conversation: his sinuses, machinery, and the glories of Fairbanks. The afternoon brought a rather heavy shower so I was relieved when Vivian, his wife, came to ask whether we would brave the weather. A little rain could not discourage me for I was eager to explore more of the island during its first summer flowering.

Already we had been informed by catty remarks of several Service people that drives were rare privileges. "There are always cars for the Natives but not for the whites," I had been told numberless times by many individuals, "except for the agent and mechanic." They needed cars in carrying out their duties but the tasks of physician, storekeeper, and the others were within pedestrian range.

Truth and falsehood mingled in the criticisms. McMillin, or Mac as everyone called him, was not a person to be bothered with planning recreation for the Service employees under him. His job as he saw it, and perhaps seventeen years on the Pribilofs had narrowed his outlook, was to get sealskins and to keep the Aleuts working hard enough to accomplish that job. He lacked the imagination to know what other people desired and the impulse to want to keep them happy and contented in order to avoid the deadly petty feuds of a circumscribed community. Mac possessed the heartiest, most infectious laugh I have ever heard, but like the Pribilof sunshine his broad smile could be wiped away by such an abrupt gust of irritation, noisy and vulgarly expressed, that timid souls shrank deep into their boots when he erupted. Yet he tried to avoid the task of apportioning cars after work hours by delegating the responsibility to Oberg. Earl likewise shrank from the duties of arbitrary judge of car sharing. Two small cars and five families, excluding Mac's and the Obergs, posed a difficult problem for the fairest judge.

People like ourselves, who stood in no awe of Mac and regarded him with tolerant amusement, were not afraid to approach him for a car. Too many of the others, less valiant, clinging to their jobs and fearful of the damage an adverse report from the agent could do their civil service rating, hesitated to brave Mac but grumbled constantly behind his back. The result of personal repressed timidity bred an unpleasant social atmosphere and paved the way for many unsavory quarrels and nasty feuds. I thought, after months of studying the behavior pattern of the official community, how much friction could be offset by equitable regulations about transportation for recreational purposes. People needed to escape the confines of the village to refresh their mental outlook by a change of scene. They should not be barred from the most beautiful parts of the islands. It was not fair that recreation should depend upon the human frailty of individual agents. Too often in the past agents had been so culpable in displaying favoritism that the island rocked with reverberations of social friction. Mac played no favorites as far as I ever noticed but he had other failings that produced discontent among the officials and made him the object of much unnecessary dislike.

Vivian chose to introduce us to Zapadni. We drove out of the village along the lagoon and past Ice House Lake, a tranquil little pond that furnished the town's water and ice. Beyond it a road broke from the main highway to Northeast Point to curve toward the southwest side of the island. I sat wedged in front with the Obergs while Sam bounced up and down on a wooden box on the open-back truck, exposed to the wind and rain.

The rain-dulled atmosphere was lit by the brilliant colors of the flowers that thronged from the road's edge down to the dark shoreline and up to the exposed rocks of the hills' rims. The sunny yellows, the lush shades of rose, and the sky-borrowed blues were refugees from an opulent tropical jungle. This was not the semi-barren hyperborean land I had envisioned. I surrendered my last faint regret for the roses of my Greenbelt garden.

We had driven less than three miles when we made our first sortie into the fields. Through the thick grass that shed its burden of raindrops upon us as we brushed through, we plodded shoreward. The delicate pinkish mauve of crowded lousewort blushed under protective parasols of grass. The deep rose and purple blossoms of beach pea vines crisscrossed the sand with so soft a web of roseate purple velvet that it was sacrilege to crush such radiance with clumsy heavy feet. Since there was no pathway we went on treading lightly, leaving broken stems and dying flowers in our wake. Sam blessed the hip boots that he had borrowed for the afternoon. My corduroy slacks clung cold and damp from many inches above the rim of my knee boots.

We emerged from a small valley between sand dunes to look along the majestic sweep of English Bay, from the strong indomitable face of the cliffs of Tolstoi to the less rugged headland of Zapadni Point. Tolstoi referred to the thick strength of the promontory and was not dedicated to the Russian novelist, unborn when the rocks were christened. A cluster of black rocks marred the rolling tossing waters of the bay, islets called Nerpski or Hair Seal Rocks. Long, long before our visit the rocks had been deserted by the hair seals. When we tired of the view we turned back and drove along a level plain of stunted sparse grasses where millions of yellow poppies beckoned the unwary who did not know what a nauseating fetid perfume they emitted. We drove up a rolling slope and looked down upon Zapadni. How prosaic rookery and cliff would sound in the English translation, West Rookery and West Point with its military association. But the syllables of the Russian word, accented on the first *a,* possess a romantic cadence that delights the ear and the imagination.

Within a curve of the shore beneath us a sluggish stream crawled through a sand flat that extended from the foot of the hill to the headland. Legend has stamped this tiny beach as the landing place of Popov and the Aleut hunters. At some place nearby after they splashed ashore, scattering the multitude of seals that crowded the beach, they came upon a charred space where a few ashes remained in crannies, testimony that they were not the first men to stand on the island's soil. Adjacent to the fire site they found a copper sword hilt of European make and a clay pipe. Further traces of the previous visitors were either not found or forgotten through the years. On a picturesque broken ridge high above us on the right a Russian cross marked what I had been informed was the cemetery of one of the earliest villages. I was anxious to climb up to seek for traces of old graves but the Obergs showed no enthusiasm so I regretfully followed the moods of my hosts.

When Elliott described the spot in 1870 he wrote, "One of the prehistoric villages, the village of Pribylov's time, was established here between the point and the cemetery ridge, on which the northern wing of Zapadnie rests. An old burying ground, with its characteristic Russian crosses and faded pictures of the Saints, is plainly marked on the ridge. It was at this little bight of sandy landing that Pribylov's men first came ashore and took possession of the island, while others in the same season proceeded to Northeast Point and to the north shore to establish settlements of their own order. When the indiscriminate sealing of 1868 was in progress, one of the parties lived here, and a salt-house which was then erected by them still stands. It is in a very fair state of preservation, although it has never been occupied since, except by the natives who come over here from the village in the summer to pick the berries of *Empetrum* and *Rubus,* which abound in the greatest profusion around the rough and rocky flats that environ a little lake adjacent. The young people of St. Paul are very fond of this berry-festival, so-called among themselves, and they stay there every August, camping out, a week or ten days at a time before returning to their homes in the village."[1]

A cluster of buildings stood forlorn in the rain, down on the grassy flats between the headland and the cross-marked ridge. There were tumbled ruins of a barabara, just a broken heap of sod and driftwood, a small shack, an outhouse, and a sturdy frame camp cottage built to house fox trappers in winter. Not far beyond the buildings Antone Lake was a small circular smudge of dark grey among the green fields. Not far in measured feet or by kittiwake wing, but the fields between the houses and the lake were studded with massy clumps of grass that demand nimble feet for steady progress from one hummock to another.

Since we women were already soaked above the knees from our first outing, we had no qualms about breaking our way through the damp welter of the higher sedges. Among the nearest grass hummocks we gathered long-stemmed, large-faced purple violets. The unfortunate beauties lacked perfume and were further afflicted by the clumsy botanical of *Viola langsdorffii Fisch.* Crowding our less hardy and lovelier vegetation stood patches of that coarse unlovely member of the angelica family, called *pootchki* by the Aleuts. When I first saw Aleut children peel off the outer skin of the thick stems and crunch the stout juicy core, my mouth twisted wryly in remembrance of my own childish exploits with rhubarb. Of the many English common names for the plant, one is appropriately "Indian rhubarb." Another less pleasing term is "cow parsnip." The scientific name of *Heracleum* is a reminder of its ancient relative, dedicated to Hercules, who prescribed it for illness, if Pliny is to be believed. Until the advent of turnips and other root vegetables imported or raised by the Russians, *pootchki* was one of the few vegetables in the Aleut diet, eaten either raw or boiled.

I left unplucked the Jacob's ladder blooms, which I could gather on the village outskirts. What pedestrian mind ever bestowed such a name, slurring the beauty of the delicate blue flower face with its golden heart by paying attention to the pinnate regular opposite leaves that are too close together to give more than a vague impression of a ladder?

One of the few sweet-scented flowers of the island grew amazingly high in the damp runlets between the hummocks, the wild heliotrope, a member of the valerian family.

Again and again my attention wandered from the search for flowers to scan the uplands. Directly behind the buildings rose a low rounded hill called *Kleba* [*kliibax̂*] by the Aleuts, a rather mutilated way of expressing Loaf Hill in Russian. Just beyond it the faint shadows of tossing antlers betrayed the presence of grazing reindeer.

July 8, 1941
We changed quickly and got up to the house for the beginning of the news broadcast. The U. S. took over Iceland for the duration. What next? Battle still raging with no definite trends yet on the eastern front.

July 9, 1941
The news broadcast last night indicated that Hitler is having a tough time. He has lost his blitz that is certain. If the Stalin line only holds. A Russian military delegation had arrived in London and was greeted by cheering crowds, crying long live the unity of the Soviet Union and the English people. If only England would take advantage of this period. But probably she will wait, hoping both sides will become exhausted and she can step in to take over. And the R. A. F. bombed Cologne and thousands were evacuated. I wonder what is happing to Crystal and her grandmother. And Franz.

Volcanic cones broke the skyline irregularly. The mist that clung gently above them seemed slow-drifting smoke from their craters. Hidden behind them was the seldom-visited terrain of Southwest Point, accessible only on foot from the

Zapadni Road cross or between those hills or by boat when a skillful steersman was willing to face the dangerous currents and treacherous maze of reefs near the peninsula of Southwest Point. Opposite Antone Lake lay the long rocky mound of Ridge Wall. Above it and along the shore the air was full of phantom birds, visitors from the vast bird rookeries of Southwest Point.

On our way home Sam dropped off to inspect the fragments of a bleached skeleton whale that littered the grass around the sandy flat. Most of the bones were vertebrae. He selected the best as a memento of our first visit to Zapadni. It was a natural footstool, not easy to sweep under because it weighed thirty-five pounds. How the imagination can run riot when one's feet rest on a massive block that is but one small segment of the huge skeleton of the masterpiece of the sea animal kingdom. What boundless oceans the mind can cross inspired by such a steed.

Chapter 9

One book we consulted before leaving the States contained a harrowing account of Pribilof housekeeping. The hungry arctic foxes, it stated, habitually haunted the villages, leaping through the windows to snatch food from the plates on the table. Reality proved less melodramatic. Actual problems were colorless, commonplace, and irritating.

The raised eyes of wives of Service employees when I spoke of a maid intimated that I was an upstart, overturning social conventions. Everyone does her own work was the social dictum. I had come willing to act as nurse without compensation, but I had no intention of forsaking my plans for study and outdoor activities. The prospect of being chained to a dishpan and a broom for my year of island recreation was enough to make me take the next boat back to the States.

Even if I wanted to be a lady of leisure, I was told, I would be unable to find an Aleut girl interested in earning money during her brief idleness between leaving school at sixteen and marriage with the first available male. I did not realize then that I was violating a very deep-rooted social taboo against eating food prepared by the "dirty natives." If I had realized the fact at once it would have made no difference to me.

Appeals to various Aleuts whom Sam was treating brought us a child of sixteen who stayed one month [Antonina Stepetin, who resigned on July 19].

Another girl [Fedosia Merculieff], extremely pretty and very sweet, left to prepare for school just the week I was expecting Tobyanne. Until she left I had been unaware of her youth, believing her to have finished her schooling. Our third applicant [Heretina Kochergin] stayed longer. Her father brought her in one noon, pushed her into the living room, said, "If she stays here she won't be running around the streets," and promptly left. Her parents had chronic organic disabilities that flared up more severely when they disagreed, which they did frequently. So bitter was the discord between them in the fall that her father remained in the hospital, gradually working his way from patient to the position of handyman and finally to the role of attendant to the patients. He continued to live in the hospital until we left the island. In midwinter his wife decided that upsetting our

July 8, 1941

At Marunich there is the inevitable mess house for trappers only as there is no sealing nearby. Hence the bad road, too. Close to the mess house is the remnant of a barabara, a Native house. I doubt that it is as old as Mrs. O[berg] says. She reports that the village used to be there and that the Russians landed there. So did the Hellbaums for the weather last Sept. would not permit the boat to come near the regular landings so they were brought in by baidar at that point and driven into town. That, if it happened often enough, might be a good excuse for repairing the road. I knew Sammie was getting an awful jouncing despite the fact that Mr. O. was crawling along with great care. For even packed in Tobyanne and I were getting some rough treatment once in awhile. And DeLee says no auto driving at all during pregnancy![1] Well, so far, since I recovered from the sea, I am feeling better than I have for a couple of years. But I ought to knock on wood. I want to be able to do things right up until labor starts. And if I can use all my energy for good things and have to waste none working at drab tasks in the house, I can seem to keep my feet and hands from swelling too much.

Incidentally, I told Mrs. O. casually that I was pregnant so as to get the word around and save them guessing.

domestic arrangements would bother her husband and perhaps rob him of our goodwill. She appealed to the Village Committee, composed of a half dozen of the most civic-minded Aleuts, to stop her daughter from working for us. The committee, with the acting agent in attendance, met very solemnly to consider the testimony of mother, father, and daughter and announced that the young woman was to continue working for us. By the grace of the community's government the domestic-help problem was solved for the duration of our stay.

Gradually the young woman and I surmounted the language barriers and established bonds of affection between us. Always in the background, alternately cajoling and beating her, was her mother. It was a long time before I learned about the whippings. When I saw the purple wheals left by a belt or strap I asked Hoverson, then acting agent, to punish the mother and put an end to the beatings. He felt that the matter of child protection was not his responsibility. All I could do was threaten the mother that I would ask the doctor to discontinue her supply of "red pills," a mild placebo that she was inordinately fond of for her "pain in my side." Sometimes the threat worked for quite long periods.

School had given the three girls a fine basic training in cleaning for which I was grateful. Whenever office hours or hospital emergencies did not conflict with mealtimes, I did the cooking. None of the girls was a successful cook as we joked about the "scorched earth policy" that produced shrunken dark-brown wooden splinters from chops and steaks. For pastries, which too often reminded us of petrified forests, we substituted canned fruit and Jell-O. Bread, fortunately, we obtained from the Company House kitchen. Carelessness when lighting the gas oven might have been tragic. Fortunately, the worst burn was no more than singed hair on the forearm and a scorched eyebrow.

Although I insisted I be called, when at home, to light the oven, the girls persisted in their attempts to conquer its temperament. A violent plop, a steaming whoosh, and a scream of fright and hurt were frequent preludes to dinner.

When Dr. Migliori had departed we had moved down from the gracious atmosphere of Government House with mayhem in our hearts against the ugliness and gloom of our permanent quarters. Shades flew to the tops of the windows and remained there. The curtains were pulled back to the limit of the window frames. The light that streamed in was only our first tiny victory. Half of the heavy bulky furniture was banished to the attic. It became possible to move through the rooms, to breathe easily. The few bits of colored antique glass I had tucked into my suitcases and our books gave us a faint feeling of home. From the shores we dragged souvenirs as decorations, fantastic coils of dried kelp, perforated shells, curiously shaped bones, bird wings, and colorful stones. Month by month I added to our pictures from the leaves of a calendar of Audubon bird prints. Magazines gave us bright maps and flower prints for other rooms. By the last autumn boat a shipment of some casual ornaments and a hundred new books, gay in their vivid jackets, brought a little more cheer. For the new books Peter Kochergin and his oldest son, Victor, made us a modernistic bookcase that Peter never tired of admiring.

> July 15, 1941
> I notice Mrs. H[ellbaum] has a very catty way of saying something nice about the Natives and suddenly adding something nasty. Such as raving about what bright children they are and then saying they do not want to [attend] school after sixteen in such a disparaging way. This was in connection with Antenena . . . although Mrs. H. grudgingly admitted that she thought A. was one of the girls who went to Mr. McMillin and asked for longer periods in school. Which doesn't sound bad to my ignorant ears.
>
> We stopped off at the greenhouse to water and I set out a few heads of lettuce that Mrs. Hoverson gave me. . . . And we took advantage of Mrs. O.'s instructions to help ourselves to a head of lettuce.
>
> I got most of the supper [while] hoping Antonina was drinking in the methods. She hung over me and after she had cleaned the lettuce, we both recleaned it. So maybe . . . ! I hope so.

Not until after Christmas did a regiment of Aleut workmen invade the house to refurbish it with the vividest blue, yellow, and green I have ever seen under a roof except in Greenwich Village cafes. The intense colors were better than the dirty ecru they covered and preferable to the lukewarm sickly hues that seemed the only alternative mixture the paints could produce. When the painters came we moved up to the little attic room that had been the darkroom of a former physician who was a camera addict. At last we could actually lie in bed and see the stars and clouds and wake up face-to-face with the sky through the narrow windows. We remained upstairs and our own bedroom became Tobyanne's nursery. She was too young to be depressed by the weird deep blue of the walls.

I collected from various storage nooks the sections of a huge rolltop desk for the bedroom, which we transformed to a study. In that room we had a miniature museum. Animal skulls, glass jars of sea specimens such as tunicates, snails, and barnacles rubbed against rocks and shells. In a dark corner of the cellar we unearthed a small homemade filing cabinet that was soon bulging with notes on our experiences and from our reading.

The Washington and Seattle offices had failed to inform us that the government did not furnish electrical appliances. Mrs. Elliott, the radio operator's wife, lent me an extra iron at first. When she packed up to leave the island, Mac's wife gave me her spare one. The girls used the dilapidated electric washer, a part of hospital equipment when laundry work had been one of the attendant's duties. A bed light found in attic rubbish was repaired by Mr. Elliott and saved my eyesight as I read steadily during my postnatal convalescence.

While I was jotting down the main portion of this chapter in my island study the sealers were at Ice House Lake cutting ice and storing it in a pit in the perpetually frozen interior of a scoria bank. I had certainly never considered ice a Pribilof necessity. In the wall in the kitchen was a narrow closet with two slits opening to the outside world. It was euphemistically called the cooler. All summer I grumbled at the waste as we threw food away after one night in the "cooler." The winter winds penetrated the slits easily. They carried such quantities of fine scoria dust that closely covered containers were little protection. Too often the food emerged covered with what seemed to be a slight powder of nutmeg. Since most of our food except for an occasional seal liver, reindeer roast, or gift of fish or fowl from the Aleuts had to be transported about two thousand miles, it hurt to throw it away unused. I was sometimes resentful thinking of the big gas refrigerator in Government House, utilized for only a few weeks of summer. At least during the remainder of the year it might protect the sera, vaccines, and medications that required steady cold temperature to retain their useful properties. Without a refrigerator we were unable to keep blood on hand for emergency transfusions.

The canned foods we purchased from the government store were principally of low-grade quality. All the families complained of grass and stones in the spinach and a moist pink mush labeled salmon. They were too timid to ask the Seattle office to keep quality in mind as well as prices in accepting bids. The *Penguin* brought citrus fruits, root vegetables, meats, and perishable fruits and vegetables in small amounts depending on the season. Service families supplemented their diet with fresh vegetables raised in the tiny greenhouse. We put in seeds of fast-growing vegetables a few days after we arrived. Until our own lettuce, radishes, and spinach were grown, we were generously supplied by our neighbors. I grew endive for salads and gathered enough broccoli for two family meals. Little green onions were gifts more appreciated than orchids. The celery plants that one family gave me failed to bleach sufficiently for my taste but added savor to summer soups and provided dry leaves for winter seasoning.

Outside the greenhouse in a small fenced area were plots for each family of employees. It was too late to utilize ours. The others had beets, carrots, and even a few hills of potatoes. Turnips and kale, which not even the monotony of canned foods could make me like, flourished. Some families made quite a fetish of eating radish tops "for health's sake." I could not follow their example. A large section of the outside garden was set aside for rhubarb for all the families. We had quite a hardy stand of it outside our own house, too.

One or two Aleut families had small cold frames for vegetables close to their houses. Otherwise the sealers were without leafy green vegetables and had only root vegetables furnished from the government stores and occasionally a few canned vegetables. No large-scale gardening attempt had ever been made for the entire community despite its cheapness and desirability as a means of improving the health of the Aleuts.

When Veniaminov visited St. Paul in the 1830s he was impressed by the wide diversity of wild plants in comparison with the few varieties at Unalaska. He added, "Among edible roots, [meaning wild plants], it is said that the yellow tubers, tho nutritious and pleasing to the taste, yet on account of blemishes, are unwholesome and their use has caused boils and other eruptions." He probably referred to the rice root or licorice root of the wild heliotrope. He continued, "Kitchen garden stuff grows well; turnips, radishes and potatoes; unfortunately it is not always possible to procure seeds for the last mentioned."[2]

Chickens seem to have been much more common in those days, for Veniaminov wrote, "Of domestic animals none but fowls are raised, these however in large numbers, so that the better householders in the fall of the year have flocks of two hundred or more."[3] When we arrived few families owned chickens, perhaps because these innocent fowl have been the source of much friction in the years after the Americans arrived. Unfortunately Veniaminov did not describe where the Aleuts housed their chickens. If the chickens shared the shelter of the owners it would have seemed ordinary to one bred in feudal Russia. American officials objected to such cohabitation. When two-storied frame houses were erected for the sealers, the top floor usually became the winter quarters of the chickens. Again and again through the years official *pronunciamentos* were issued ordering all chickens to be housed in outbuildings of their own. The recurrence of the edict is evidence that the Aleuts were rather deaf to the order. Only in recent years have the villagers complied with the law. Chickens kept outside the house in stormy weather require more attention, special heating arrangements, and extra fuel, which accounts for the subsequent lack of enthusiasm for chicken raising, once the order was obeyed.

There have been experiments in raising chickens for the government employees only. Both the chickens and the experiments were short-lived.

Milk for Service families, for the sick, and others only when there was a superabundance came from the small herd of cattle. We had been puzzled at first by the large proportion of veterinary texts in the medical library. Reading fragments of old medical records still intact we came across such tidbits as "Sally Rose died today. Post Mortem revealed . . ." Sally Rose we discovered was either a cow or a mule. The physician had once been, and probably still is for all we know, responsible for the health of the domestic animals. Such duties were not alien to the vanished horse-and-buggy doctors. Today knowledge in the fields of both animal and human care is too broad for any physician but a genius to be an expert veterinarian. Had Dan Shabolin, the Aleut dairyman, not been able to cope with most of the symptoms of his charges, we might have been very glad of those dusty books in the attic and the huge fever thermometer decorating the office. Fortunately Sam had only to provide Dan with disinfectants for cleaning the stable, soap for bathing the animals once or twice, and cathartics.

July 14, 1941
I forgot to relate that Sam got ill with his cigar smoking Saturday. We had lots of fun over it once he felt better but he looked so pale and was awfully dizzy. He has a cold that is nagging him a lot and a little infection in his nose that is irritating him considerably.

We found some interesting old reports and papers in his office today-including a will and receipts for gifts to various churches of Alaska to which Xenia Krukoff had willed fifty dollars each. And a lovely report about a post-mortem on a bull that began with an apology that it had been impossible to get Tony's complete body into the autopsy room.

Not many years ago a physician made the following humorous report entitled "Autopsy Report on the Bull (Commonly known as Tony)":

> Due to the difficulty of getting the entire body of "Tony" into the Autopsy Theater, the examination was confined to the contents of the thoracic cavity. The verdict was death caused by lobar pneumonia.

Almost as soon as we disembarked we were regaled with vivid narratives of cold winters that made us shiver. The accounts were surprising contrasts to the advice of Washington officials. The clothes we had brought were certainly not adequate for outings in zero temperatures.[4] Some of our first letters to the States sent our friends scurrying over the hot pavements of New York in August searching for winter garments. Not all of their purchases caught the last autumn boat. From a chance remark we learned that we might "borrow" garments for the duration of our island stay from the still large stores of Army clothing left from the last war. As a confirmed disciple of the slacks cult, I had no objection to facing the wintry blasts in the heavy masculine clothing. So we were outfitted with thick woolen undershirts and drawers, canvas parkas fringed with wolf, and canvas trousers that barred the wind. There were some extremely large gauntlet gloves excellent for covering the cracks between ordinary gloves and sleeves. I never minded wearing soft woolen mittens inside them. Sam acquired a pair of brick-colored suede gloves trimmed elegantly with hair seal cuffs. I chose a pair with muskrat backing and cuffs, the last complete pair of the kind. There was a large packing box full of left-handed gloves only. In the spring wandering along the north shore I lost my right glove too and on a few chill days walked about keeping warm by wearing my large left glove on first one hand and then the other.

The word *parka* disturbed me. Everyone on the island said "parkee." Invariably I found the word spelled with a final *a.* I was extremely grateful to Ivan Petroff, enumerator of the Tenth Census for the Alaskan territory, for including in his report the information that *parkee,* spelled as generally pronounced, was a Kamchatkan word that had lost its correct spelling in English usage but retained its alien pronunciation.[5]

Our food, clothing, and shelter shared none of the picturesqueness of the real Arctic. No igloo, no seal blubber lamps, no dried frozen fish for us. We had a gas stove, electric light and appliances, steam heat, modern plumbing, everything but a refrigerator. It was only outside our home that we could be aware of our separation from the runways of man known as twentieth-century civilization.

Chapter 10

For half an hour we had been bumping up and down over the sparse plain that lies across the center of the island, following the faint traces of infrequently traveled road track, rising and falling into abrupt hollows in the earth, like a ship beating her way through heavy seas. At the road's end lay Marunich, marked by three small buildings huddled in the tall grasses above the shingle. Here, I had been informed authoritatively by the oldest "white" inhabitants, was a picture of man's way of life on St. Paul, an objective history of the developing civilization of hundreds of years. Nothing dramatic in the scene evoked memories of the bloodshed and suffering of the Aleut people. Yet here was the external record, the crude barabara, the small flimsy wooden house of the earliest days of American occupation, and the sturdy trim bungalow camp house for the present fox trapper.

The early Russians introduced no immediate change in housing to the Aleuts. Because no trees grew on the windswept Aleutian archipelago, the only wood for any purpose was chance gifts of sea currents. Since the time of their occupation of the island, the Aleuts had utilized driftwood for timbering their houses and their grave pits. Usually, however, the supports and framework of their huts were the more easily obtainable bones of the whale. The first Russian hunters could barely carry a cargo of food and ammunition in their vessels ample enough for journeys of uncertain duration, dependent upon such factors as weather, hunting success, and the cooperation of Aleut hunters. They could not overburden their small boats with lumber for shelter. Instead they adopted the living habits of the Aleuts, glad to share their partly underground huts. When necessary, particularly where the traders were attempting permanent settlement, the Russians even copied the Aleut mode, utilizing either driftwood or whalebone. Very slowly, as more and more ships plied between Kamchatka and Alaska, while the Russian-American Company strove to build up their fur empire, was enough wood imported to erect buildings. First for the church, then the company storehouses, and then the homes of officials. Not even when that great dreamer and builder Aleksandr Baranov became the pilot of colonial

Russian America and had established a sawmill at Sitka was there wood enough to supply the needs of all the settlements. In time the Russians might have brought the age of wooden houses to the various peoples whose destinies they determined, but they sold their possessions to the United States before that could come to pass. Even under American control, on St. Paul where changes in housing made greater speed than in the Aleutian islands, two decades passed before the barabara became a historical relic.

The barabara at Marunich, I had been informed, antedated the arrival of the Americans and was considered nearly a hundred years old. The wooden skeleton of the frame had sagged under the amassing weight of plant roots in the sod roof. The sodded walls were tilted inward. I looked long at it and thought: Now this reminder of early times is beginning to crumble and in a few years no one will remember its exact site. It will be only another indistinguishable hollow in the earth, a pitfall hidden in the grass to trip unwary hikers. I am glad I have seen it before the grass has completely conquered it.

Months later Peter Kochergin shattered my romantic illusion by narrating proofs of his natural fastidiousness: "I can't eat where it's dirty. When I came back from Chemawa School I went to stay at Marunich in Elary Stepetin's barabara. It was all right the first morning but at noon we went inside to eat our lunch. There was dirt all over the floor and those crawly bugs and dead grass and I couldn't eat! Elary and Dorofey Stepetin laughed at me. I could not sleep there either. They had to bring me home that afternoon."

At the word *barabara* I pricked up my ears. And then I learned that John Misikin, John Emanoff, Elary Stepetin, Dorofey Stepetin and some other men had constructed the barabara, revered as a link with the distant past, in 1925 for a shelter on hunting trips. Elary and Dorofey claim the area as their hunting ground but apparently permitted others to share their province.

But when I next visited Marunich and surveyed the ruins of the barabara, for the winter frosts and winds had left it a debris-choked hole, I felt that my romantic impressions that Peter's accuracy had deflated had not been in vain. While the ruins still stood side by side with examples of later building, though not a real fragment of the past, the scene truly symbolized the growth and progress of living conditions on the Pribilofs.

Marunich shores filled us with delight. The stillness was broken on that first visit only by the soft wash of the sea. No seabirds winged against the sky. The silence we hesitated to shatter with our voices created a poignant atmosphere in which to stumble across pieces of an old whaling vessel, wrecked in an April storm in 1892. Captain Shovey and his crew escaped safely from the sinking *Alexander* and cheated the sea of human prey. But death hovered over the scene of the tragedy until it claimed a victim. As long as the brig held together, the crew assisted by Aleut villagers worked busily to salvage as much cargo and as many ship parts as possible before the waves destroyed the wreck completely. One night as the men were coming back from the village, they missed one of their fellows. Some retraced their steps to Marunich but though they called and searched the immediate shore, they found no trace of him. When morning came the man had still not returned home. At Marunich the men of St. Paul tramped the shores and searched inland among the dunes. At last they came upon their friend, who had walked toward Vesolia Mista to enjoy the contents of a bottle of gin stolen from the *Alexander.* Having helped himself generously he had become drowsy and curled among the dry grasses to sleep. The cold had killed him stealthily as he lay clutching his almost-empty bottle of gin.

[Written following the rescue of three men who went missing after their fishing boat's motor had failed. They were able to drop anchor but drifted in place through a long night.]

July 17, 1941
Mr. East came by and when no one answered his knock quickly dropped off two copies of the *Saturday Evening Post* that contain heartbreaking articles about starvation in Spain. I read those while I had tea and cake. Then only I took my bath. I wanted to type but was afraid of waking Sam. I waited until nearly noon before I closed his door and tried to put down something adequate about last night. I made a pretty poor job of it. I shall have to try another version a little later. Odd how the news of the lost men yanked us straight from an atmosphere that was like a pleasant intelligent evening of good talk at home in the States right back into the realities of the dangers of island life.

But the story of the shipwreck achieved a happy ending. When Captain Shovey left for San Francisco he took with him a new daughter, Feodosia Kozlof, fourteen years of age, whom he had adopted with the consent of her mother and the government agent.

No such happy chord appears in a tale of an earlier tragedy that began near Marunich before there were roads on St. Paul. In 1876 Dr. Meaney, physician, James Gill, meteorologist, and a Mr. Washburne, tempted by fair weather, set out with two Aleut companions to explore the far reaches of the island adjacent to the north shore beyond Marunich. They had a rousing walk and enjoyed a picnic lunch. Just after they started villageward, a sudden *poorgah,* a terrible gale, swept in from the sea. In just a few minutes their thick clothes were drenched. Soon they were miserably cold. They tried to walk quickly in their soggy clothes, but the rough terrain and their wet clothing hampered them. The wind gave them no respite. When they reached the house at Marunich, they decided to push on because there was no stove. At some point beyond Marunich, Gill began to insist that he could walk no more. The two Aleuts went ahead to summon aid. Unfortunately when they reached the village in the evening they were so storm worn and exhausted that they could not speak intelligibly. A half hour slipped by before they could direct rescuers, who set out immediately on foot. A second party with the mule cart met Mr. Washburne stumbling along near Ice House Lake. Before he collapsed he could just mumble that Dr. Meaney and Gill were not far behind him, on the uplands of Tolstoi. A few minutes later the rescuers came upon Dr. Meaney leaning over Gill, who had fallen and been unable to rise again. The doctor was weakly rubbing Gill's hands and legs to restore circulation. Gill died a few minutes after he was brought to the village. Dr. Meaney and Mr. Washburne recovered from their exposure in a few days.

Gill, the victim of the weather he had come to study, was interred temporarily in the churchyard. Permission for his body to remain there depended upon the approval of the Russian priest, who was absent. Apparently the priest offered no objection to the grave of a nonmember of his faith in the church grounds. For just above our home in the shadow of the church stood a simple granite monument to James Gill, which says: "Born in Brooklyn in 1855, died on St. Paul, 1876."[1]

His death inspired the government agent to send workmen to Polovina a few days later to patch up an old salt house and install a stove to provide, belatedly, haven for storm-besieged walkers. In 1941 the fox-trapping cabins near all rookeries not adjacent to the village, at Marunich, Tasmania, and Southwest Point, offered stout roofs, stoves, and fuel for storm-harried travelers.

Strange that Marunich should have been the scene of so many human happenings, of violent shipwreck, of tragic deaths. For the luminous atmosphere, the hushed serenity of the gently waving fields that lie between the high dunes of North Point and the steep copper red slope of Marunich or North Hill suggest a world freshly created, a pristine land of tranquil innocence undefiled by man's violence and his tragedies. Nothing finite and flawed belonged there. Here time was not and space was limitless. Even the cluster of buildings sinks back into the ground as if a natural part of the earth instead of the product of man's toil. Now the land belonged to itself once more, strong and unaltered by the progress of human feet across its surface.

My first visit to Marunich is starred in my memory because on the long road to the shore I first glimpsed the fallen patches of sky that botanists call *Eritrichium*. It seemed as if thousands of miniature butterflies from the tropics had invaded the north and alighted to rest with outspread wings. The minute exquisite blossoms of this dwarf forget-me-not, the perfection of each incredibly tiny four-petaled flower with a golden heart, form a mosaic of jewels lying softly upon the silvery setting of the mosslike foliage. The world contains no more beautiful flower than this shy bloom that, having brought the blue of the sky earthward, colors the more barren surfaces of the earth far from human popularity. Had it chosen a more temperate home, its human admirers might long ago have uprooted it and destroyed it forever. It is not a flower to be picked for it is stemless. It is a flower to be visited almost as one approaches a shrine, reverently grateful for such color.

Every trip to Marunich increased its fascination.

All winter I dreamed of spring when I might return there to spend a few weeks in an enchanted realm.

Chapter 11

I postponed witnessing a seal killing as long as I could, but I went to watch a seal drive as often as I had permission. I missed no opportunity to visit the outskirts of rookeries where I could watch the seals without disturbing them. Occasionally I reminded myself that the sealing season was nearly over and unless I wanted to neglect an important piece of Pribilof activity I had to steel myself to see murder done.

I was learning many things about the seals. I knew that like Milne's "Pooh" the seal was an animal of "very little brain." Yet I had a sentimental affection for them that curdled my admiration for sleek fur coats. It was not a new emotional reaction to me. There was Jane, a pet rooster, which my family ruthlessly slaughtered in his old age. I mourned his loss by abstaining from chicken dinners for most of my adolescence. There was Fomka, a calf who grew too formidable for a pet. For his memory I avoided veal for many years when I was supposedly adult enough to accept the brutalities of life. Now the expectation of seeing my capering little flippered friends killed filled me with resentment against woman's vanity that robbed them of life, not for warmth but principally to be dressed smartly and luxuriously.

I might have found excuses not to visit the killing field indefinitely but one grey afternoon the cutter *Atlanta* dropped Ruth Gruber, Secretary Ickes' special Alaskan investigator on our doorstep.[1] She had less than twenty-four hours to spend on St. Paul and wanted to see everything on the island in that period. The next morning's drive was scheduled from Tolstoi Rookery, across Village Cove, and from Lukanin Kitovi opposite Tolstoi on the eastern shore.

We talked so much about everything in the world that it was nearly two a.m. when we persuaded Ruth, who had been battered by the Bering on her trip down from the north, that she ought to take a nap. Sam and I stayed up and wakened her an hour later. We breakfasted with the sealers in the warm bright kitchen of the Aleut bunkhouse that I hated so. Johnston was our guide as usual. A substantial meal of hotcakes and fried eggs fortified us for the drizzly morning, the perfect sealing weather.

At Tolstoi we stood on an embankment looking down into an abyss of grey mist. Not until autumn, when we tramped at liberty over the tenantless rookery ground, did I acquire a true picture of the shoreline. Nor could I ever locate the spot we stood that morning. If I had not spent too many fall mornings in the Catskills I might almost have believed every exaggeration of the fog legend that morning. As we gazed down into this gulf of swirling haze, dark shadows began to move within the nebulous greyness. The shades became darker, posed briefly like graven images against the mist, and became the flurry of moving seals and men. Shepherds of the fog I thought romantically to myself.

We stood on our pinnacle and watched the seals scramble across a narrow plateau and come plunging up the short steep embankment to our level. When the last pod had passed us we followed them toward the grassy slaughter space.

At first the furious activity of the killing field seemed a chaotic brawl. Only gradually did we grasp the pattern of swiftly coordinated divisions of work and recognize that the automatic rhythmicity of the assembly line of the twentieth century had extended its influence to the north.

A pod of seals was driven to the edge of the killing field. The clubbers went to work at once. A slight blow on the head is sufficient to fracture the seal's thin brain case and kill it. The clubbers swung their long cudgels quickly and usually accurately. Although the bachelors piled up on top of one another in squirming masses, they seemed stampeding in accordance with their natural tendency to rush together when disturbed rather than in response to a definite fear of the sealer's club.

One man constantly twirled a large bright tin can at the end of a six-foot pole. One moment a curious clown playfully brandishing his strange toy in the air, the next he was expertly thrusting the can into the wriggling heap, separating the seals so the clubbers could strike them down one by one. The clatter of his pole against the sides of the can rang out clamorously above the snorting whistling of the bachelors and the sharp cracking thuds of the fractured skulls. The bright revolving pail pursued each rejected seal for the animals' sole desire in life seemed to be to throw

July 28, 1941
But in came a young woman. I woke up enough to hear Dr. Gruber, and then Sam and I were both exclaiming over her notoriety when Congress recently had a battle about the appropriation for her study of Alaska because she had written a book about the Soviet Arctic and ended up by saying that someday she hoped to go back and swim in the Arctic Ocean.[2] [Ben] East looked surprised to see how we seemed to know all about her.

She is certainly a charming and swell gal. We sat and talked and she took some notes. She had been invited to the tea party being given for Mrs. Grover and Mrs. Schetzel and so had I.

So we talked and talked and finally Bob Scott came in to help Sam make solution for his X-ray films and added some facts about the fur end of the business. We went up to the tea after three. It wasn't bad at all. I sat on the floor and smoked and made everyone who wanted to smoke happy.

cont.

themselves under the clubs of the killers. Almost every other animal would flee for safety when a chance occurred. The rejected seals, whether males too young or too old, or truant females caught accidentally by the drivers, fought stupidly to remain in the midst of the confusion. The inexorable glittering noisy pail frustrated their suicidal notions. It was astounding to see these refugees, forced to safety from the pack at last, calmly sitting in the grass a few yards from the bloody steaming carcasses of their brothers nonchalantly fanning themselves with their flippers or idly scratching their fur.

Hardly had a seal collapsed from his coup de grâce when hands were dragging the limp body to make one of a row of ten corpses. The stabbers immediately plunged their knives accurately into the seals' hearts. If the blow on the head had not killed the animal he, except very rarely, remained unconscious until the knife made death certain. Simultaneously with the lining up of the bodies and the stabbing, one man was swiftly passing along the row, measuring the warm palpitating bodies. As he called out the measurements a co-worker stationed at the side of the skinning area jotted the numbers in a notebook. Only three-year-old bachelors are killed. Their average length is between forty and fifty inches.

> I had already asked Ruth to stay with us. Johnston came for her to take her down to the boat to collect her belongings for she had decided to stay over and go down with the *Penguin,* hoping that the *Penguin* would not leave for a couple of days . . .
>
> I told Johnston I would like her to stay with us and he thought that nice. So Fedosia and Sam brought down the single bed from the attic and put it up between the desks. Fedosia was busy cracking the crabs for supper. I tried to copy the most important bits from the *History of Alaska* since J. had warned us the *Penguin* was apt to sail at noon.

The cutters followed in the wake of the stabbing knife, slitting the pelt around the flippers and straight down the abdomen. Their knives moved up lightly to the lower jaw and around the head. If necessary they cut down through the thick white blubber to loosen it.

Other sealers wielded large two pronged forks with which they pinned down the neck of the animal and held the body in place with the aid of their feet. As they established their grip, two men attached a tool called *nippers* to the pelt at the head. A few quick steps backward and the carcass was stripped bare. The sound of ripping silk whipped the air as each skin was removed. The nippers have eliminated the danger of cutting skins in the wrong place. Such accidents were frequent when the sealers attempted to skin a large number of seals at one time with knives. Kneeling on the ground, bent in awkward positions, the men were cramped and tired quickly and then the knives slipped easily in the wrong direction. Cut skins have little or no market value.

A special clipper resembling overgrown pruning shears was invented to cut the leathery flippers from the body. Flippers must be discarded before the carcass reaches the cooking vat in the processing plant, for they stew up into a gluey mass that clogs the machinery and ruins the meal and oil. The clipper men worked right behind the skinners.

A few men and young boys, serving their apprenticeship on the sealing gang, pull the denuded carcasses to one side to provide a wide land for the trucks. Very small boys picked up the skins and spread them singly on the grass to cool. When the trucks moved up this macabrously bordered highway, two men on each side speared the carcasses with salmon pughs and threw them up into the vehicles.

Once the first row of seals was stretched out, work went on continuously with no interruptions. Each man performed his task over and over with regular rhythm. No one paused for a second.

Clubs rose and fell with uniform drumbeat tempo. The tin pail flashed and shrieked in the air. Row after row, ten seals to a row, the bodies were stretched out neatly, one behind each other. They were dealt out as smoothly as cards dealt on a table surface. The knives rose and fell and a red fountain rose from the quivering bodies. The cutters knelt to slip their knives under the soft skins and rose to hurry to the next bodies. The men with the grim forks stepped into position, deftly imprisoned the neck of the carcass, and brought their booted feet down on the seal's head. The pair of skinners bent simultaneously to affix the nippers, straightened up and walked backward in unison, denuding the bodies neatly. The clippers worked steadily, snip, snip with their weird scissors, severing the flippers just in time for the busy hands ready to drag the carcasses out of the center. The boys darted back and forth with the pelts, spreading them on the grass so that no two touched. The trucks rolled up and only the chauffeurs had an idle moment as the steel prongs of the pughs tossed their grisly burdens up and swooped down for another load.

After my first tense moments of repugnance, when my nausea and disgust were conquered, I could appreciate the coordination of the workmen. The killing lacked the fever of the slaughterhouse because the seals were so acquiescent. No odor of blood stung them with fear and foreboding. So far scientists have not ceased wrangling over the acuteness of the seal's olfactory organs. But rookery life, with its constant bloodshed, must have accustomed them to the smell of blood. Like sheep, seals follow a leader blindly, even to the death blows of the sealing clubs. Were the seals to panic in fear from their executioners, I know I would have left the islands transformed into a crusader to persuade women to forego such winter wraps. There have been protesting outcries by organized groups of tenderhearted people and to prevent further agitation, no cameras are permitted on the killing field. A black-and-white photograph of the carcasses would evoke images of animals suffering acute pain and mental anguish and rouse more kindly souls to try to stop sealing. Such an impression would be false. It was the seal's indifference to bloodshed and death that stilled my own sympathy and made the hours on the killing field bearable. The meat I normally eat in one week probably represents more suffering than a thousand sealskin coats. But we must have meat to nourish our bodies and must overlook the emotions of the animals that feed us. We cannot all turn vegetarian. I doubt if I could ever wear a sealskin wrap with an easy mind but I have no real objection to other women's enjoyment of such garments. I do eat chicken and veal today. I cannot swear that I shall never forget and pick out a sealskin coat someday.

But standing beside those pathetic skinned bodies, no matter how numbly the seals accepted their fate, I was upset and cursed my earlier poetic flight. Not shepherds of the mist but butchers was more fitting. Something about the prostrate limp bodies from afar brought to mind the battlefields on other continents. I remembered sprawling blurred bodies under the trees of Madrid's University City, which I had seen in 1937.[3] As long as man killed man, it could not be rational to expect the seals to escape the butcher's knife.

The gory factory in the field had exhausted its raw material. Men collected their tools and climbed into trucks. Off we all went to Lukanin Rookery. On the way Johnston explained how tradition protected the Pribilof Aleuts, who alone possessed the rather dubious privilege of clubbing and skinning seals. A promise made to them soon after the American occupation when the islanders were beset with worries as to how they were to make a livelihood had been kept inviolate. Only the chauffeurs who spent their waiting period snipping off flippers and measuring bodies worked beside the resident Aleuts. This minor assistance from "white" men did not count as infraction of tradition. Johnston was proud that the men could handle, from the clubbing to the final skin laid out to cool, eight hundred seals an hour.

The Lukanin area rises in a pleasantly rounded hill of the same name. Seaward the grassy sward ends abruptly at the head of ebony terraces. The mist had disappeared when we reached the hauling grounds and a fine rain had begun to fall. We watched the pods of seals climbing the shorter stairs of the terraces and then slipping and sliding as they scrambled up muddy channels between the rocks. We leaned over rock walls and looked directly into the harems. Half-grown pups, gazed back from their popping, thyroidic eyes. Concluding they had nothing but contempt for us they sniffed and snorted their disdain. They slithered up slippery muddy inclines and enjoyed sliding down.

Despite our sleepless night and the blood we had seen spilled on the grass, our morning outing exhilarated us. Back home we had a second and lighter breakfast seasoned with much wit and laughter. Johnston and Stitt, the mate of the *Penguin*, regaled us with Alaskan yarns. Sam took Ruth out to inspect the village. Wan but striving to be alert she followed submissively in his energetic footsteps and took voluminous notes. I started out with them but returned to superintend household activities. At noon came the summons from Captain Knudsen. I sent messengers through the village for Ruth and packed part of her baggage. In an hour she was gone and with her went many other friends who had added to our enjoyment of island life.[4] But of them later.

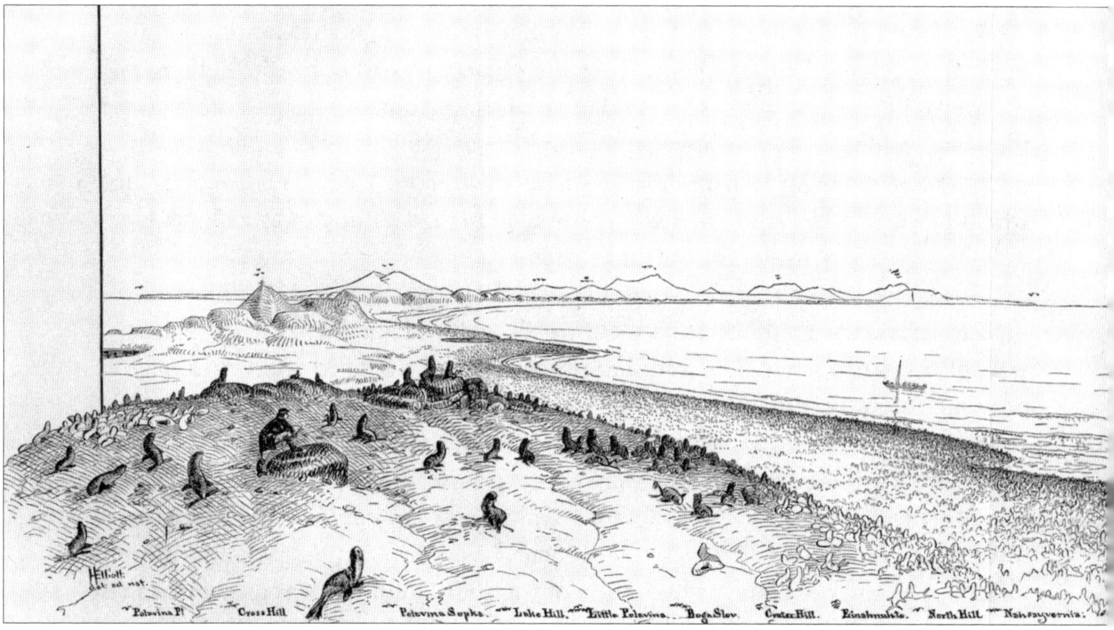

Henry W. Elliott's drawing "The North Shore of St. Paul Island." This was drawn from the summit of Hutchinson Hill. The line of mountains in the background is across the center of the island (*Fur-Seal Fisheries of Alaska, 1889,* Plate 8).

Chapter 12

On no other single stretch of land in the world do so many mammals congregate at one time as on the shores of Northeast Point on St. Paul in early summer. Henry Elliott first labored to describe the view from the central point of Hutchinson Hill looking down at only one side of the peninsula where three quarters of a million seals were engaged "in moving in one solid mass from sleep to frolicsome gambols, backward, forward, over, around, changing and interchanging their heavy squadrons of mighty hosts that it refuses to analyze any further."[1] No pen will ever succeed in delineating that picture for a reader. Only a natural-color sound film can capture the immensity of animal life, the ceaseless movement, and the tumult of so many throats.

In 1941 from the same vantage I gazed wonderstruck, turning my eyes slowly from Morzhovoi rookery on the east to Vostochnie on the northern shore, taking in twice as much shoreline as Elliott groped to depict. Along this three miles of uninterrupted beach a half million seals bewildered my eyes. I was stunned. My incredulous eyes looked from the east to the north and back again. It could not be true. My mind could not accept the eye's testimony. A dark brown flood rolled at my feet, churning, bellowing, ebbing, and flowing. I tried to rest my eyes by looking at idle bulls and small harems near at hand, where I could see distinct body outlines, recognize seals. When I looked beyond I was again rocking with the surge of pulsating life, too blinded by mass and movement to discern individual patterns, to separate single gestures from the whole throbbing sinuous undulation.

Whenever I revisited the hill I always succumbed to the same bewildered sensations of incredulity and awe.

The presence of so many hundreds of thousands of seals at Northeast Point dramatized the implacable natural laws that govern them. Every one of those amphibians had left the seas to sojourn on the rocks in obedience to the instinct of reproduction.[2] Each female had returned to bring forth the life she had been carrying for nearly a year. The adult male who awaited her had arrived earlier compelled by a mating instinct he could not disobey. Impressive and independent in demeanor, he was merely a passive instrument of the sexual drive. Not his the freedom of will to make a choice between spending a summer sporting in the seas or accepting harem responsibilities. He was riveted to sleepless, hungry sentry duty on his rocky station for from two to three months, obliged to fight bloody combats to protect his prison, his duties.

Only when the last female had arrived and been impregnated could he relax. Then his brown coat hanging limply around his shrunken body, he could turn back to the sea for rest and nourishment. When he chose, he might return probably not to the stone-strewn margins of the sea, but to the softer comfortable grassy areas behind the rookeries, there to drowse at ease as long as he desired.

By the end of July the rookeries were no longer a patchwork of definite, irregular blocks, each conspicuous because of the dark furry sultan of the seraglio. Gone was the plunging, snorting beachmaster, with the manners of a fiend, replaced by frowzy, untidy old animals wanting nothing but privacy, snapping halfheartedly at romping pups who came too close, scuttling seaward at the approach of man, like a frightened rabbit. Pups of varying ages roamed freely through the rookery and hauling grounds, playing games that were practice tryouts for the poses and actions of adulthood. They paddled in the low, brackish pools, ventured carefully into the sea, and skipped squealing back when large waves pushed them. Day after day their confidence increased and they struck out a little farther from shore, moving their small flippers clumsily. No kind parents coaxed them to practice swimming lessons. Each pup had to learn the art alone.

Intermittently females climbed up out of the sea, steely grey until their soft fur dried in silvery shades. They wandered back and forth, in search of their own pups to nurse. Resting between their long journeys for food the females strolled at will about the beach, no longer dominated by tyrannical males. Life moved and cried out on the beach but its movement was fluid and easygoing, its sound was duller, enlivened only by the shrill weak bleatings of the lamblike voices of the pups.

On Morshovi the seals had interesting neighbors with whom they mingled pleasantly, a few hundred tawny-coated sea lions. *Eumetopias jubatus,* the Steller or north sea lion, was first described in the pathetic documents received in St. Petersburg after Steller died in Siberia on his way back from the island of Bering's death. Steller's reports, written in picturesque eighteenth-century zoological Latin, were first published in the 1749 reports of the Imperial Academy of St. Petersburg. Linnaeus studied and respected this work. But poor George William Steller, whose star had led him to strange, unfriendly shores on Bering Island and destined him to be the first scientist to have intimate contact with fur seals, sea lions, sea otter, and the sea cow, the latter long since wiped out by man's weapons and known principally from Steller's ancient text, savored none of the rewards for the knowledge he had risked his life to obtain. His name lives again for a moment when men mention Steller's sea lion.

My first contact with the sea lions of St. Paul was unpleasant. As we were tramping through high vegetation to visit the sea lion rookery, our noses were assailed by the horrible stench of decaying flesh. Not far from us a mass of bloated, ugly carcasses, blackened with greedy swarming flies, steamed under the sun. We ran quickly to windward. These lions we were later informed had been killed because they were mixed in with the seals during a drive or drives.

In a few moments I had forgotten the evil odor and ugly scene. Directly in front of me two magnificent golden figures with heads flung back disdainfully posed facing each other in identical postures against a blue background of sky and sea. So still they remained that they seemed bronze statues flanking an entrance to the blue realm beyond. I stopped in mute rapture. How must Steller's heart have pounded when he first observed these lions of the sea's reaches. How dull and insignificant is the photographic memento we secured of that scene. Only my mind retains the leonine majesty, the superb dignity, the burnished sheen, the carven outlines, of that pair of sea monarchs.

The sea lion, never to be confused with his little California cousin who sports in zoo and circus, is a huge animal. The weight of full-grown males varies between fifteen hundred and two thousand pounds. The females carry their smaller bulk of five to six hundred pounds more lithesomely. Each female bears a single pup, a lusty youngster of about thirty-five pounds, about the middle of June.[3]

When we reached the borders of the sea lion purviews, we saw the water crowded with animal life. Seals and sea lions, old and young, swam busily and playfully and noisily together. Many mother sea lions were turning and twisting about in the waves accompanying their young. The mother seal lion was more affectionate than the neighboring female seals. Young sea lions like seal pups possess no instinctive knowledge of swimming. Throw a young animal of either species into shallow water, as Steller did long ago on Bering Island, and they bolt for shore in fright. First they must paddle in tidal pools until they have won enough courage to venture into the sea. Day after day they experiment in deeper water, becoming adept at keeping afloat, then attempting diving and leaping out of the water. It is not long before they are more at home in the sea than on land.

Since the sea lions breed earlier in the summer than the seals, by the time we saw them the harems were broken up. The average harem of the sea lion contains ten to a dozen cows.

Northern tribes valued the sea lion highly. The firm white flesh was sweet to eat; the thick white blubber gave odorless warmth in the stone lamps. The strong, tough smooth hide made the stoutest seaworthy covering for boats. Shoes, clothing, and pack straps made of the skin were very durable.

Steller wrote ecstatically of sea lion fat, "The blubber as well as the sweet flesh is well-flavored and highly prized and the gelatinous flippers are considered a prime delicacy. The fat is not greasy like that of seals and whales, but it is stiff and resembles that of sea boars in color but not in flavor and smell. The fat of the young is sweeter than mutton tallow and resembles the marrow of leg bone."[4] Perhaps the coarse, unpalatable, often wormy and moldy fare of the explorers accounted for Steller's enthusiasm. I cannot judge its excellence for the only time I had the opportunity to taste sea lion flesh, the meat was scarcely cooked and my over-fastidious appetite made me bolt a few unchewed mouthfuls washed down with very strong tea.

The vast ancient herds of sea lions have long been gone from the northern seas. The European hunters harried them mercilessly once they discovered their haunts. It seemed as if the sea lion were to follow the sea cow into the musty obscurity of old scientific reports. Just in time laws were passed to protect them. Like the walrus, only Alaskan Native tribes who need them for food and clothing, or scientists who can prove their valid need for specimens, are permitted to kill them. Uninhabited Bogoslof Island, the youngest of the Bering Sea islands, shelters the largest known herd. Small rookeries similar to the one on St. Paul are scattered throughout the northwest.

The sea lion once inhabited both the large Pribilof islands. When Elliott was collecting data, he heard from St. George Aleuts that their island had been so overrun with sea lions that the Russian hunters used to drive thousands into the sea, hoping that untenanted coastline would tempt more seals from the sea.[5] Choris, a gentleman traveler in search of novel material for a travel book, touched at the Pribilofs in 1820. He discussed the sea lions on St. George without alluding to the presence of fur seals. It may be assumed that the throng of sea lions was so great that the few seals seemed unworthy of mention. There were thousands of sea lions in rookeries on St. Paul, too, in those days. And even on the inhospitable stone block of Walrus Island.

Now only a few hundred return yearly to Vostochnie, to the neighborhood of Sea Lion Neck, swimming through Sea Lion Bight, familiar haunts that have long borne their names.

Russian hunters slaughtered sea lions for their own food, for boat covers for themselves and their Aleut henchmen, and exported the stiff, smooth whiskers to China where they were mounted in gold to serve as toothpicks for the elegant upper classes.

When the Treasury Department leased the Pribilof sealing rights to the Alaska Commercial Company in 1870, the company did not receive permission to kill the sea lions. Yet the company wanted the hides badly for boats for their freelance hunters along the Aleutian chain and on other Alaskan coasts. No other skin was quite as satisfactory for either the large baidars or the small baidarkas. Since the Pribilof Aleut retained full right to kill as many sea lions as they wished for their needs, the company could buy excess skins. The price of forty cents a skin seems little enough for the labor of skinning and partially preparing the hides for use. Since the ordinary hunts for sea lions for food for the village provided fewer skins than the company required, its island officials practiced many artifices to induce the Aleuts to kill more lions than they could possibly utilize for food. Government agents were not always aware of these tricks. Some of these agents did not know that the sea lions belonged solely to the Aleuts. Others did not seem to care if they were.

Far-seeing Aleuts resented being coerced whether by gentle bribes or by threat to decimate the herd of animals that provided so large a share of their livelihood. But whether through ignorance or indifference, these Aleuts received little support from most government employees, sworn to protect both seals and Aleuts from any violation of the sealing contract. Disputes frequently arose over equitable division of payment for sea lion skins. Since the animals belonged to the whole Aleut community, men who had not assisted in the actual driving and killing still felt entitled to a share in the monetary proceeds. The company was inclined to pay only those who took part in the hunting.

Big-hearted, vitriolic Colonel Marston, who was the assistant treasury agent in 1875, bitterly condemned the company's ruthlessness in trying to rob the Aleuts of their rights. He combated the efforts of one or two favor-currying Aleuts who sought excuses to make unnecessary drives at the company manager's prompting. He railed at a company that, unsatisfied with the enormous profits of sealing, cared not whether the Aleuts' property were wasted and offered inadequate prices for the peltry. The Aleuts treasure many stories of his outspoken rebellion against the sharp and petty practices of the commercial company. It is pleasant to remember him in contrast to the tacit acceptance of many small injustices by his successors.

Elliott's almost-forgotten report on the Seal Islands contains a graphic picture of a sea lion drive. In 1941 when trucks ran freely along the island roads it would have been a simple matter to drive the lions a short distance inland to a level grassy field and bring the meat and hides back to the villagers. Long before our arrival, the annual sea lion drive for food had become a memory.

In 1872 a journey to Northeast Point was either a slow twelve-mile trudge over grass hussocks and boulders or a hard, long pull at the oars to bring a baidar from Village Cove. In 1875 William J. McIntyre, assistant treasury agent at the time, though soon to be on staff of the Alaska Commercial Company with his relatives, after eating supper, ran to Northeast Point from the village in one hour and fifty-nine minutes, winning a wager against the scoffers who said it could not be done in two hours, eleven and five-eighths minutes. This feat probably few people could or would want to repeat.[6]

Certainly the poor sea lion, who was forced to pack his own skin on his back from his rookery to the village, could not emulate it. The drives took from six days in damp weather to three weeks or longer when warm dry weather overheated the animals too quickly. The big drive took place every autumn. A gang of Aleut hunters moved out to barabaras located at the site of the oldest villages of that area. Close by stood a building known as Webster House, in which Captain Daniel

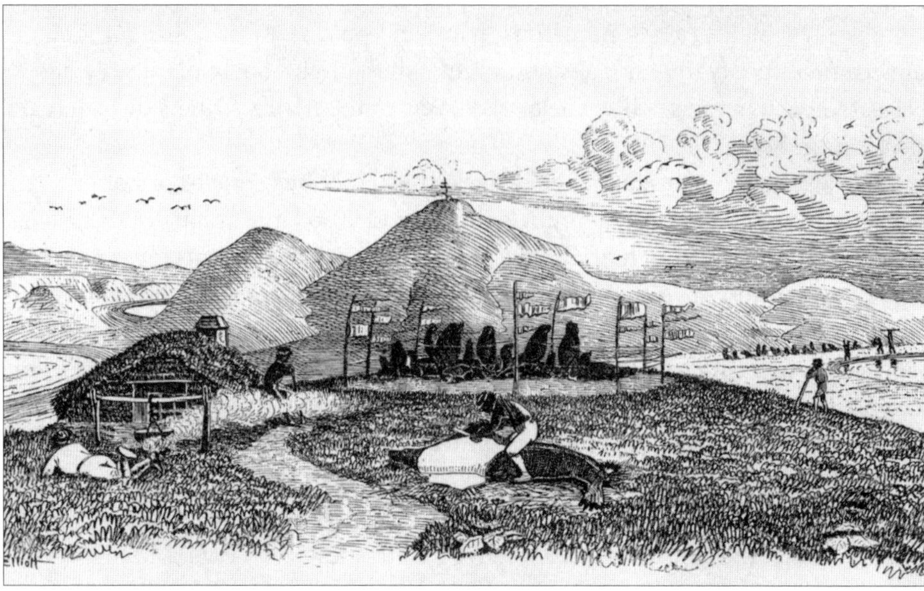

Henry W. Elliott's drawing "The Sea-Lion Pen" was made at Northeast Point. Note the barabara with its deep-set window and the cooking fire outside (*Our Arctic Province,* 1886, opposite p. 365).

Webster, one of the most famous of the old American sealers, spent many summers supervising sealing operations of the immense northeast rookeries for the Alaska Commercial Company. His name still lingers there, attached to the pleasant bungalow reserved for government employees, to a pretty lake, a hill, and a small cape.

Night after night when the wind blew off shore and the moon's betraying light was hidden, the hunters crept on all fours over the rocks until they were between the lions and the sea. Then a wild hullabaloo started. The hunters shouted and fired their revolvers at the sky. The startled animals drew back from the shadowy, brawling foes at the water's edge and fled inland. Occasionally a terror-crazed beast would plunge right past or over hunters. The great bulk of the beast is more than sufficient to crush a man. Hunters often received slashing bites or other serious injuries but tradition tells of no greater casualty than the castration of one luckless man. Elliott witnessed one incident when a lion plunged over a crouching hunter. The hunter bounced up miraculously unharmed while the lion escaped safely to the sea.[7]

Near the camp by Webster Lake a rude circular corral of driftwood posts linked by strands of sinew, usually sea lion sinews, was prepared for the captives. Rags dangling from the sinew strands were sufficiently alarming to keep the sea lions penned in although guards kept constant watch lest the strangeness of the fluttering cloths wore off.

Days or weeks might pass, waiting for friendly winds and nights sufficiently dark for hunting before the number of lions for the winter's supplies had been gathered together. When the quota was at last filled, the long arduous trek commenced. Men hemmed in the sea lions, leaving only a narrow opening toward which the beasts were urged. Young males and females, whose light bodies permitted faster travel, usually headed the march. As the line thinned out almost to a single file the drivers had to be alert to keep the procession intact. The old bulls were the first to sink to rest. Prodded, they often showed a willingness to fight. The drivers ambled along, clapping their hands or sticks and bones together (the broad scapulae of the sea lions make excellent, resounding clappers), firing their revolvers, waving strips of cloth in the very faces of the exasperated animals. One device that was extremely successful on Elliott's trip was a blue gingham umbrella shoved close to the face of a recalcitrant sea lion and opened and shut quickly. Elliott asks, "Is it not an amusing coincidence that while lions are hunted under umbrellas in Africa, their marine namesakes are chased with them in Alaska?"

The lakes and ponds that string along the length of the island gave welcome refreshment to the weary sea lions. Big Lake was the first long pause. All the animals were secured in a temporary corral similar to their prison at the Point. When released they were driven in single file into the water. The drivers, traveling in baidarkas, kept the animals swimming and wading in the right direction. In less than twenty minutes two miles of the journey was done and the sea lions had been reinvigorated by their bath. The small lakes gave them briefer respites. The causalities of these long drives were enormous, even when drivers took care not to hurry the herd. Too often the hunter's intense desire to reach home after the long absence tempted them to goad the animals unmercifully, no matter how many died.

It was a relief to both man and beast to reach the village killing field. But the sea lions had little time to enjoy their journey's end before the killing began. The troublesome old bulls who never lost their will to fight their captors were dispatched first by a shot in the head. The less dangerous young males and cows were killed by a skillful thrust of a stout lance, directed behind the foreflippers, piercing them to the heart. As death pursued them the panicked lions crowded together, piling up on top of one another, but finding no escape from man's weapons in undefined unity.

In contrast to the seal killing, Elliott found the scene "dreadfully cruel and bloody." He makes the carnage almost too real: "The natives spear the cows on top, which, as they sink in death, are mounted in turn by the live animals underneath; these meet the deadly lance, in order, and so on until the whole herd is quiet and stilled in the fatal ebbing of their heart's blood."[8]

When the butchery ended the Aleut women set to work. Their granddaughters have never learned the tasks their female ancestors performed so skillfully. For it was then customary for the women to assist in skinning and dividing the meat of the sea lions. The intestinal and throat membranes were carefully scraped clean. Raincoats generally called *kamleika* since the Russian hunters introduced the Siberian term were made by sewing the intestinal tissues in circular strips with sinew. These garments weighed little, lasted longer than rubber coats, and shed water perfectly. Before civilization blighted Aleut art by substituting Sears Roebuck fashions as standards of beauty, the Aleutian *kamleika* was a gorgeous garment, each encircling seam decorated by gaily dyed wisps of bird feathers. Only occasionally is such a garment seen today and never on the Pribilof Islands, even without decoration. Only on remote islands of the archipelago or among the Eskimos of Nunivak or St. Lawrence are there a few old women who possess the skill and patience for such dressmaking. But in 1872 such garments were still worn on St. Paul and each family took a share of membranes. One throat tissue usually was enough for the upper part of a waterproof boot, soled with a piece of lion flipper and stitched with its sinews. Extra tissues found a ready but poorly paying buyer in the company, which needed them for hunting garments for their other hunters.

Little of the animal was discarded. The sinews were stripped from the spinal column for thread and pack lashing. The stomach was saved to serve as an oil container, for oil rendered from the hard white lion blubber or the softer, ill-smelling seal fat. Gall bladders, carefully extracted from the fresh carcass, were dried and used as poultices for scrofulous lesions so commonplace among the Aleuts then.

Cooking was still a gesture with the inhabitants of St. Paul. Choice bits such as liver and lung and fine flakes of blubber were eaten raw, often steaming fresh from the carcass. The meat was hung in the open air from wooden forms called *laabas*. It would serve as food from autumn until May, even if it became tainted and ill smelling.

Although a refrigerator preserves meat now, I noticed some of these *laabas* in the yards the first time we walked through the village. Several of them were laden with dangling, shriveled gobs of dark red flesh. When we inquired what was hung out to dry, there was an amazing lack of knowledge. At last one man drew Sam aside and whispered that the objects were the genital organs of the male seals, being dried for shipment to San Francisco. Chinese pharmacists paid three cents apiece for them, grinding them into conçoctions supposed to restore youth and virility.

Salt beef and salt pork from the government stores and canned foods have replaced the enormous amounts of sea lion flesh that was once consumed in a year. In the 1870s, in addition to thousands of young seals killed especially for food, three thousand sea lions were considered a fair winter's supply for a population about half the size of the 1941 census, about 130 to 140 people. Not today could the Aleut slaughter enough of these animals to satisfy their needs.

The rotting sea lion bodies we stumbled upon were also explained to me as animals killed for food and neglected. Gossip claimed this was merely official language for cutting down the number of sea lions that became mixed up with seal pods on drives. I heard the officials fulminate about the sea lions often as "darn nuisances" because their bellicose defense tactics delayed seal killing. Why ever they were killed, thus further depleting the small total of these magnificent leonine marine animals, I do know that the carcasses were left to rot, providing food only for the big bluebottles, the foxes, and the maggots.

Aleut hunters killed an occasional sea lion during the winter but since the villagers needed not only a change from their monotonous rations but also supplemental food, I refrained from begging a portion when the body was divided. I did so want to sample some that I cooked myself. I wonder how many lions are shot that are never recovered for use. The hunters, stationed along the shore, waiting for birds or mammals, fire at their prey and then wait for the tides to wash the game ashore. I met one boy returning disconsolately from hunting one night. He told me he had shot eleven birds but all had floated away instead of inshore. When we made a circuit of the coastline in spring we counted fourteen bloated, rotting corpses of sea lions, all or most of them victims of a hunter who had no way to bag his catch.

There is an intangible charm about the sea lion's poise and the fluid ease with which he moves his huge body on land as well as in the sea that fascinates human observers. If *Eumetopias jubatus Steller* is wiped out by gradual wasteful killing, or decides to desert Morzhovoi rocks, the last link with the wildlife kingdom that owned St. Paul before man came, the bond between prehistory and history, will break. The Pribilof Islands will become merely a huge stock farm for breeding fur seals and foxes. The summer air of Northeast Point will be quieter if the sea lions' resonant cries are stilled.

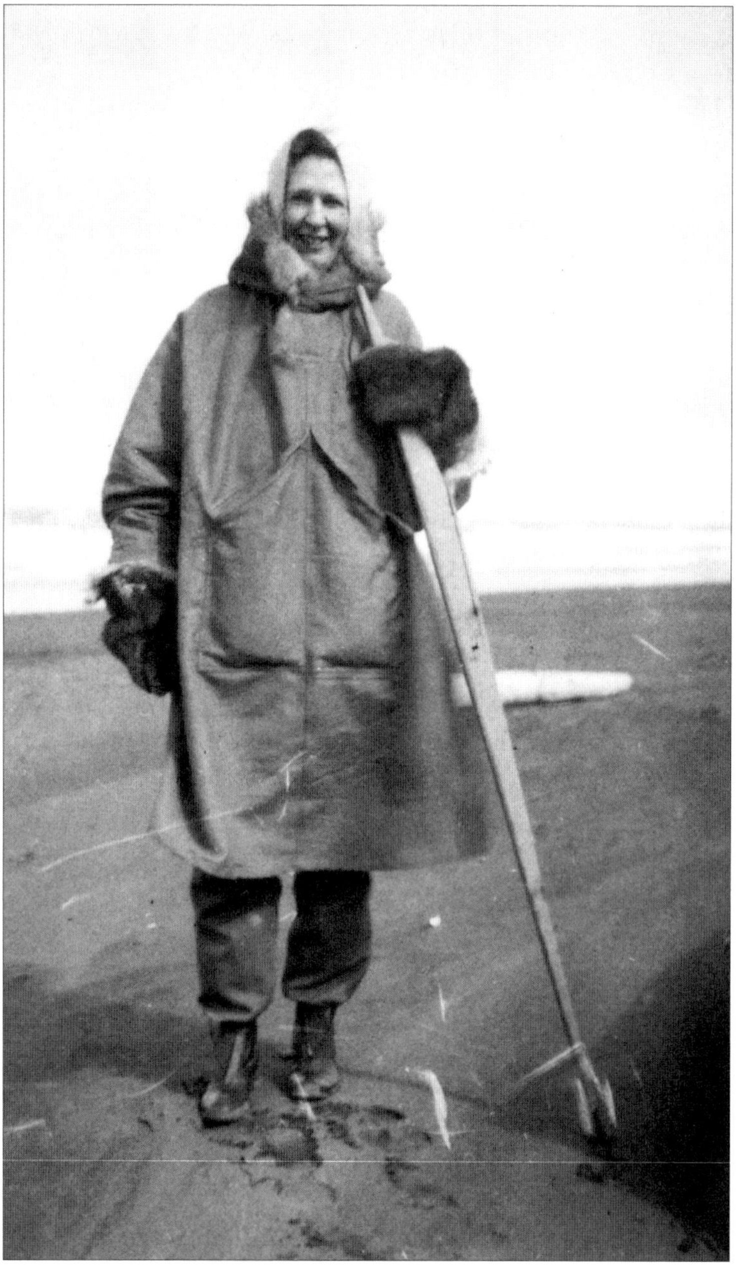

Fredericka Martin dressed for hiking (from the Martin Collection, USUAF210, Archives, Alaska and Polar Regions, Rasmuson Library, University of Alaska Fairbanks).

Chapter 13

When I count over the hours of our island stay, I recall wistfully how little of our time was spent exploring. Some days I regretted the professional halter that kept us indoors, days when the wind cried at the window for our companionship, when the sea's voice called as someone opened our door. But we were no tourists free to spend our hours as we liked. Sam's skill and knowledge were the passports that had admitted us to the island. The sealer's need of his services came first. Whether we tramped the sands beyond Marunich or walked only to the top of Village Hill, someone knew where we were and was prepared to summon us if an emergency arose.

Though there are as many ways of practicing medicine as of doing any other work, there is but one right way. It is a profession that demands constant striving toward perfection of technique and wholehearted sympathy for those who are distressed no matter their social station, the color of their skin. Prejudice of any sort must be alien to the good physician. Neither personal fatigue nor pain can be allowed to mar one's services. Carelessness, callousness, and irritation at human foibles cannot be permitted to affect one's helpfulness.

Other doctors before us had struggled alone with the tasks of pharmacist, laboratory technician, nurse, and cleaning woman as well as their own duties. In vain they had begged deaf officialdom in their annual reports for the aid of a trained nurse. Sam, at least, had my assistance. And because I shared his work, the *we* I use in discussing Pribilof medical practice is no vague editorial pronoun.

It was not easy to know where to begin restoring order in the littered rooms of the dispensary. I just began pulling dirty empty jars and bottles off shelves and sorting piles of rusty instruments. When a space was cleared, I rolled up my sleeves and scrubbed and arranged cleaned and useful articles in convenient order. After several days of strenuous housekeeping labors, the dispensary had a new face. It was light because the shades were rolled up and the dust-catching curtains had been stored away. There was space because useless furniture, obsolete drugs, and broken, unrepairable equipment had been stored neatly in the cellar. The three rooms of the dispensary, a part of the building in which we lived, were as efficiently prepared for the treatment of patients as our combined skill could effect with the resources and appliances available. Sam, who had scrubbed at my side, had won a new respect for nurses.

> July 24, 1941
> We are trying to establish a routine of living so that we can really accomplish something in the way of study. Office hours are from eight to nine in the morning. We decided that if we were to be disturbed to inspect men who reported ill for work we might as well make it a steady business. And again in the afternoons from five to six. In the morning after hours, Sam attends to his hospital patients and I fly to my typewriter. I've had a difficult time trying to get everything down on paper that we have been experiencing. Because so many different types of things are crowding upon me. And when I do get caught up I start a letter so that I shall have a lot of fat envelopes ready to leave any time a ship comes in. We do get visitors and chances to send out mail at odd times—and if mail has been sent via Dutch Harbor it arrives here by similar methods. So we have had about five letters to keep us in touch with home.
>
> *cont.*

A revolutionary change had taken place. The office door stood wide open. No longer need patients huddle timidly in the narrow hallway. There were freshly painted white chairs in the first office for them to sit on. The freedom of entrance and the luxury of sitting comfortably while waiting to see the doctor overwhelmed our first patients. Embarrassed and frightened they sat tensely on the edge of the chairs, gripping their hats in nervous hands. In a few weeks the novelty of such a simple innovation disappeared. Patients came in confidently, greeted us warmly, and relaxed at ease while they waited their turn. When the seats were occupied there were the chairs in our living room across the hall. In one respect we were adamant. Save for emergencies, the islanders had to observe regular office hours from eight to nine in the morning and five to six in the afternoon. Since our predecessors had not insisted on definite office hours, it required several weeks of patiently and gently turning away the visitors who arrived at odd hours for such "emergencies" as refilling their cod liver oil bottle.

My nursing standards were an innovation hard to adjust to for our janitor, Paul Merculieff. From no supervision under previous doctors to observance of a typed schedule of daily cleaning duties was revolutionary. "No other doctor," Paul grumbled one day as he performed the monthly sweeping of the attic where drugs and medical supplies were kept, "ever said sweep attic. Maybe you too clean, eh?" I assured him we were still a long way from cleanliness and he finished his job with alacrity and disappeared before I should demand further improvements.

Paul was a gentle lovable chap, possessing fundamentally a great deal of pride in his work. He was subject to violent bouts of ambitious frenzy when he scrubbed so vigorously that he endangered the paint. From time to time he would make suggestions for improving or decorating the office. However, sometimes Paul lapsed into moods of defiant indifference to dust. Every time I grew weary of Paul's negligence he would restore my faith in him by performing a task not scheduled for him. Once, at the beginning of 1942 when the dispensary shone with new white paint, the dust threatened to engulf us again. Just as in despair we were about to request the agent for a new janitor, I heard a clatter in the dispensary basement. Paul was on his hands and knees painting the floor. Sweat pouring down his face, he looked up at me with a shy smile. "It don't look so good with everything else painted. I like everything clean," he explained.

We always had an announcement of good mornings. From the hallway would come a sharp sound of rattling tin. Paul was vigorously beating the metal doormat. "Paul is rattling his antlers," one of us would comment. "All's right with the world." No need then to take our own maid from household tasks and have her clean yesterday's mud away from the dispensary floors.

Our inventory of usable equipment was disappointing. The confusion in the office had hidden the defects of so many articles that it gave us a false impression of the number of tools to work with. I almost wept over the ruined instruments, rusted for too many years to be salvaged. That nurse other doctors had begged for would have paid her salary by maintaining the equipment for a long useful life. When every nook and corner had been investigated and every box of rubbish explored, except for some unsharpenable, monstrous-sized knives, there was no scalpel. Visions of opening an abdomen with scissors or a sharp kitchen knife haunted us every time a patient complained of a slight abdominal ache until the *Penguin* brought us new knives in late July.

> And every time I start a letter I do not know where to begin. I have made a few copies of my diary notes of a seal drive that are quite rough so that I do not have to repeat that stuff and waste time for I know everyone is curious about them. As for me, I don't like seal coats anymore. I like to see them flopping around over the rocks on the backs of the original owners too well.
>
> I could write a book to every friend if I had time and strength to pound the keys. And paper. We did not bring any paper because Sam thought he could continue his habit of using what the office provided. . . . Stationery supplies are non-important here. So we got some of this thin paper that despite my efforts to pad it slides around in the machine.

One piece of office equipment I came to hate. Even in my dreams I wrestled with the vagaries of the little pressure cooker, our sole means of sterilizing linens and rubber goods. One day I came across the physician's copy of the order of goods received that contained the notation "autoclave." The physician had requisitioned a real autoclave and opposite the notation he had written in protest, "Toy!!!" That was his reaction before he became its jinni. I wonder what he might have liked to write later. Nothing printable I am sure. My own expletives were far less gentle. At the mildest when I saw it gleaming on its shelf in front of the window I grimaced and snapped, "You devil."

The diabolical conspirator with the deficiencies of the pressure cooker was the electric plate. The current fluctuated so often that I frequently had to repeat the process of sterilizing three or four times to be able to assure my conscience I had fairly germ-free packages. Months of experimentation gave me no sense of timing in controlling the machine. If I dared to bring a book into the office while I waited for the gauge to reach the temperature I desired, the cooker took a diabolic pleasure in reaching the maximum pressure quickly. The safety cock would open and with a whoosh that sounded like the end of the world to me the room would be filled with my precious steam. Then I would have to wait for the cooker to cool before beginning the long process over again.

To provide the minimum of sterile articles for a clean, safe delivery required several days of constant sterilizing. If I had time I recooked as many packages as possible as soon as I heard that a patient was beginning to have labor pains. I had become so bewitched by the satanic personality of the cooker that I used to talk to it, threaten it, and challenge it: "No matter how badly you behave I won't let you beat me. The patients are going to be protected by sterile goods even if you and I both blow up in the process."

It was easier to cope with on the nights when, while a woman in the hospital sobbed softly from the wrenching pains of birth, I resterilized the packages of rubber gloves and towels and umbilical tape and dressings. The current was steadier at night when it was shut off in the Aleut houses and the only lights in the village were the few flickering street lamps and the bulbs in the hospital, our house, and the power plant. Then the cooker purred placidly like a metal kitten. At such moments I remembered to be thankful that I suffered none of the inconveniences of other isolated communities, the roasting of bed linen in the range oven, the heating of water in washtubs and buckets on top of the range. On such nights I found a certain companionableness about that cooker that might be warding off death from that pain-wracked woman in the hospital or the terrible ravages of puerperal fever. But I could not be consistently Pollyannaish about it. So much money had been spent for equipment that would be wasted and ill spent if the pressure cooker failed in its purifying task. X-ray apparatus, shining chrome instruments, the enamel cabinets, and operating-room table represented thousands of dollars tossed away if evil bacteria resisted the heat of the cooker. The value of all other equipment depended upon the pivot of hospital hygienic success, the modern autoclave. I can honestly say that no other single object has devoured so much of my peace of mind and actual time for the results achieved.

Sorting out useful drugs from the boxes, bottles, and cans accumulated in the past fifty years was an amusing game. Who ordered the vast quantity of Glover's Mange Cure and why? Was this strange name a patent nostrum known to our grandparents or to their parents? What was the vintage year of this ancient cure-all? Probably we were pouring down the sink the last fluid ounce of a once highly regarded painkiller.

One afternoon Doc Moore, an employee of the fur company, and I were in the dispensary laboratory when we heard an old woman in the waiting room request a bottle of castor oil. We listened for Sam's reply with special interest. All during lunch that day we had listened to Sam's picturesque descriptions of purposes toward which he, slightly hipped on the dangers of constant usage of cathartics, would like to utilize a goodly portion of the island's colossal supply of castor oil. Sam overrode the old lady's distrust of his suggested substitute ruthlessly. She marched out with a mild cathartic muttering her disapproval under her breath. Doc Moore reported to the supper table at Government House that Sam was a man who stuck to his convictions. Alas, two days later Claudia Kochutin returned lugging back the empty mineral oil bottle. "This stuff is no good," she shouted at Sam. "Gimme castor oil." Meekly Sam filled the empty bottle for her.

All of our first patients were as demanding as Claudia. They came as if to a drugstore ordering a drug, requesting aspirin, castor oil, Epsom salts, some "red pills," a bottle of "white medicine." Patiently Sam counteracted this approach by gentle questionings. It was a bright day when a woman actually came into the office and said, "Doctor, I've got a terrible pain in my head. What can you give me?" instead of ordering her own prescription. Sam's eyes shot a gleam of triumph in my direction. Gradually everyone learned to explain their symptoms and await the doctor's advice and instructions.

We traced this attitude to its source, the fairly rapid turnover of physicians. One doctor stayed a year, was sympathetic and anxious to help his patients, maintained the highest standards of examination and treatment. His successor might remain on the island for two years, interested in nothing but saving enough of his salary to open an office when he returned to the States. The latter type of physician felt it unnecessary to take too many pains with Aleut customers, who paid only indirectly via the check from Uncle Sam. There had been St. Paul physicians so victimized by deep racial prejudices that they did not want to handle the Aleuts like human beings, who were careful to protect their clothes from contact with the patient by donning a white gown but had no compunction against making patients lie on the dirty sheet on the examining table that had been used for weeks. There had been others unable to cope with the physical difficulties of maintaining cleanliness and order without trained assistance and who crumpled up when their ideas for medical reform crashed against the insentient wall of official indifference.

Dr. Migliori had warned us that Service families on the island had an innate contempt for the physicians. I think he was correct in his analysis and that this impression trickled down from the seats of the governors to the everyday level of the Aleuts and gave them a fundamental distrust of their medical helpers. In addition the islanders had suffered from physicians whose treatment bore out the skepticism. There had been doctors who had run away from the pressure of life and found the solitude of St. Paul unbearable without alcoholic solace. As a result of several scandals, medicinal alcohol was kept under lock and key by the agent and doled out in small amounts to the physician. Who could soothe the bitterness in Dimitri Tetoff's heart when he said truly, "My baby daughter died because the doctor was dead drunk in bed."

> January 25, 1942
> Apolon B. was called Jim Crow because some Native started a joke about him being a crow, in Aleut, because he made so many visits to Unalaska—whether traveling like a crow or because there are so many crows there that he was going to see. A white man added the national touch of *Jim.* And the name stuck, being used in the records for years before there was a clue as to the real identity.
>
> Dr. Richstein, John [Hanson] says, was taken off the island because he tried to dope old Jim Crow and the people caught on to it and complained. Supposedly his intention was to release the old man from suffering. Richstein, in addition to being a drunkard, was a terrible gambler. Dimitri Tetoff said one of his children died because R. was too drunk to deliver aid. John adds that when he was drunk he used to come to the villagers' houses fighting mad and everyone was frightened of him and would run for safety as fast as they could.

There had been other doctors who were drug addicts and some who had affairs with Aleut women. But there had been doctors who had been hard-working, earnest physicians. If I read the old records correctly these doctors were a majority and, although handicapped by the lack of trained cooperative help, sought not only to cure the immediate ills of their patients but to better their living conditions. There had been saints, like Dr. Hunter whose deeds illuminate the yellowed pages of his medical records and his reports. Blackguards are commonplace everywhere. So are the careless, the stupid, the shortsighted, and the indifferent. People afflicted with race prejudices are not rare in America. But the saints in the world beyond St. Paul are extremely rare, and St. Paul's proportion of them seems more than average. As for ordinary diligent, kindly physicians, they exceed the unworthy on the roll call of St. Paul as elsewhere in the world.

But we could not convince our neighbors and patients, whether officials or Aleuts, by philosophizing and calling upon the records to bear out our contentions as to the general fine caliber of past physicians. Only by our reception of patients, by sympathy and kindliness, could we win their confidence and obedience in order to truly help them. It did not take long. If my diary were not full of accounts of those first few weeks of timid skulking in the hallway, of abashed faces and downcast eyes, I would probably have forgotten most details of that period. I would remember only the longer period when patients walked in briskly, hung their wraps in the hall, took a seat without invitation, and greeted us warmly. It is a better memory to hold, but it would not be as bright or valuable if we forgot the earlier atmosphere of nervous servility and the expectation of brusque, abrupt treatment.

Some of Sam's predecessors had struggled to inculcate a few principles of preventive medicine. The lessons had apparently taken root in one direction very thoroughly. Lacerations and animal bites might be called the industrial accidents of St. Paul. As a result of the emphasis on immediate treatment of open wounds, some amusing cases interrupted our program between regular office hours. Strong, brawny males would dash madly into the house, exclaiming, "Doctor, I'm cut bad." Far too often it was difficult to find a slight scratch. Exaggerating his mien of professional seriousness in an endeavor to check his laughter, Sam would study the outstretched hand intently, poring over a dermal scratch too slight to draw blood. Sometimes he could not forbear teasing a little. "Now just where is this wound," he would inquire as he reached for a Merthiolate swab and painted a large area of the hand or decorated it with a futuristic design.

I only saw Sam lose his patience once. At the time he was worrying over a four-year-old child suffering from an infection of the forehead whom he had just admitted to the hospital for the third time for the same affliction. Twice before he had released the girl with the wound clean and almost healed. Each time the child became reinfected. That afternoon Sam had gone to the home and discovered that the area was more seriously infected than before. Sam gave the young mother a severe scolding. All evening he went back and forth to the hospital, checking for himself the child's reactions to a sulfa drug. At nine o'clock the father came to the house door. I thought he wanted to inquire about his daughter. But no. He had scratched his cheek with a pin he said. Sam surveyed his face under the glaring bulb in the hall. Not a shadow of a scratch showed. He got no Merthiolate decoration. Sam sent him out reeling under a deluge of advice about caring for children.

Then Sam paced the floor for half an hour puzzling over the tricks of the human mind that could rush for treatment for an invisible pinprick and neglect a child until she was close to death's door.

Later we revised our opinion of the parents. He was a mere lad, burdened with marriage, who wanted to play basketball instead of do housework and care for his lively children. She was a woman suffering from the abrupt curtailment of childhood by marriage before she was sixteen. Neither was capable, because of youth and inexperience, of coping with parental problems. He told us he had hurried down to see us when he pricked his face because he was afraid he would get infected like his daughter. He had been impressed with the scolding Sam had given his wife and thought he was doing something the doctor would approve.

Chapter 14

Wne warning we had received had been exaggerated. Once the Aleuts had confidence in Sam there were few incidents of disobedience to his orders. Aleuts proved to be neither better nor worse than any average group of patients encountered elsewhere. Certainly their ancestry had not made them naturally and instinctively doctor-defiant. Their response to various clinics that Sam set up exposed the fallacy of the charge that they were not concerned about their health. When the women realized that Sam actually wanted them to come in for regular prenatal and postnatal examinations month after month, they were only too glad to keep appointments. Regular examinations of children delighted most mothers. If the weather were too stormy, someone would come streaking through the rain to ask for a postponement and a new date.

Because the sera and vaccines Sam had ordered did not arrive until the last autumn boat, it was winter before Sam could set up immunization clinics. Some wrathful anti-vaccinationist seemed to invoke storms each day set for the clinics. Just ten minutes before our first anti-diphtheria clinic for the preschool children a gale swept out of the sea and the air was choked with masses of falling snowflakes. Before we could find a messenger to ward off the parents, the first adults were swarming into the office carrying huge bundles of blankets. Out of the heavy wrappings they produced slightly stultified offspring too glad to emerge from their cocoons to protest much at the doctor and his needle. The only children who stayed at home that day were those whose mothers had lugged one down to the office and planned a return trip to get another. They were told to go home and get warm and dry and come another day.

The office was mobbed when adults were requested to come for tuberculosis skin tests. There was much good-natured shoving and pushing. It was more like a mob scene in the movies than a well-regulated clinic. The job was done in a quarter of an hour. Sam had learned a necessary lesson, which made him space appointments for reading the results of the tests. Despite the crowding and noise Sam explained the reasons for the test and just what the reactions would mean so well that not one person became alarmed over a positive redness at any point in the skin under the patch. Except, I blush to admit it, the anxious wife of a government employee who fretted and fretted until an x-ray disclosed her child's freedom from the disease.

One fact Sam omitted from his lectures. As a result of the oversight and also as a result of the date of the test, a Friday afternoon, the door was almost worn out with constant knocking. Every visitor said, "I forgot, Doctor. Can I take a bath? Will it spoil the test?"

A few males who had been working at the hour of the clinic dropped in the next day to ask for their "plaster." How I wanted a picture of some of the older men with their droopy Russian-styled mustaches or flowing beards baring their chests as proudly as if they were to receive medals. A month later in the early morning a man who had completed serving a jail sentence for assault came into the office. "When can I get my TB test?" he inquired anxiously.

Height and weight clinics interested the adults, too. People memorized the figures and most of them had to be pretty sick to refrain from asking if they could get weighed every time they came into the office.

When the schoolchildren came for their diphtheria injections we saw the influence of the movies on island mores. The youngsters crowded around the table looking with big frightened eyes at the array of needles and syringes. I lined them up one behind the other and showed them how far to roll up their sleeves. The wriggling imp at the head of the line I had chosen deliberately for his swaggering bravado. As he thrust out his arm he wisecracked, "Me not scared. Me, Cisco Kid." I tried to revive the weakening courage of two little youngsters by asking whether they too were Cisco Kids. "No," piped one of them in a quavery voice. "Me, Amigo." For those who avoid Westerns at the movies, I should explain that Amigo is the man Friday of the dauntless hero and champion of the distressed, the Cisco Kid.

Another morning we were plying hypodermic needles. One youngster, Sally Kochutin, looked up politely and said, "Thank you, Doctor." The next victim echoed her remark. The refrain caught on and Sam finished to the rhythm of "Thank you, Doctor," an irregular tempo to keep time to because of the tremulous tone of children who felt anything but grateful.

"All the Natives have tuberculosis and venereal diseases" is a commonplace indictment on the lips of the "white" population of Alaska. Sometimes I wondered whether the incessant trumpeting of that charge and other accusations of immorality and alcoholism were not an instinctive protective diversion from the unsavory truth that the tubercle bacillus, the spirochete, and the whiskey bottle were introduced by traders and adventurers. When the missionaries and teachers followed commerce it was almost too late for them to make spiritual and intellectual goals as attractive as the already well-established alcoholic civilization. The yellowing pages of the census records of St. Paul showed the triumph of tuberculosis. The total number of deaths openly credited to its ravages are appalling and incomplete. To such diagnoses as "general debility," "bronchitis," and "pneumonia" as the cause of death, there was added a note, "Has been ill for years with lung complaint."

A study made by Dr. Lutz in 1889 revealed that the population of St. Paul had decreased from 218 in 1872 to 147 persons. The arrival through the years of nearly a hundred women who married St. Paul sealers and brought children of previous marriages with them maintained the census at an artificially stable level. The years in which deaths did not exceed births were rare. Until a few years ago, the death rate and birth rate have been almost always even. In the past two decades the birth rate is sluggishly gaining over its opponent.

The majority of the deaths can be accredited to the tubercle bacillus. It is not strange that records and reports reveal that old age was one of the "seven ages" of man that Aleuts seldom experienced.[1] Even in 1941 the few old people in the village were conspicuous. Slowly better housing, better diet, improved medical service, and many years of education made a dent in the death rate, halted the sweeping progress of tuberculosis. After performing skin tests on the entire population and checking and rechecking by x-rays of the lungs all who showed suspicious symptoms, Sam discovered only four active cases out of a population of 285. An astounding number of chest plates showed extensive healed lesions of the disease. Such people are very susceptible to a reoccurrence of the illness and needed the periodic examinations that Sam introduced if the disease is to be exiled from that community forever.

Many names that appear on the first American census lists are no longer heard on the islands. The "white plague," its horror not to be disguised by a poetic name, has exterminated family after family. The ecclesiastical rule that forbids a fourth marriage to an Orthodox Russian communicant, probably rarely affecting people in most parts of the world, became an oppressive ban on the Seal Islands. There it meant loneliness, an empty home, or the breaking of other moral laws. In 1872 for instance, there were three men on St. Paul who had each buried three wives and could not remarry because of the church law. The nine females who had died were probably all victims of tuberculosis. Many years went by before such occurrences became rare. The last man who had been widowed three times died by his own hand in 1938. He had tried to build a family by adopting children. They, too, preceded him to the hill above Black Bluffs.

Dr. Hunter, physician for two periods of several years during the decade of the First World War, was a tireless fighter against germs, dirt, and ignorance.[2] He made a survey of the homes, the little dingy buildings like the hut across the street from our dispensary. He measured the cubic feet of living space and inventoried beds and bed clothing. He studied the dietary deficiencies, both quantitative and qualitative, of the government-supplied rations. He learned how many men went breakfastless to work and how many children started off to school each morning before eating. His neat numerals evoke a tragic shameful picture. Few families possessed more than one blanket. The fortunate household that owned four numbered eight or ten individuals. No one possessed adequate bed coverings, much less such luxuries as sheets and pillowcases. Dr. Hunter repeated, whether he realized it or not, a less thorough survey in the 1890s when tenderhearted assistant treasury agent [James] Judge bought with government money flimsy blankets from the sealing lessee's store. He regretted that he had to waste the taxpayer's money on such poor thin material, but he could not wait to import better once he realized the long-neglected misery within the village houses. He bought all the beds the company had for sale but there were still many people who had to sleep on the floor. He purchased unbleached muslin of which his wife and some Aleut women made sheets. They also sewed thin flannel capes for the schoolgirls, slight protection against the wind. Judge comforted himself that the capes were better than going coatless to school. The [North American Commercial] Company suddenly remembered that according to the terms of the lease, it was responsible for providing to the needs of widows and orphans. Accordingly they generously donated a few yards of unbleached muslin to the community sewing bee, for the husbandless only.

Tuberculosis was also transmitted when the whole congregation at a funeral kissed the dead on the lips. Many priests and government officials had fought over this practice. Somehow Hunter secured the cooperation of the resident priest. The teachers, Dr. and Mrs. Haley, were enthusiastic co-workers in all of Hunter's campaigns.[3] They lectured to the schoolchildren about tuberculosis and demonstrated the existence of the bacillus with a microscope. Dr. Haley and Dr. Hunter haunted funeral services and felt triumphant when they saw that even the eldest relatives or village elders only kissed the corpse on the forehead.[4] Kissing the corpse only on the forehead by family and intimate friends seems to be the general tradition now.

Hunter's reports to Washington undoubtedly woke up some lethargic bureaucrats. Shortly after his second stay and second impassioned report, the erection of larger, warmer homes for the sealers commenced.

Long before we arrived on St. Paul the slight decline in the death rate had made overcrowding an evil again. Too many married couples lived with in-laws. The lack of privacy engendered quarrels and upset family relationships. Since more children were growing up to be adults, beds and bedroom space were filled and overflowing. Sam's studies revealed numerous houses where too many children not only slept in one room together but actually in one bed. Two children in bed with the parents was common. Some people still stretched out on the floor at night in the style of the 1890s.

Not only did Hunter strive to wake up officialdom to the plight of the Aleuts under their charge but he toiled to awaken the sealers themselves. His love for them was deep and full of understanding patience. His opinion of agents who insisted on dispensing wormy dried fruit after he had begged them to throw out the boxes before they crawled away is absent from his reports. I saw a scrawled note on a memorandum to the office, "Of course, nothing has been done after two years."

> July 9, 1941
> I was not quite ready when Mr. Hoverson called for Sam to go inspecting houses. Sam told me that last week they began at the end of the village toward Reef. So I went walking up and down those three streets and nary a sign of them. I was back at the head of the steps near Gov. House when I ran into Mr. Hellbaum to chat a bit. I looked up and Sam and Mr. H. were hailing me from the school. They had reversed the order of attack today so as to catch people unawares. So I went back over the way I had been searching for them. Only going inside this time. Some of the houses are really very nice. Large airy kitchens with modern built-in cupboards and sinks, which are mere symbols because there is no running water. These brightly painted rooms made me envious. A few of the houses were ill furnished and bare and drab. None of them were dirty. Just that bare look of poverty. So many houses had electric washing machines, radios, even connected with record players. In Antonina's home, I met her older sister, Justina, who is twenty and unmarried . . .
>
> It is cold out today and there has been no sign of rain nor of sun. It is hard to write "July" in this atmosphere.

He became ill. He began to spit blood. Fearing that the bacillus he was fighting had selected him for a victim, he requested a long leave of absence or proffered his resignation. He obtained the leave. When he came back he took up his program of social improvement with the same gallant loyalty. I wish he could know, if he is still alive, how many Aleut eyes kindled with affection when they mentioned him and how great a compliment it was for Sam to hear, "You are just like Dr. Hunter. He was a good man."

During the same decade weekly sanitary inspections were inaugurated, kept up spasmodically, and finally officially set into a permanent mold by an edict of the Washington office. So every Wednesday after lunch Sam and the agent or his substitute set off to visit every house in the village, except those of the Service employees. We wives were trusted to keep our houses in order. If Mac went, I knew Sam would return within a half hour. On such days Sam would run breathlessly at Mac's heels, pop his head into front doors, nod or say hello, and back out. Many houses Mac would not enter because he disliked the family. When Sam was not rushed by authority, he went into the homes, chatted with his patients, checked up on delinquents, examined chronics and convalescents. The farce of entering the kitchen in the front of the house, looking at the housewife posed in a clean dress with the floor still damp from mopping, makes the word *inspection* too strong a term. Perhaps a few housewives would not mop their floors often enough if the weekly visits were stopped. But to ensure actual sanitation and cleanliness inspection should include bedrooms to see if beds were made and the slop jars emptied and should be made at unannounced intervals. Tradition had decreed that it is not sporting to arrive without advance notice. If for any cause the tour were postponed, the office messenger went through the village notifying each household when to be ready. If the sportsmanship were to be consistent the whole practice would be terminated, but the custom has grown hoary enough to be a ritual that nothing but a complete reversal of the Service policies would alter.

Sam's final conclusion about housekeeping, based on the inspection tours and home calls on the sick at other times, was that most women did a wonderful job. He took into consideration the lack of running water, the ever-invading mud carried in by the children, the coal and ashes that had to be carried in and out the only door. Some of the housewives could satisfy the tidiest New England dust chaser. At the other extreme there were a few families who were never clean, always families with the largest number of children.

Despite Sam's descriptions, the first time I accompanied him I was amazed. Some kitchens looked like magazine advertisements except for the bulky coal range. They contained glass-doored dish closets, enameled modernistic cupboards, gay dishes posed ornamentally on the shelves, frilly curtains, shining oilcloth on the floor, and flowering plants on the windowsills. Some contained beautiful sinks, very different from the worn old ones in the homes of the officials. The gleaming enamel and chrome trimmings were ironical. Our old faucets poured our water copiously, sometimes rusty, sometimes a bit muddy, but water. Their shining spigots were only ornaments. The drainpipes were serviceable, and the soiled used water drained out into the earth under the house.

Outside each door stood the water barrel, with a wooden cover. The men wheeled the barrels down to one of the two village faucets on a barrow over the rough scoria road and trundled the heavier load back. Some Service people told me the Aleuts would not be cleaner if they had running water, that they did not even know enough to want such a convenience. When Sam sent out his questionnaire in the spring to gather information about housing and household goods, almost all of the families wrote a note in the blank space on the paper begging him to assist them in getting running water and indoor toilets. The official excuses were that the Aleuts were wasteful people who would leave their faucets running and that Ice House Lake could not supply enough water for the actual daily need of the people. The excuses do not withstand the most superficial examination. No one has ever complained that the outside faucets have been left leaking. Let one of them run idly the whole night and Ice House Lake would be depleted. The Aleuts felt the entire village should not be penalized for a few shiftless individuals whose carelessness could be averted by installing spring faucets that close automatically.

Certainly, considering the number of other lakes within a few miles of the village, the sealers should not be penalized and condemned to a choice between backbreaking toil or being filthy by the officials taking advantage of the very human inclination to avoid hard work. Official economizing of the water by making it difficult to obtain should at least not hide behind false charges of the Aleut's natural filthiness. One agent actually stated that in his annual report. To supplement the sources of fresh water, seawater could be piped inexpensively for toilets and even bathing water just as it is run to the Fouke Fur Company washhouses.

Perhaps a farmer's wife in North Dakota trudging back and forth to the well in the bitter cold winter could sympathize with the Aleuts' reluctance to use water lavishly. The winds from the Bering can be unpleasant enough without pushing a heavy barrel-laden barrow up the hill. If I had to go in and out of the house in winter, dipping pails of water out of the barrel, I imagine I would use no unnecessary drop of such hard-won fluid. And if I had used half a year's sealing cash to buy a beautiful Sears Roebuck sink that stood tauntingly in my kitchen, I would turn violently anarchistic.

Two families had rigged up indoor toilets, with equipment purchased by themselves from Sears Roebuck. One man taped the village main for running water. A second had a barrel on the roof that was filled by hand with buckets. Homemade cesspools took care of the drainings.

Privies stood near most of the houses. One day I pointed out to Sam that most of them were padlocked with very rusty locks. He received very frank answers from his patients about using outside toilets. Dr. Hunter had pleaded, begged, and gathered mountains of statistics in order to bludgeon the officials into building privies and cesspools. The spring questionnaire gave us a full picture and showed how his work had been futile. A few families said the males of the families used the privies in winter. The majority said frankly that they were used only in summer. The frankest admitted that theirs were never used.

Just before Sam relinquished his responsibilities, he had completed blood tests on the adult population of both islands. The few cases of old untreated syphilis that he discovered gave the lie to the canard about venereal diseases. Had the figures been high the fault would have been principally that of the carriers who came from the outside world and not the islanders.

Hygiene, sanitation, and the health of the islanders have improved more rapidly under direct government control (since 1910) than during the forty years the private commercial companies dominated island life (1870–1909). However, the rate of improvement has been shamefully slow and the present situation remains deplorable. The changes have not been commensurate with the devotion and labor of many well-intentioned officials, both doctors and laymen, nor with scientific advances, because of social factors that constantly counteracted the efforts of individuals. Although we recognized that the fundamental policy of island management needed overhauling, we too tried to make our small contribution for the improvement of conditions for the islanders.

Chapter 15

For a long while on St. Paul when I said "hospital" my voice hesitated because the term was farcical. The building where the sick could be given bed care lacked everything that makes a hospital more than simply a structure of wood and cement. I had been led to expect too much when Mr. [Ward T.] Bower in Washington had described the fine ten-bed hospital, staffed by two Aleut women, trained by previous doctors. Undoubtedly the word *hospital* has a connotation to me that Mr. Bower did not share. To me a hospital must be a quiet, shiningly clean, efficiently run institution that imparts confidence to those in pain and their anxious friends.

> [From a letter dated July 24, 1941, incorporated into the journal]
> Being here means we have a hospital. At least we have a fair building with eight beds and two bassinets and some odds and ends of equipment and a good x-ray machine. To date there have been quite a few hospital patients. Thank goodness none of them have been desperately ill and in need of real nursing care or I would not have seen the island. For we have two females who are termed nurses, who really do a lackadaisical job of keeping the place cleaned and give food and water to the patients and can be entrusted with minor medications. They do make beds after a fashion. But they are not apt to be good material to train and we have not found a young woman who is unmarried who is interested in becoming a nurse.

The hospital was closed when we arrived and my first impression was not too hopeless. Dingy walls, grimy floors, shabby beds could be transformed by soap, paint, and elbow grease and we had been promised painters as soon as sealing was over.

When the first patient, old Metrofan Krukoff, was admitted we went through the familiar routine. Up went the shades, the curtains were pushed back, the sound of scrub brushes in action commenced. Metrofan was a charming old gentleman. His heart was too battered and worn for Sam to do more than prolong his life for a few months. Installed on the top floor in the room with the best view of sky and sea, conversationally close to the curving path

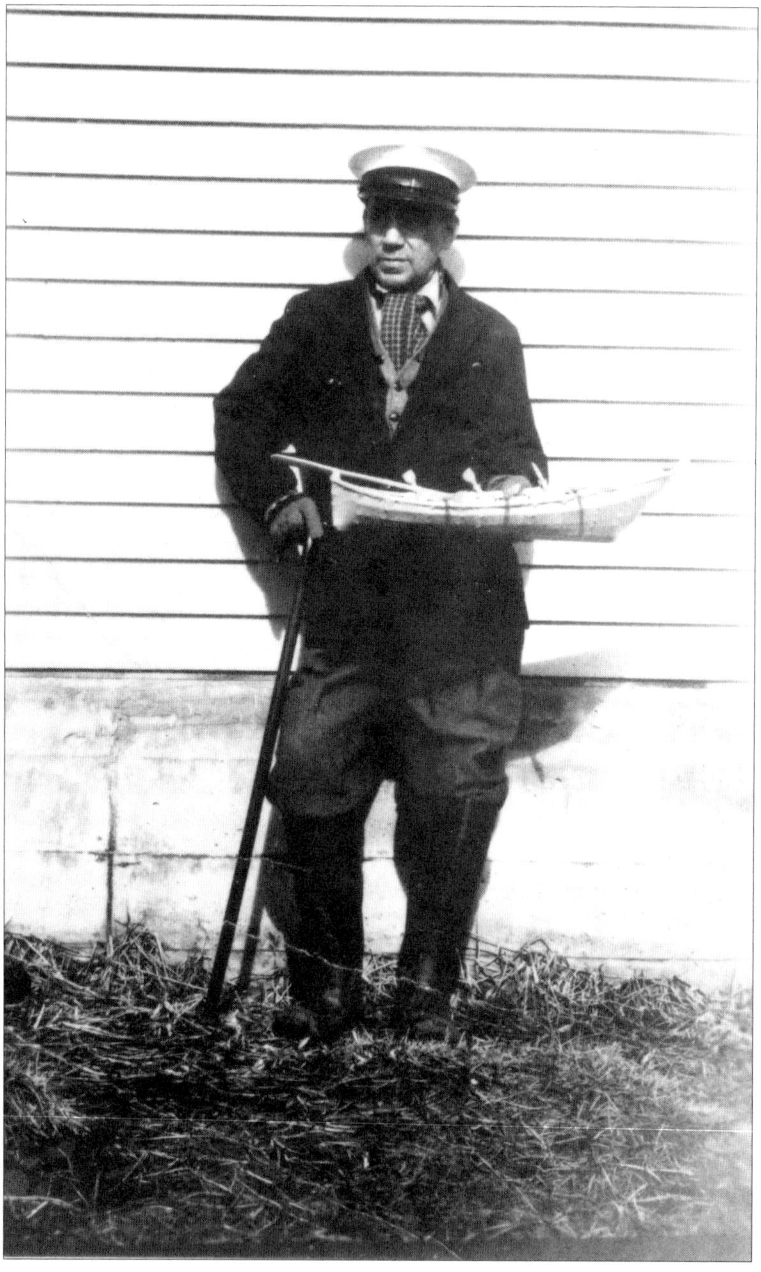

Metrofan Krukoff holding a model baidar (from the Martin Collection, USUAF210, Archives, Alaska and Polar Regions, Rasmuson Library, University of Alaska Fairbanks).

that led to the next village terrace, Metrofan settled back to enjoy life and provide us with joy although he was unconscious of the latter.

Rocking back and forth on the edge of his bed, he sat for hours telling stories. He seemed to have stepped out of a Chekhov play. He became our first link with the life of the Aleuts, which was far removed from the rarefied atmosphere of the Service families. From his window gossip he kept informed of every event and relayed many of them to us. He kept his radio playing day and night. While his village news was accurate, his versions of English broadcasts were weird and wonderful. He was almost as content to listen to foreign-language programs as to try to understand the rapid flow of English of an American commentator.

When we made morning rounds in the hospital, Metrofan reported how many seals had been killed and the number of road skins, which he had known since the first sealers came home. When we had become trusted friends, he confided who had quaffed a cup or two of forbidden kvass the night before and described just how and why some luckless individual won the black eye he or she was sporting. To encourage our frequent visits he kept a large box of cigars on his bedside table for Sam and Lucky Strikes for me. He was a gracious host in his small kingdom.

Once Sam gave him a six-ounce bottle of a mild, tastefully flavored Petrolagar and was shocked to find the bottle empty that same evening. Metrofan praised the taste but regretted distressing Sam. "I won't need more for a few days," he said comfortingly. While he resisted the temptation to imbibe more cathartics, he often fell victim to the bouquet of his cough medicine and drained the bottle at a sitting.

He was a typical elder, delighting in an attentive audience, to whom he could discourse on the theme "the younger generation is going to the dogs—or seals." He would describe his own disciplined youth, the long hours of each day spent at work, the evenings spent indoor practicing his cornet lessons. He professed admiration for his stern father who had kept him home practicing instead of permitting him to attend parties and stay out late. Alas for the young men of 1941. Metrofan would sigh like an old sea lion. They were idle, pleasure-loving creatures doomed to eternal wrath. They wanted to do nothing but dance until three o'clock in the morning. (Unfortunately for the satisfaction of their desires, dances at the Community Hall actually ended at eleven, except on very special occasions when they continued until midnight.) They never spent their evening practicing music.

"Worked hard?" snorted Johnston when we mentioned Metrofan's opinions. "Why Metrofan was one of the laziest men on the island."

Metrofan was still nominally chief of police and the bandmaster. Someone had given him a naval officer's cap. His passion for that hat was extraordinary. It was never out of sight. Sometimes when I came upstairs softly I discovered him sitting on the side of the bed gasping for breath, clad in his bathrobe and THE

HAT. Perhaps it was his talisman against the attacks of his rebellious heart and crowned with it he could more bravely fight off the pain.

Metrofan was all alone the evening in November when he died.[1] The nurse was busy with other patients. When I closed his eyes and tied the bandages around his wrists the tears ran down my cheeks. Our first island friend was gone.

When it was necessary to send Metrofan to the hospital, we had called in the trained assistants of whom we had heard one account in Washington and a sadder version from Dr. Migliori. Mary Oustigoff, the day attendant, was a middle-aged woman who met our friendly overtures with evident distrust. The sweet smiling face of Natalia Nisikin, who stayed in the hospital at night, was reassuring. Anxious to obey the doctor's orders and sympathetic toward people in pain she did her best, and it was refreshing to come into the hospital in the evening and meet Natalia's welcoming smile after enduring the hard unyielding face of Mary all day long.

During the day the hospital rang with Mary's clumping tread. Her feet were expressing her resistance to the new doctor and his meddling wife and their absurd orders. We began to search for a substitute at once. No women were interested in the job. For working twelve hours a day and a seven-day week, for doing the heavy housework as well as attempting to give some nursing care, the reward was fifteen dollars a month. Before our time the hospital was used little except for some obstetrical and surgical cases but rarely for medical patients. The attendants were sent home when the building was empty and enjoyed a respite from heavy work, without pay. The hospital was never closed for a day after we opened it. It was constantly serving the needs of the sick who certainly could not be well taken care of in their own crowded homes that lacked so many sanitary facilities.

No young girls wanted to slave for such miserable pay during their brief waiting period between completion of school and marriage. We might have been able to persuade one of the girls to accept the job after we were able to arrange alternate Sundays off and a half day of leisure a week. By then we knew that no one dared to take Mary's job away from her.

Yet Mary did improve. Before Christmas she actually smiled occasionally. She made efforts to carry out her work. Through Heretina Kochergin I learned that Mary respected my own willingness to pitch into disagreeable tasks when need arose. She was pleased when Sam arranged for time off for her. She was most impressed because both of us really cared what happened to the patients. She gained, as the hospital redecorating progressed slowly, a surly pride in the changes, a pride fed by the praise of the villagers and of Sam and myself. When reports from the villagers came back to her repeating that I had said she kept the new colored curtains clean, she grew a bit warmer.

In the autumn the problem of providing better care for the patients improved when Heretina's father, Peter, began to make himself useful around the hospital. For a long while he forgot his pains and his family problems as his paintbrush transformed dark melancholy dens into bright pastel-tinted rooms. The novelty of light and color in the hospital intrigued the villagers, who flocked to see the style of painting opposite walls in different colors to create a more spacious atmosphere. The dainty curtains, wrung from water tinted with cake coloring, kept out no light. Peter worked madly to have the hospital dressed up for Christmas. He and Mary and the four permanent tuberculosis patients on the top floor were proud hosts to most of the village during the holiday season. And Mary, for once, did not mind running around behind the visitors with a rather cleanish looking mop, wiping up their tracks.

Peter's delight in his workmanship and the praise, which was pleasant incense, spurred him to new duties. He wanted nursing books to read and he attempted to study them seriously night after night, greeting me each morning with a list of words to interpret and an exposition of the knowledge he had absorbed. "By golly," he would say with a grin, "You know, you was right about . . . It says the same thing in the book. You must be awful smart." One morning his grin was wider than ever: "I read in the book last night that patients s'posed to have baths every day in bed so they don't get sore. I told Mary but she swear nasty words to me so I give Frances bath." Apparently our many words to Mary about bed baths had been falling for weeks upon deaf ears.

But the situation was novel. A few days before, Peter had helped push Frances' stretcher into the operating room as she was nearing the end of her labor. She had clung to his hand. "Stay with me, Peter," she had begged. If she wanted him at the head of the delivery table we had no objections. But a male nurse performing intimate services for a female patient was so untraditional that I opened my mouth to protest and then clamped it shut quickly. What actual difference was there between his action and my own care of sick men? Were not objections merely conventional expressions of the old feeling that nursing is a degrading work and therefore fit for women only? Had we demurred when Peter stood beside us helping care for Frances' baby, day and night for forty-eight agonizing hours until, despite oxygen, stimulants, and blood transfusions, death conquered? Were not Peter's careful, gentle ministrations comforting for the sad young mother? So Peter's ministrations were no longer confined to male or children patients and invariably women patients preferred his nursing attention to Mary's.

In April we secured a new night nurse. Before Christmas Natalia had to change her role from nurse to patient. An ugly ulcer was eating away at one of her swollen legs. For a time Peter stepped into the breach. But the novelty wore off. No wonder his enthusiasm did not endure. During these months he slept only at odd moments, rousing at night to make rounds on the sleeping patients, getting up by the aid of the alarm clock to take new infants to nurse. For weeks he was a hero. We canvassed the local unmarried girls and no one wanted night duty.

Our janitor, Paul Merculieff, had an eighteen-year-old daughter, Julia, whose right arm was malformed and withered from birth. He had wanted to secure an artificial arm for her for years but the agent had always frowned upon her going to Seattle for the necessary fitting. Sam and Johnston arranged that Julia should go to Seattle with her father in October and return early in November. In February she visited us and asked if Sam would permit her to attend his English classes in order to earn a Girl Scout Merit for herself. He had a couple of young people over sixteen whom he was trying to assist and he agreed. Weeks later, toward the end of March, Julia lingered after class and confessed the real cause of her interest in learning English. It was an amazing yarn. She had wanted to remain in Seattle to study to become a missionary. Johnston had withheld permission on the grounds that she lacked money. He had suggested she return to the island, get some nurse's training from me and work at the hospital until she earned three hundred dollars. Then he would permit her to study in the States. Julia considered that Johnston expected her to have the money by the end of the summer. Since it would take almost two years to earn the required sum, we doubted whether Johnston had made any definite promise. We were curious, too, why she had waited four months to apply for a nursing job. The current village rumor that the *Penguin* would soon be at St. Paul might have reminded her of her dream. And she had begun English classes to enable her to study before she tackled the problem of earning the funds.

Julia had striven to overcome her affliction. She had learned to make beds, sew, and cut out patterns. It seemed that she could do some simple tasks for the patients at night, carry a nursing baby to its mother, and permit Peter to get much-needed sleep. She could at least remain awake at night and summon Peter when patients called for aid she could not give. Natalia had been able to do little more for weeks before she resigned.

I left a woman who had just given birth to a baby in Julia's care one night. I repeated over and over again that Julia was to remain at the bedside, keeping constant watch of the woman whose uterine muscles were inert and sluggish. I stressed the dangers of postpartum hemorrhage. Julia listened with a smile. How glad I was for my trained conscience that sent me back two hours later to find the room aflood with light from the ceiling bulbs. Julia sat indifferent to all but her Bible and the woman was bleeding profusely. I lost my temper as I began to massage the woman's abdomen, shouted to Peter to bring ergot and pituitrin and then get Sam out of bed. I don't know what I said to Julia at the moment. When the danger had passed, Peter sat down to guard the woman and I took Julia into the utility room. I tried to tell her more calmly about her responsibility to the patients. Her airy attitude kept me boiling in spite of firm efforts to control myself.

It was futile to scold her. And cruel. From that night on we regarded her as a useful sentry whose presence allowed Peter to sleep and any attempts to teach her nursing procedures were abandoned. In respect, the standards of nursing care we achieved with our trio became more and more miraculous.

Chapter 16

Many of our patients were in the hospital for months and months. Among those who came and went within a brief period, the majority were either obstetrical cases or the victims of abscesses and accidents.

Peter's son Moran, just passing into adolescence, jumped playfully out of the upper window of his home one night while acting out a movie-inspired western drama. Unfortunately, there was no saddled horse waiting under the window and he broke his ankle. He enjoyed his hospital stay because of the food.

> August 19, 1941
> Simeon always pricks our superior knowledge quite completely. The first time I saw him a friend had driven him down to the hospital for an x-ray of his chest. He had been diagnosed as a tb. by Dr. Migliori and been told to stay home in bed early in May. He had a history of night sweats, I believe, loss of weight, fatigue. Apparently no chest plate had been taken previously.
>
> Sam, with his charming habit of putting patients at ease by chattering a friendly explanation of whatever process they must undergo, was explaining the various features of the x-ray machine and the steps of the picture taking and making. When he donned his big leaded apron and gloves, he let them feel their weight.
>
> *cont.*

From autumn on, the four tubercular men discovered by the village survey inhabited the top floor, fretful, idle, and bored, but gaining a little weight, the progress, at least, of the disease checked by bed rest. Old Vlass Pankoff was too ill to be rebellious and almost happier in the hospital than living in bachelor quarters with an adopted unmarried son. He did miss the movies very much. Chatting with him was impossible because he knew scarcely a half dozen English words. His wrinkled face made him look more like a death's head than the state of his lungs warranted. Lavrenty, whose infection was seriously advanced, tried earnestly to learn more English and grasp the political and military state of the world as presented by the radio. "Sometimes I think it's just as easy to understand them Japs as it is them guys speakin' English fast," he confessed.

Abie Merculieff brooded resentfully that he had been cajoled by Sam into what he considered a prison. For Abie was desperately in love. The brief visiting hours for the top-floor tuberculosis ward hardly satisfied his longing for his sweetheart's company. Simeon Kochutin, Abie's room partner, contentedly tinkering with his own radio, was a seemingly more cooperative patient. One day Sam noticed an enormous quantity of wire and radio parts under Simeon's bed. Then he learned that Simeon had been earning a little pocket money running a radio repair shop in bed. When Sam ended the project, Simeon rigged up some apparatus so that Lavrenty in the other room could learn code. They filled many tedious hours sending messages back and forth to each other.

Magazines and newspapers went to the top floor only when the other patients had finished with them. From the tuberculosis ward they journeyed swiftly to the furnace. No one could meet the demand for fresh supplies. Since none of them could read English well, they soon tired of scanning headlines with print large enough to puzzle out fairly quickly and advertisements in large type. Pictorial magazines were their favorites. Had they been able to read, their morale would have been better and their response to treatment more swift. Individually they had moments of striving to learn more English, jotting down lists of words that they did not understand. We intended to send out for small dictionaries on the spring boat. Waiting for Sam or me to define the words was a nuisance. Such a tedious dull method of learning soon palled. Setbacks like Abie's discomfiture over mistakes in reading killed ambitious attempts quickly. Once Abie drew Sam's attention to an advertisement for diamond cuff links that he wanted and for which he planned to mail a money order for thirty-two dollars. I suspect it was not so much shame at being unable to read the price correctly as thirty-two hundred dollars as a repugnance at learning more of a mad world where mere cuff links could cost the equivalent of many years'

> Simeon's friend asked, "Are they what you call x-ray proof?"
>
> I was much amused by this sudden technical term.
>
> Then Sammie explained that he would not have the plate ready for a few days as he had to clean the developing tanks and get clean fixer, etc., ready.
>
> Simeon asked, just as he was leaving, if he might get up around the house, and Sam said a little while each day.
>
> A couple of days later as we were passing the Aleutian bunkhouse, out dashed one of the boys to give Sam a picture of himself and some of the lads grouped on our front porch. He had taken the picture with a simple box camera and the result was very good.
>
> Sam enquired who had developed it.
>
> "Simeon Kochutin," was the answer. Sam looked at me in speechless amusement. Here he, the amateur in developing Kodak shots and x-ray plates, had been talking to a good technician who probably knew more about such things than he. And again today when Sam was being most careful about his language being simple as ABC in explaining reading a thermometer, Simeon piped up and said, "It's just like the thermometer I use in my developing tank."

sealing shares that turned Abie away from reading for a while. Toward spring the empty hours drove Abie to learn crocheting.

> August 12, 1941
> Mrs. Oberg dropped in and her husband followed up a little later. We had lunch here, went driving over to the top of graveyard hill and walked about looking for mushrooms. We found only a few toadstools. But we wandered over to Ketovoi rookery and spent a pleasant hour watching the seals. Sam took a lot of pictures, some of pups huddled in the cracks of the rocks at three feet. But since it was a poor greyish day, the results may not be too good.
>
> Back home with a huge bunch of purple monkshood and a couple of lupine, I made up two bunches, one for Metrofan and another for Anna Stepetin, and pressed a few choice specimens, leaving a small vase for myself. Spent a few minutes with Anna but did not practice my Russian because her daughter was visiting her. Her daughter lives on some island, possibly Unalaska, and is back here after a fourteen-year absence to visit her mother. She, the daughter, had a youngster with her who was very attractive. He is her tenth adopted child. She had had none of her own but was probably a good mother to those she took under her wing. She was bewailing the fact that this boy, Mike, who is four, had not picked up any Aleut because they spoke English at home and she thought he ought to learn it. He has been picking some up playing with the other children.

On the ground floor among our more permanent patients were sweet-faced Elizabeth Tetoff, sixteen years old, a victim of rheumatic fever, and Anfosa Melovidov, a youngster of seven who need orthopedic care for a diseased hip.

Anna Stepetin, a merry laughing old lady, was our star boarder, vacationing fitfully in her son's home when her troublesome heart behaved quietly. Anna and I fell in love when we first met. Her gaiety despite her pain, her birdlike grace, her trilling laughter that was invariably choked off by a bout of coughing, were so refreshing under that roof. She listened for my footsteps on the basement stairs. She scolded me when I missed a visit to her for a single day. She crocheted innumerable gifts for my baby and for everybody else's baby. No matter the color of the yarn she could get, dark blue, lavender, whatever ugly shade the Canteen had in stock, she utilized them all for baby articles, caps, booties, and mittens.

At home she was not supposed to go outside except to attend church or the movies in a car. She was not to be restrained by a mere doctor's order. Often I would hear the door open and a little gust of giggles and coughs. Then Anna would peek around the door frame into the living room. As soon as she had her breath she would beg me not to tell the doctor or her son that she had run away and walked down "just to see you." Her English was very weak but she and I knew about similar amounts of Russian so we could converse easily. "Oh, the Babeeeee," she would coo rapturously to Tobyanne. "You won't forget your old Anna, will you?" There is a snapshot, a fine linen handkerchief, the baby clothes, and a worn old brass cross that Anna gave the baby as an Easter gift. Someday they will tell Tobyanne of Anna's love and devotion.

All children loved Anna. She always had a sweet morsel in her pocket or a song for them. The officials, of course, had nothing good to say about her, but Anna who loved life and laughed at the pains that menaced her breathing could not be stained by stale, purulent, and false anecdotes. The laughter that welled within her, spilling out in tinkling tones, was her immunity.

The lack of a common language was a constant handicap in all medical work, a high wall over which we could barely communicate with our patients.

If our problems nagged us ceaselessly as we struggled to improve medical conditions we were horrified as we collected stories of the circumstances past doctors had been faced with. As we cleaned up filthy piles of paper from dark cellar corners, from the bottom of a woodbox in our furnace room, from the nooks under the rafters in the attic and cleaned and sorted them in an effort to preserve a portion of the island medical history, we found the first hints of past tragedies. The memories of the older of our Aleut friends furnished stories that made us see too clearly the misery, the drabness, the callousness of the past illuminated by so little humaneness and mercy. A history of the ills of a community and the care given the sick is more revealing often than conventional history. On St. Paul even their stern patron saint would have blanched at the prospect of enduring the Aleuts' long martyrdom as revealed in the scraps of evidence we collected. The plight of many physicians who came to alleviate the sufferings of the islanders is also distressing to contemplate. They endured personal privations and discomforts and suffered even more from the obstacles that hindered the full practice of their skill.

Chapter 17

How those first St. Paul physicians would have envied our spacious quarters, office, hospital, and residence. The first "surgery," as a tiny shack was dubbed, possessed little except the historical distinction of being the first wooden house built in 1869 under the American flag by Captain Pomeroy of Hutchinson, Kohl, and Company. In 1876 it was torn down and the equipment moved to a slightly larger building.[1] If later reports describe improved conditions, the instruments the first doctors worked with must have been even more unsatisfactory than the cramped space.

During the Russian period the sealers had to depend on native remedies, crude ideas of their Russian associates, and occasionally the ministration of a *feldscher,* a Russian medical worker neither doctor nor nurse.

For the first forty years of American control, the physicians were the employees of the sealing companies. Neither firm could honestly boast of fulfilling the spirit of the clauses of the lease that made them responsible for the general health and welfare of the Aleuts, particularly the orphans and widows, the aged and infirm. Both companies complied with the letter of the contract by maintaining physicians on each island. They paid them very low salaries and quartered them in the Company House. A bachelor physician sometimes lacked privacy and had to room with other company employees. A married doctor had a single room for his family and no homelike surroundings.

The routine medical practice of those days will remain a secret. The reports submitted to the company have been lost. Many more details of the doctors' veterinarian pursuits, such as postmortems done on seals or cattle, survive in government reports than about the treatment of human beings. The fragments of facts are almost too much. Some conditions reflect the low level of medical practice before the commencement of the advancement of the profession fifty years ago. But even bare vital statistics betray social deficiencies inexcusable on that ground. Buttressed by the accounts of tragedies too shocking to be forgotten, the past speaks loudly.

For example, a frightful accident in 1877 expunged the name of one family from island records. Michael Bachoff, his wife and child, and a visitor were found dead in bed one morning, in a smoke-filled house.[2] During the night the kerosene lamp left burning had exploded. The rags and old papers with which the walls were covered had caught fire. The damp woodwork effectually halted the flames but the smoke was as deadly as fire. The bodies were buried in a single grave. The dampness that checked the fire indicates that the two-room, ill-ventilated, poorly warmed house was a barabara. It reveals the unhealthy atmosphere of the shelters and helps to explain the success of the tubercle bacillus.

Three years later among the causes of death the word *scurvy* appears. Two women died of this easily preventable disease because diet determined by government and company officials lacked essential foods. In 1869 hard bread and bread flour, sugar, and tea were the main rations supplementing the seal and sea lion and the occasional fish and game birds. The first lessee contracted to supply smoked and salt salmon and salt beef, for which the Aleuts acquired a taste very slowly. Gradually the shelves of the first company store were stocked with a wider assortment of foods and other merchandise. The prices, however, were high and the purchasing power of the sealers low. No wonder that for years the Aleuts spasmodically petitioned the government agent to permit rival traders to land and open stores. Competition, they argued, would lower prices and introduce better quality merchandise.

Government agents were instructed to make sure that prices were not more than twenty-five percent higher than San Francisco retail prices. How many agents were experts in judging the quality of food and clothing? How were they to keep watch of prices in a changing retail market three thousand miles away? When a brash agent exposed an example of the company's overcharging, it was always evident that the abuse was of long standing and had been neglected by previous agents.

Early physicians or agents made a habit of introducing their sketchy annual reports with the statement that the health of the village was "generally good," a peculiar phrase compared with the figures of the high death rate. In 1882 an optimistic individual, not a physician, rashly wrote that the general health of the people was improving. That very day two people died. The death toll that year mounted to the staggering total of fifty out of a community of two hundred and seventy-five people. The final census summation revealed a population of two hundred and thirty-one souls, the loss being but slightly compensated by the births of the year. Did that writer recall his optimism at the year's end and blush?

Severe epidemics of coughs and colds that incapacitated most of the community were commonplace and difficult for the physician to cope with. The first boats of spring imported a vigorous brigade of germs that swept triumphantly from one crowded household to the next. In 1883 Dr. Hungerford tried in desperation to combat a cold epidemic by administering medications during school hours to the children well enough to come to classes. Almost every villager was ill and five people died.

A more serious epidemic flared up in 1890. A woman who had been visiting relatives in Unalaska was taken ill during her return trip. Her family was soon infected. Soon the grippe had invaded every house. School shut down for the teachers as well as the majority of pupils had succumbed. Church services were discontinued. As the disease spread there were not enough healthy people to tend the sick. Poor Dr. Lutz worked day and night with no trained and very little untrained assistance. At one period not one adult male was able to be out-of-doors. Six people died, mainly tubercular patients who could not combat the additional infection.

When the epidemic subsided Dr. Lutz encountered other troubles that he finally took to government agent Murray. He begged him to prohibit Nicholas Krukoff from treating the sick with a device known as the "cupping scarificator." The villagers regarded cupping and bleeding as the universal omnipotent cure-all. When the doctor prescribed treatment that did not include one or the other torture, the sick called on Nicholas and his infernal-sounding instrument. Nicholas beat his breast and swore that he had never, never practiced his avocation without the permission of the doctor. In the same breath he vowed never to use the scarificator again unless the doctor ordered him to. Murray, unimpressed by eloquent denials and exuberant promises, confiscated the offending machine. Later that day Nicholas sold the scarificator to the Alaska Commercial Company for five dollars. It was handed over to the guardianship of Dr. Lutz. No purchaser appeared for a second scarificator, owned by Katherin Nedazeroff, which came to light during the investigation of Nicholas.

Dr. Lutz had more serious complaints to lodge with the agent concerning the activities of the village midwife, Ellen Volkoff. "Blind Helen," as she was familiarly called, had been sightless from birth. The villagers, particularly the women, turned more readily to her for help than to the physicians. A belief against the presence of men at childbirth lingered at St. Paul and supplied Ellen with an opportunity to dominate village obstetrics and extend her ministrations into other medical fields. Dr. Lutz had charged that Helen countermanded his orders to patients and advised them not to take the medications he prescribed. Ellen stoutly denied her guilt and was warned to obey the physician's orders without questioning. She promised vehemently.

Three years later Dr. Perry Pond submitted a lengthy blistering report against her and condemned her practice of manipulations. He reminded the agent of the child who had died during or just at the conclusion of a dose of Helen's "manipulations" shortly after he came to St. Paul. The agent penned a letter to Ellen, forbidding her to go near a sick person, threatening to deport her from the island if she as much as gave advice to a pregnant woman. He informed her that he had made his decision a perpetual injunction by entering it in the official log for his successors to read and enforce.

In 1900 a spring boat brought the grippe to the islands once more.[3] During a terrible thirteen days seven people died on St. Paul. Doughty old Captain Daniel Webster, who had spent most of his life as an employee of the sealing companies and resided for a quarter of a century on the islands, was one of the four who died on St. George.

Later in the summer, before the villagers had completely recovered from the effects of the epidemic, a more terrible malady invaded the island. Agafia Kochergin developed a rash that the doctor tentatively diagnosed as smallpox. Accompanied by her husband, Mrs. Kochergin was removed to quarantine in the watch house at Polovina Point until developing symptoms would permit certain diagnosis. Her home was thoroughly fumigated. Blind Helen still acted as chief nurse. Dr. Ross asked permission to vaccinate the whole village with serum that had, fortunately it seemed, just arrived from San Francisco. The Aleuts, summoned to a community meeting, were informed of the possible danger and agreed to submit to vaccination. Hardly had the doctor completed vaccinating the townspeople before he was able to decide that Agafia had measles, a disease incoming boats reported rampant throughout the north.

There had been a measles epidemic on St. Paul in 1888 with no fatalities. Perhaps the earlier epidemic had not been true measles for the importation of the virus twelve years later spared few. In a few days all normal activities in the village had come to a halt. At least one member of each household was ill and often more than one. The first to die were a mother and her prematurely born infant. A few days later in house after house whole families lay stricken with no member well enough to tend the others. The government and company officials began a door-to-door distribution of boiled rice cooked in the company kitchen. The few healthy Aleuts assisted them. Metrofan remembered how a knock would thunder at the door that was then swung cautiously open only a few inches. A hand would appear putting down a bucket of cereal. None of the distributors were exposing themselves to infection.

When Mrs. Kochergin's quarantine was lifted and she returned home, Blind Helen was released from the care of one patient to tend many. But not for long. She herself fell ill. Five of the healthy men succumbed the same day. Only four remained to carry soup, cereal, and medications to the houses. That day too, Vasilii Sedulik died, the last of the "baidarka" men, as Aleuts skilled in hunting sea otter and other animals from their small craft were labeled. While one Aleut dug a grave for Vasilii, the others continued their messenger duties. Mr. Allis, the company manager whom rheumatism had kept bedridden for days, bravely limped to the shop and built the coffin. Only four Aleuts and two officials saw the old hunter to his last resting place.

The next day two more deaths occurred. Two women suffering from tuberculosis had been unable to win the fight against the measles infection. By this time some convalescents were trying to prepare nourishment for their families and groceries were delivered to their homes. But the carriers still brought prepared food to most of the houses. Two more Aleut messengers had to join the quarantined. Only George Kochergin, husband of the woman who had brought the disease from Unalaska, and Zahar Tetoff were left to carry on the relief. Zahar, who was monarch of the village laundry when we reached St. Paul, was still fond of boasting of his male physique and good fortune and describing the distress of those he toiled day and night to assist.

Aggie Kushin, who had come from the Kurile Islands to join the St. Paul sealers, was the next to die. Others left their beds too soon and suffered relapses. Dr. Ross, worn from constant labor and lack of sleep, was bitterly discouraged. There was another death. The next day still another. Two people died the following day. That afternoon the burial squad trudged wearily back from the cemetery to find that a woman had died during their brief absence.

The agent cried out in despair that smallpox would have been preferable because there was a vaccine to protect the people and there was nothing to control the spread of measles or arrest its deadliness. Nothing, because the houses were too crowded and sanitary facilities absolutely lacking. There was either inexperienced nursing or none at all in most stricken homes. The sealers were too undernourished or too wracked with other diseases to have the hardihood to combat the measles. The agent seems not to have recognized the underlying causes of the severity of the epidemic.

The day after the agent appealed in vain to heaven for surcease, a young child died. Two days later another woman. At least enough Aleuts were convalescent and strong enough to bury her without the aid of the overworked officials. People began to creep out of their houses, pale, weak, coughing loudly. Blind Helen was the next to die, just a week after her nearest relatives, her brother and his wife. At last her fight against the officials, her struggle to maintain her prestige, was over.

Eight more died before the epidemic ran its course, twenty persons in all. The mounds of raw earth choked the cemetery space. In the autumn workmen fenced off more of the hillside, preparing for the casualties expected during the next season.

Chapter 18

In 1909 a combination of circumstances seemed about to revolutionize the social policy decided in Washington. Understanding and consideration were about to speed up the social regeneration of the sealers. Leasing the islands to private commercial firms, first the Alaska Commercial Company from 1870 to 1890 and then the North American Commercial Company until 1910, had ended. With the cloven hoof of private lessees exiled, the sole administration of the people and the seals was transferred to the Bureau of Fisheries. A visionary social-minded commissioner of fisheries in Washington outlined a plan for collecting knowledge necessary to alter official policy and improve living standards. A government employee already stationed on St. Paul, Harry D. Chichester, was assigned to handle this survey because he had received some medical training.[1]

The commissioner's demands for information covered a great variety of matters. He requested a thorough description and analysis of housing, clothing, diet, and living habits. He was as curious about parasites that bothered both man and beast as about diseases suffered only by human beings. He ordered the thorough investigation of each disease that had occurred on the island, a detailed history from the date of its first appearance, including the age groups affected by it, the treatments carried out, and their results. As if he knew the chaotic state of the medical records, he recommended that a permanent file of health cards be instituted to ensure continuity of efficient care by future physicians. He sought suggestions as to the best solution to the drinking problem and the continuation of illicit manufacture of kvass despite severe punishments. He was anxious to follow the destiny of the 265 gallons of alcoholic beverages requisitioned for the islands for the next year, enough, he estimated, to provide each male over sixteen with three gallons of spirits, although it was prohibited to the Aleuts, or twenty-six and a half gallons for each "white" employee.

I wish someone had satisfied the commissioner's curiosity so I need no longer wonder about its ultimate fate. Several of the older sealers told me that after a day of hard work, particularly during bad weather, a company official would say to the work gang with a broad wink, "Now boys, go up and see the Doc. He'll take care of you." The doctor would be waiting in his office, bottles and glasses prepared to give each man a good swig of whiskey or rum. The company—and after all the physician was the company's employee, not the government's—considered this open violation of prohibition a means of keeping sealers obedient and docile.

The commissioner's outline is still socially progressive. Investigations based on it would have unearthed many unpleasant facts even in 1941.

Mr. Chichester began his studies while carrying on his routine duties, which, that winter, were those of the acting agent. He was sorely disappointed at the medical records, not written up for years, meagerly factual when chronicled. Physical examinations, already under way after the commissioner's hint, were being duly recorded on cards. We found some of them in boxes of rubbish or under a heap of filthy bottles in the cellar, which we cleaned and filed. They were so few as to have little value to medical history but we felt as if we were erecting a little monument to one broad-visioned official by rescuing them.

It was a busy winter for Chichester. Suddenly it was spring. A fresh Sunday morning in May tempted Harry Chichester and Dr. Walter L. Hahn, the resident naturalist, to go sailing on the Lagoon with their wives and Neon Tetoff. John Hanson told me the day's tragic outcome.[2]

Villagers then walked nearly a mile along a path that curved beside the Lagoon to get water from wells near the present by-products plant. John, young and unmarried, lived with his mother. She asked him to get her a barrel of water although it would make him late for church. While he was filling the barrel he watched the sailing party. Halfway back to the village he paused to rest. Glancing toward the Lagoon he saw the boat had overturned. He ran directly to the church to summon aid and helped launch the first rescue boat. Neon Tetoff lay safely on the broad overturned keel. Hahn and Chichester were clutching projections of the boat with one hand each and helping their wives to keep afloat. Dressed in cumbersome fur coats the four had been unable to climb out of the water even with Neon's help. The exhausted quartet were dragged ashore near the well. The women, John said, could talk but "the men kept rollin' around like dying animals, like the seals that die on the road in a drive." The men were carried to the Company House where hot blankets and stimulants were waiting. A second hospital had been set up for the women at Government House. Suffering shock, exhaustion, and severe chill Mrs. Hahn began to undergo premature labor pains. By the time her baby was born, both her husband and Chichester were dead. The men's exertion in assisting their wives had fatally sapped their strength. Lucky Neon whose poorer clothing had not hampered his limbs was back at work in a few days.[3]

The projected survey seems to have died with Chichester. A few of his opinions jotted down as notes indicate how scathing would have been his indictment of social conditions and medical care and how dramatically he might have illustrated his findings. He had helped Dr. Morgan attempt to operate on a child for a strangulated hernia. That day rain, snow, and sleet storms took turns besieging the village. Nevertheless the child wrapped in blankets was carried through the storm and placed on the crude table in the surgery. When the hernia was uncovered, the operation could not be satisfactorily completed because several necessary instruments were lacking. The incision was sewn up. The child lived through this almost insane ordeal to die a few weeks later from tubercular meningitis.

As a consequence of this experience, Chichester ridiculed the term "surgical equipment" as applied to the homemade operating table and sterilizer, the few shell- and wooden-handled knives that could not be properly sterilized, and the few glass and enamel articles. Operations had to be performed either in the seven-by-ten-foot surgery where doctor and assistants could barely move or in the doctor's heavily carpeted and curtained living room, described as having dust everywhere. Perhaps some of Chichester's notes or oral reports were relayed to Washington because a few years later a small building was assigned the official title "hospital."

Peter thought the building had been one of the old salt houses. The toilet was a makeshift affair in the *kalador* [the entryway chamber], leading to a small hole in the ground. Later a real toilet seat was installed but the sewage system remained primitive. The single room introduced a perplexing game of switching male and female patients back and forth between hospital and home in accordance with which sex was most seriously ill. Screens were often used when the conditions of patients of both sexes made hospitalization a matter of life or death. A small room was added for a nurse and eventually one for a kitchen. Kondrat Krukoff was an attendant there for years. His principal function seems to have been bringing trays of food from the Company House.

A fresh attempt to stabilize the custom of annual physical examinations began in 1915. Dr. Hunter, as might be expected, missed no individual and gained the distinction of being the first to overcome female reluctance to examination by a male. He found no evidence of venereal disease. In the light of previous known medical history, a slight but actual improvement in village health had been achieved already, due to some improvement of general living standards once the dual control of government and commercial company ended. Friction between the agents of two masters had hindered progress. One set of officials had been able to explain away island defects by blaming the other group.

In October 1917, during Dr. Hunter's second period on St. Paul, an influenza epidemic invalided the population for days.[4] The rapidity with which the majority of villagers contracted a contagious disease as soon as it was introduced was an unassailable demonstration of the consequences that Dr. Hunter's painstaking measurements of the small houses had hoped to ward off. Fortunately, the Spanish influenza pandemic did not strike the Pribilof Islands.

In 1924 Dr. Davis turned in a thirty-three-page annual report so thorough, so damning of the government's inadequate safeguards for the people's health that the agent felt obligated to submit a six-page accompaniment, half apology and half explanation of conditions.[5] His arguments limped badly because he could contradict no more than a few minor points. The doctor had made the usual complaints against drinking habits because of the health hazard. The agent thought drinking could not be controlled by officials because the Aleuts observed the frequent law breaking of temporary, non-Aleut officials and were aware of the widespread contempt in the States for the Volstead Act.[6]

Dr. Davis, appalled at seeing children eating refuse from garbage cans and at the haphazard unbalanced meals prepared by the housewives, suggested a common mess hall until such time as the villagers understood the importance of regular meals. The agent's retort was a tirade against the lazy women whom even beatings, administered by their husbands, could not bestir to tidy housekeeping and civilized eating habits. He offered no counterproposal for supplying schoolchildren and working men with food to enable them to carry on their studies and work, except the vague hope that someday education would awaken the women to a sense of duty. The agent apparently agreed that beatings were a fine means to win a women's love and inspire her to cherish her family and tend her home. What a brutal picture he unwittingly uncovers, supplemented in old case records by a number of fractured arms and clavicles due to husbandly affection. And the doctors were probably summoned only when the beatings wrought serious injuries. How could any sane person expect the women, who were drudges and beaten like dumb helpless beasts, with official approval, to act normal, to have any pride or joy in homemaking or desire to be loving wives and mothers?

Although Davis merely stated that the old, overcrowded houses and the long trip to the lagoon well for water were conditions that made it almost humanly impossible to keep houses very clean, his comments goaded the agent into a virulent attack on the Aleuts. He accused the Aleuts of being naturally dirty and weakened this false premise by the claim that a great change would take place as soon as the contemplated new houses were constructed and the water piped closer to the village. He blamed the delay in fulfillment of both projects on the weather.

Dr. Davis illustrated his report with photographs: open trays of food being carried through the snow to the hospital, a man drawing a barrel of water on a crude wooden sled, and a close-up of the doctor's house to demonstrate his written description of cramped rooms used interchangeably as office and home. The family's living room was the dispensary. When patients came the family withdrew to a leaking, unheated bedroom. The agent wailed that the doctor meanly showed his house at the most unpleasant time of the year, that the building was much more impressive when not contrasted with a big snow bank, and that furthermore the doctor had been unfair to mention the matter at all since plans had been in existence for a long time to erect a new residence and dispensary. In 1924 the erection of the house we occupied was begun.

Both Hunter and Davis pleaded for a resident dentist. Since their day dentists have been stationed on the island at infrequent intervals. In 1942 Sam found himself repeating their plea in his report. His independent survey was based on facts he collected and experiences he underwent. Yet his lengthy annual report is filled with echoes of the other brave doctors who appealed to the infinitely distant powers of Washington.[7]

In 1936 Dr. Collins diagnosed and quarantined three cases of scarlet fever in one household and checked its spread through the community. To enforce that quarantine on the night he discovered the disease, he had to go over the head of the indifferent agent and make a personal appearance at a dance at Community Hall to appeal to the people to disperse. He was indeed a courageous man.[8]

The last epidemic, an outbreak of German measles, was just ebbing when we arrived. Fresh cases were cropping up only among the Aleut workmen from the archipelago, our neighbors across the street. Custom demanded that each new patient should pick up his blanket and hike over to the tiny jail. The bunks became crowded and the overflow was installed in the little historical souvenir shack across from us.

The convalescents were expected to take care of the very sick. I went inside the jail with Sam one day and nearly wept in front of the men. Sam's clamor had resulted in removal of the panes of glass from window frames never supposed to be opened for the comfort of the malefactors. Even so the smoke from the small stove and the odor of canned fish were overwhelming. Crowded and smoked like fish, the men lay fully clothed on the hard bunks. Nevertheless, their abode was palatial beside the dirty hovel known as the Aleut bunkhouse. Official eyebrows rose in amusement when we protested against such squalor. We were crazy newcomers who did not know that the Aleut was indifferent to dirt and discomfort. Had the epidemic arrived after we were more familiar with the island not one of the men would have had to enter either building, even if we had to take them into our own home.

Dovetailing the fragments of information together and comparing the whole with the measures taken to safeguard the seals, one conclusion is unavoidable. On the Pribilof reservation human beings, whether government employees or Aleut sealers, are of secondary importance because they do not grow fur. The unnecessary misery of body and mind are largely the result of a haphazard approach to the needs of the Americans who tend American property, with the main emphasis on the commercial aspects of the island. No one can ever know whether the conscious desire to keep a sealing gang conveniently at hand has been mainly responsible for this social backwater within the jurisdiction of a government agency or whether the combination of isolation, the inarticulateness of the sealers, and the individual agents' ignorance, prejudice, and other character defects has been most to blame for this dark spot on the record of American government.

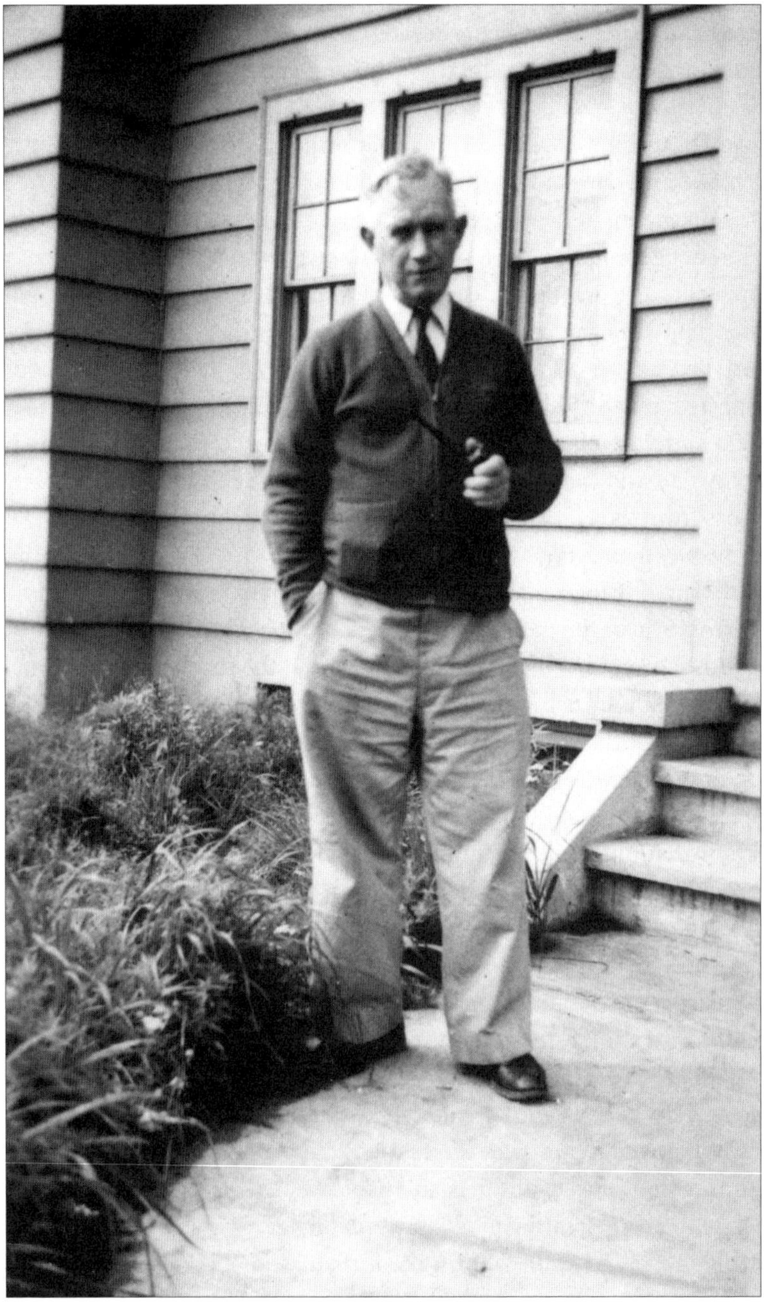

Edward C. Johnston (from the Martin Collection, USUAF210, Archives, Alaska and Polar Regions, Rasmuson Library, University of Alaska Fairbanks).

Chapter 19

The Seal Islands are as difficult to visit as the Grand Llama. On a few occasions the Alaska Steamship Company has obtained permission to land a few summer cruise passengers for a brief glimpse of a seal rookery. To secure a visa from the Department of the Interior a person must present credentials that show his motives are those of a scientific observer. The novelist Edison Marshall spent three weeks on St. Paul in 1925, the only one of his craft so fortunate.

The summer of our sojourn brought an unusually large number of visitors, including several individuals with whom we established quickening bonds of friendship deeper than the casual bonds of passing travelers. Several of the temporary summer employees were persons who made the weeks much happier socially.

Edward Johnston, a little, greying man whose weathered face crinkled into such wry attractive smiles, introduced us to many Pribilof interests and acted as guide to many beauty spots. His summer duties were onerous. Present at every drive and every killing, supervising the search for road skins, his most important function was "counting" the seals. For a couple of weeks at the peak of the breeding season he tramped over the rookeries of both islands, counting bulls by their noses, estimating by a complicated and not wholly reliable system the numbers of other classes of seals.

Although he was out of bed every morning at two thirty for the drive, the problems of seals, Service personnel, and Aleuts beset him all day and late into the night. Yet I never as the weeks wore by saw his placid kindly demeanor ruffled although his eyes dulled gradually from fatigue and his face became grey and drooped from sleeplessness. Toward the end of his stay he learned that his only child, a young boy just approaching manhood, was suffering from a fatal disease. He bore evil tidings with quiet courage and met his obligations with the usual unfailing outer calm. My obvious admiration for him kept petty Service gossip about him out of conversations when I was present until months after he had left the island. One night a woman boiled over into vituperative nasty criticism that sickened me and I was glad when she caught my glance and choked on a word.

It seemed to me if anyone escaped the tar brush of local slander it should be he. Since he seemed to be singled out for the worst kind of filthy scurrility, I decided to evaluate all further gossip I could not escape, as the more false the more vehement and coarse it was. The worse the gossip the better the man became my yardstick.

Johnston was a naturalist who found himself more at home in the island world of plants and animals than behind his Seattle desk. He regarded the seals he walked so easily among as ordinary men regard a batch of playful puppies snapping at their heels. Having studied and collected the flowers of both islands during the years before and after the First World War, he taught me much about St. Paul flora, especially where to look for rare species. In 1941 he was collecting beetles. When he had a moment of leisure, armed with a gallon bottle of his "juice," a mixture of molasses and water seasoned with a dash of asafetida, and empty tin cans, he drove from one collection spot to another. He gathered in his cans full of squirming sticky captives and put out cans of fresh bait. Then he hurried back to the laboratory in the basement of Government House to bathe his specimens and preserve them.

His absorption in nature and acceptance of her law that is called the struggle for existence may have been principally responsible for his blindness to the needs of man. He forgot as many do the other natural law that is a better pattern for man than the fierce law of jungle beasts, the example of the cooperative interrelationships of species for the common good. He lacked what is called social consciousness. He considered us fanatics when we caviled against outdoor toilets and faucets and the faulty education system. He argued that he had had to lug water a long distance for his family when he was a boy and that the Aleuts were incapable of rising above a fourth-grade level. Judged by his conversation, he was harsh and prejudiced, but he met every individual case brought to his attention with sympathy and whatever relief he had power to provide. I loved him for overruling Mac's surly resistance to Julia's Seattle trip for her artificial arm, expressed as "They ain't got no money," with the definite, firm-voiced statement that if the father had no money, money would have to be found.

The little things he did for people endeared him to me. He remembered always to bring me the first bloom of a species I had not yet seen. He was forever rooting in the dirty library in the Government House basement to locate odd bits of information for people, such as the number of vertebrae a whale possesses.

Harry May was a jolly companion. He had been coming north for the fur company since 1928. He spent an inordinate amount of time vowing the summer was his last on the island. His jovial attitude would have seemed humbug in any one but Harry. As I heard someone say, "You know he is just slapping you on the back for the sake of the Fouke Fur Company but he makes you like it." He enjoyed those duties that turned him into Lady Bountiful. He was in charge of giving out the traditional sack of oranges to each sealer's family on the Fourth of July and on the last day of sealing. I was astounded the day before Independence Day when Harry came in and dropped a book and a box of candy in my lap and tossed a box of cigars toward Sam. I had no idea the fur company felt it necessary to notice island officials.

Harry presided over the games and entertainment of the Fourth, distributing sacks of candy and ice cream cones high with double scoops. He also chose and had tastefully wrapped the individual Christmas gifts for each Pribilof child. He wrote a note on Tobyanne's gift, "Sam, this is for the kid. Don't you break it."

There was a tendency among Service families to deride the company's gift with the remark, "Fouke Fur gets enough out of the islands. It is only right to give a few pennies back." Some went so far as to term the presents "conscience money." Whatever the motive behind the gifts, one man's heart was in his job. If Harry had any objections to the custom it was probably the regret that Independence Day and Christmas come but once a year.

Doc Moore, soft-voiced and sympathetic, cherishing the young student blubberers like a fond mother, won everyone's heart. It was a sad day when in early August the *Penguin* left taking the three of them from us. Part of the happy camaraderie that had been St. Paul went with them.

Opportunities to know all the working students were limited. Jack Frost and Bob Scott, medical students from St. Louis, came to see us frequently. Discussing social problems and the modern doctor's approach to medical care kept us up until long past the hour all good blubberers should have been in bed.

Pleasant visitors who spent only a few days with us were Dr. Cole of the University of Wisconsin, a former member of the Harriman Alaska Expedition, revisiting the scenes of that earlier journey, and his brother-in-law, Edward Mulliken, a retired businessman traveling for his health. Dr. Cole busied himself collecting seal pituitary glands for a fellow scientist while Mulliken prowled leisurely around the village dispensing sweets to the children from seemingly inexhaustible pockets. He seemed more interested in the Aleuts than most visitors and accompanied Sam to some homes. He was brimming with anecdotes of his travels to odd corners of the world in pursuit of health.

August 10, 1941
So between office, hospital, letters, and social affairs, I have neglected records.

Yesterday was a saddish day for the *Penguin* started back for Seattle, carrying away Johnston, Harry May, and Doc Moore and our two favorite college lads, Jack Frost and Bob Scott.

Saturday night we were up for our last little get-together around the radio at seven and came back with a few treasures. Harry gave Sam some large paper, carbon paper, a few notebooks, Scotch tape, a whole box of paper clips, cord, pencils. Doc Moore contributed blank sheets from his large notebook. Also, Sam acquired shoestrings, a pair of boots, and a promise of a choice of the records that the company has here. Doc Moore left a box of lab stuff, including two bottle brushes for which I am very grateful.

Ben East, wildlife editor for a number of Michigan newspapers, and his wife, Elinor, stayed longer than the other travelers but not long enough. Ben was following the coast of Alaska and the Aleutian Islands photographing wildlife for his newspapers.[1] Elinor, whose appearance called for the permanent background of a decorative drawing room, maintained her daintiness amidst all the discomforts of non-passenger boats and chance lodgings and upheld the standards of exquisite femininity constantly. We had many mutual interests ranging from a whiff of garlic in our salad dressing to favorite authors. The Easts possessed an enthusiasm for living that made them charming companions. Limited to no specialized field of study they were absorbing all the facets of Alaskan life, floral, animal, and human.

> July 8, 1941
> We met the visitors. Dr. Cole . . . a very charming old man who reminded me of Dr. Bethune. A Mr. Mulliken. A Mr. and Mrs. East who are bouncy and are equipped with all sorts of movie cameras, etc. Mrs. East is very dressy in her sport clothes and wears tremendous earrings and a huge elephant pin on her blouse. She seems a sketch. Mrs. McMillin came down to go to the movie with her. I heard Mrs. East tell her, of all people, "My husband said this afternoon that I looked as if I had had a drink. But I told him I had had a bath." I wish I had a picture of Mrs. M.'s face. . . .
>
> Dr. Cole is the professor of genetics from Wisconsin and he is collecting flies, I gather not for himself alone but for others, and also pituitary glands from the seals. He said last night that he had taught Andre Mandregan how to open the skull with an axe and Andre was quicker and better at it than he, cutting down quickly so that it was possible for Dr. Cole to get the gland easily.

Beyond Zolotoi across the narrow nook to Reef Peninsula was a slight elevation named Gull Hill. We spent a bright morning there with Ben East as he photographed the bird dwellers of the cliffside. Despite the name, no gulls nested there. The solemn clowns of the bird world, the puffins or sea parrots, sat back on their salmon-red splay feet, indifferent to the chirping gossip of neighboring bevies of auklets. Both species of puffin seem something nature contrived of leftover scraps. Both wear somber bodily raiment befitting affected pedantic prigs. Huge swollen lemon beaks mar their mien, transforming them into cliff-dwelling Cyrano de Bergeracs. The vermilion stains of the tufted puffin's beak suggests that his raven plumage conceals the nature of a libertine who had drunk too deep of the grape and deserves the pallor of the white circle around his eyes. His diminutive yellow plume only accents his melancholy rouéism. The horned puffin simulates innocence with an immaculate white bosom. The narrow black strip between his snowy breast and his white face imparts the sly coquettish airs of the bygone belles with velvet bands below deceivingly demure chins. His gayer topknot rakishly dropping over one eye gives the final lie to his pretensions of respectability. If puffins are not schizophrenic, they are probably mentally protected with a shield as thick as their tough dermal covering of which the ancient Aleuts fashioned stout parkas. I suspect their immobility, their rigid silent stances are defense measures. I surmise they are self-conscious and very vulnerable to ridicule.

Our morning companions took turns at stationary sentry duty and flight patrol. One would waddle forward and plump his stocky body off the edge of the rock. His short stubby wings beat the air frantically as if unaccustomed to flight. Yet he forged through the air rapidly, passing back and forth in front of us as if performing prescribed exercises none too gladly. Swimming in and under the sea, puffins are more at home. Breeding duties bring them ashore. They are among the few large seabirds to burrow deep in the earth, if natural rock cavities are not available, to lay their eggs. Their broad feet are useful for nest digging. Their horrendous bills are savage weapons against the nest robber. Both male and female take turns warming the single white egg, mysteriously inscribed with dark lines on the inner side of the shell. Nature gave puffins more to endure than a bizarre appearance. Their primary feathers molt at one time, leaving them helpless and deprived of power to fly.

We lay in the grass above them watching patiently for the graven images to perform for Ben's camera. No gesture foretold the decision to fly. Occasionally one shifted from one broad foot to another. I found myself listening for the rasp of a nervous throat. Usually the puffin settled back to blink solemnly seaward. *Ipatok* or *ipatka,* as the Aleuts called him, was a favorite game bird despite the stringy dark flesh and unpleasant fishy taste.

Least auklets and crested auklets sunned themselves, fidgeting continuously. Auklets are gregarious and playful fellows and born chatterboxes. They lay their eggs, a single one to each couple, deep in natural rock interstices. The parents share brooding duties. We used to love to loiter over

July 18, 1941

The Easts . . . were the ideal guests. We had such a grand evening of good talk. . . . We also learned about sea otters. . . . One island that they visited when traveling on the *Brown Bear,* either Amchitka or Attu, had no guards there—just buildings from previous years at both ends of the forty-mile island. And [Ben] East said there were so many otter there that he was not at liberty to name the figure, since if poachers hear where herds are increasing, they may undo all the conservation work done to date. We saw, a while ago, some stills he managed to get of a sleeping otter. . . .

He reported that a Native here [on St. Paul] had found a dead otter and had turned in the skin on which there was no suspicious mark indicating that human means had killed the animal. In this one place in Alaska, the government will sign a quitclaim to the skin and give a legal stamp to it and permit the Native to dispose of the pelt. In other places, when a Native voluntarily hands over the skin of a dead animal that he has found, it is he that signs the quitclaim and the government takes the skin with a mere thank you. There are some odd contradictions about here. Which brought up the question of the status of these people here, whether mere government

cont.

wards or citizens with voting rights. According to East a law was passed granting full citizenship to the Natives of Alaska and these ought to come within that provision. Also, once they voted—but the wrong way to the desire of the Bureau of Fisheries, so never again.

One of the most delightful stories concerned the redlight district of Unalaska: a house, very small house, on an island between Unalaska proper and the naval base.[2] Three girls at present, or two and the madam, Mary. A boatman runs a small launch back and forth, day and night, fare fifty cents. The fee for the produce is five dollars.

In 1899 Prof. Cole had visited this spot and had photographed the only clump of trees growing around that section, a clump of cedars [actually Sitka spruce] that he estimated were about a hundred years old today, although barely above the roof of the house that stands there now. Incidentally, the island has been christened "Treasure Island." He wanted to secure pictures of the same stand of trees. He took Mr. Mulliken with him and they found, after a few inquiries, that there was a boatman who would take them there. While they were crossing, something went wrong with the motor and this took some time to repair. They suggested that as soon as it was repaired they return to the land. But the Native grinningly indicated that it would not take long now, so they continued on their way.

cont.

shingles where *chuchki,* as Aleuts call the least auklets, using the Russian nickname, dwelt underground and listen to the confused murmuring and twittering of domestic conversations.

A group of six crested auklets, their dainty tasseled plumes bobbing in front of their eyes, were skimming up and down a tilted basalt slab with short running steps. These *canooski* or little captains came to a full stop, slid slightly, and propped themselves against further descent with their tails. Occasionally as we lay in the grass a Pacific kittiwake darted by scolding loudly, deserving the Russian term the Aleuts clung to, *gavarushka,* the talkative one.

A cormorant perched somnolently on a jagged outcropping. He permitted Ben to descend close to him to take pictures. A consistently natural poseur, the shag, as the bird is rudely dubbed, is a perfect camera subject, preening and stretching his long glistening neck in graceful patterns. His flesh is the toughest and fishiest of the birds the Aleuts hunt.

The morning was a moment that was quickly interrupted by the faint tolling of the village dinner bell. Ben had to obey its summons. The car had taken advantage of our absorption in birds to develop a flat tire and condemned us to walk home. Ben's lunch time was fixed but someone kindly saved food for him. Elinor scolded him for being a blind male who had not observed the fourth member of our party and had permitted me to lie on the cliff's rim so long on my stomach. As if he could have forbidden me. For unborn Tobyanne and I were seasoned hikers who had learned to scale steep cliffs and curl up comfortably in rough spots in direct contradiction to all textbook directions to the expectant mother.

There is only one Jack Eggis in the world. To tell about him requires a special book. He is the sailor of the enchanted yarns we all hope to encounter someday. But Jack is more than a spinner of fine tales. He is the most generous, kindly soul, a person whom children throng about, whom stray curs follow. *Good* is a curious adjective to apply to a retired ship's engineer who has knocked about the seven seas since early boyhood. Frankly, I know no better descriptive adjective for him. Jack is a short, round man with a Norwegian tang to his words and a hearty laugh that rumbles alarming in the depths of his capacious abdomen and wells up geyserlike. It is hard for Jack to think evil of a fellow human, much less speak evil. He regards tough, hard-drinking seamen with a kindly paternal eye as just bad boys who can't help themselves. He could flare into a terrible anger with a bully or someone injuring a woman, child, or helpless kitten. He was untainted with the island taste for indulging in petty gossip, although a veteran summer worker.

> They landed, went past the house, and took their photos of the cedar trees. Coming back to the beach there was no sign of their boatman. But they noticed a man working and asked him to locate the boatman. He got him from the house. The Native seemed puzzled and asked peculiar questions—earlier he had seemed most skeptical when they explained why they wanted to go to the island—but they were actually coming away without having done anything but photographing the trees. And the Native was very mystified at this glimpse of a new kind of white man. Not until the next day did Cole & M. find out what the house was for and why the Native was so confused by their interests

Jack was spending his sixth summer on St. Paul, officially as a plumber and socially as a healthy jolly leaven. It was impossible to credit him with sixty years but he had retired from the sea because of his age. He spent his winters on Bainbridge Island near Seattle with a much younger wife and four children. How they must have missed him summers. When he said "my kids" the listener's heart would quiver in response to the pride and love in his tone. Describing their childish exploits tears would begin to spill from his eyes, even while he chuckled over some comic detail. His love was not restricted to his own children.

The autumn before we met him an Aleut child was sent to Seattle to have a safety pin extracted from her lung. There were wives of officials traveling by the same boat, but not one of them seemed inclined to play nursemaid to an Aleut baby still in diapers. Mac had a few troubled moments until Jack volunteered to nurse the baby. "Them women," he told us, "they come round to watch me wash the baby but I didn't let them touch her. She was a fine little fellow all right." It was possible to see the scenes as Jack talked, the sudsy baby gurgling and warring against the waves of the bathwater as the *Penguin* plunged and bucked in the waves of the greater bathtub, and Jack cooing in reply. His discourse on the technique of laundering diapers left me stranded between the desire to shed tears for

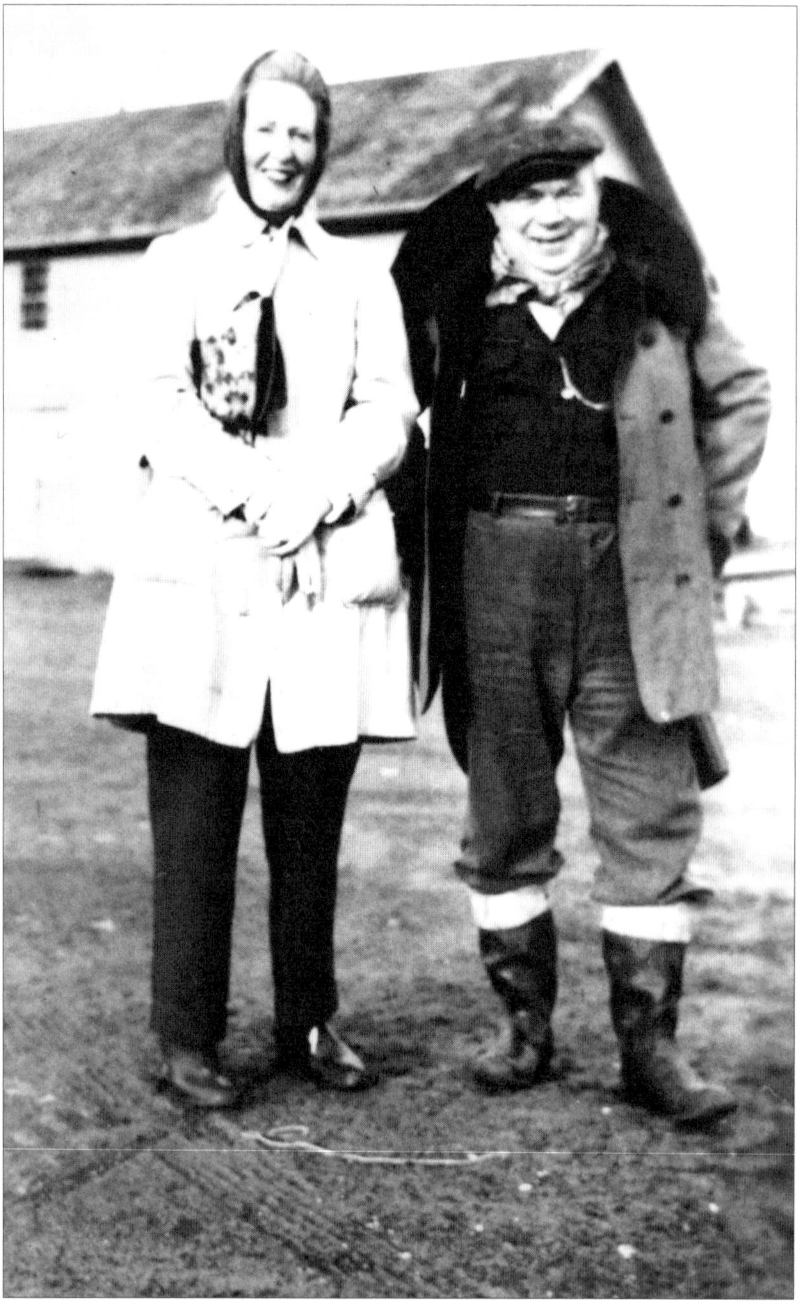

Fredericka Martin and Jack Eggis (from the Martin Collection, USUAF210, Archives, Alaska and Polar Regions, Rasmuson Library, University of Alaska Fairbanks).

his painstaking tender care of the baby and laughter at the thought of rotund Jack bent over a bucket of seawater scrubbing clothes.

Jack's sea yarns ranged from gory descriptions of naked corpses in the grasses of the Kamchatka peninsula, souvenirs of the Russo-Japanese war, to tales of pet harbor seals whom he fed canned milk and clams. A favorite of his was the account of a rolling storm that tumbled the ship so vigorously that at noon the pound of butter slid from the table and stuck on the wainscoting. As long as the butter lasted the men simply reached over and cut off a portion for themselves.

Andy Holland, head cook for summer employees, lived at his range from early morning until late evening. Of Scandinavian origin, he very proudly sported recently acquired American citizenship papers. His duties included apportioning meat and baking bread for the Service families. Occasionally he sent out other baked stuff with the bread. When the other wives were model housewives, needing no additions to their own pastries, he sent them occasional offerings of cookies and doughnuts, but he flooded our house with pies and cakes lest the doctor suffer from my negligence or Heretina's less digestible concoctions. The doughnuts were very mysterious. At the Government House table on a doughnut day I first heard speculation whether the dessert were to be cake doughnuts or bread doughnuts. The difference proved too subtle for my palate. Only a veteran of many summers of Andy's cooking could judge. I enjoyed dunking them all.

Andy's wit was quick with a stoical philosophic twist. He was much amused by the elaborate costly investigations of seals and was prone to expatiate on the difference between official interest in seals and that of the Aleuts. When we were all looking forward to the arrival of the *Black Douglas,* a schooner scheduled to follow the seals south to discover the boundaries of their southern winter feeding grounds, Andy would ask, "And when is the Flying Dutchman coming?" And add, "Them seals had been coming here for hundreds and hundreds of years without benefit of political and financial advice, coming right up on the front doorsteps and it is a shame that they cannot have some privacy in their lives."

His humor blossomed in regulations he had posted in his kitchen domain for his Aleut staff to read, laugh over, and obey.

1. English will be the language spoken by all kitchen employees while on duty.
2. All noncommissioned officers of the culinary staff must report for duty not later than 6:15 a.m. (Sundays and Holidays one hour later) and must leave the premises at 2 p.m. to report for duty again at 5 p.m. and stay until the job is finished for the day.
3. Cleanliness and speed are the best qualifications for a kitchen officer—anyone appearing with a greasy-looking uniform will not be permitted to work and as punishment he will be given 10 days on Walrus Island

without shelter. If the charges are of a graver nature, the offender will be turned over to the proper authorities for a hearing.

4. No shouting or unnecessary noise will be tolerated during meal hours or at any other time. If you feel like singing or hollering get down to sea lion beach and you will have lots of company. Don't let outsiders get the impression that the kitchen is an institution for mentally unbalanced human creatures.
5. This is not the Hog Island Navy Yard nor a stone quarry or any other noisy place. Always bear in mind that you are employed in the dining room and kitchen for the WHITE MESS of St. Paul and conduct yourself accordingly.

A. A. Holland.

"And a *white mess* it is," he would often say ruefully. "I don't know where them Fouke Fur boys come from. They yell about the food. Then they eat it all up and yell for more. They make the tablecloth dirty and yell for a clean one. I only get clean linen issued to me three times a week. Sometimes they spill soup on the cloth so I will give them a clean cloth but I don't have it to give them. And here I am trying to get these poor lads in the kitchen to be clean and learn some manners. They won't do it if they copy the manner of them Missouri cowboys in the 'white mess.'"

Once I intruded upon an indignant meeting in his kitchen. A scurrilous article about the immorality of St. Paul Aleuts had just appeared in the *Alaska Sportsman.* It was written by a former clerk who had graduated to a better position in the Washington office. He was credited with carrying on some rather sordid affairs with Aleut women to whom he promised much and gave nothing. "The ————," chorused Andy and Jack. "And —— was just telling me that he ordered this fancy author to leave his wife alone and was knocked down by him. And imagine going outside and writing bad things about them on top of it."

Jack reached into his pocket for his flat tin of snuff and administered a soothing dose. Andy was thoughtfully stirring some cake dough. He looked up and grinned. "Sour grapes. I'm safe from the girls. My face is so ugly no girl would marry me even to get to the States."

Andy alone bore the *Penguin*'s autumn delay without fretting. Sam jokingly asked how he would like to stay on as our cook. Andy looked at him seriously and sadly.

"This island is all right in summer when the people get their money but I couldn't stay here all winter with hungry kids coming round for dry bread and hawk eyes watching from the office to be sure I didn't give them a crust," he said. This was our first inkling that the regular weekly rations, supplemented by a small weekly credit for food purchases at the Canteen, were inadequate in quantity during the winter months.

Andy adopted two cows to whom he carried choice tidbits of cabbage and apple peelings. His largesse was limited to the two who waited regularly across from his kitchen. He drove off stray visitors. "If the rest of them are too lazy to walk up a little hill every day," he would say, "they needn't be coming around just once in a while to steal the sweets from others."

The preceding winter Andy had shipped as assistant cook aboard a ship loading apples for oriental markets. Unfortunately a box of "apples" split open, revealing TNT. The head chef and the other assistants left quickly as if assisted by the explosive. Andy alone remained. The captain rewarded him with the salaries of all absconded help. He also showed him where he kept the key to his personal supply of beer. I suspect that Andy is now aboard another ship carrying equally dangerous cargo to a distant battle point. If the ship goes down, I know that Andy will face death calmly "without benefit of political or financial advice."

Chapter 20

It required the United States Navy to escort us through the industrial buildings of St. Paul. The salt sheds and blubbering room were still mysteries to us when the slim grey *Charleston*, flagship of the Alaska waters, pulled into Village Cove one drizzling late July morning.[1] It was a pleasant invasion. Trucks filled with sailors plied busily between the dock and a nearby rookery. Officers lunched at Government House and the Company House, throwing Andy into culinary convulsions and necessitating excessive watering of the soup.

> July 30, 1941
> So Sam is now off in the village. I think he went down to see a naval ship that came in and I have let her [Fedosia] go down to look at it because I have a great deal of work for her to do this afternoon. I also have to worry about Sam's shirts and see what arrangements I can make about getting his collars starched.
>
> Fedosia just came back from taking a look at the ship and is trying to make some starch. I don't know what the result will be since I'm not a good guide, knowing nothing about starching clothes myself. I guess I am pretty inadequate. Other women have done lots of work and managed to write at the same time. But I can't make the grade. If my mind is cluttered up with domestic problems, it can't function at writing very well. I am so envious of gals like Ruth Gruber who can float around experiencing and taking notes on her experiences and
>
> *cont.*

The ship's surgeon and the dentist were entrusted to our hospitality in accordance with the tradition that medical personnel like nothing better than hospital inspection. But we liked each other and sidestepped as much shoptalk as was humanly possible.

Because of our social responsibility we were included in the officers' expedition to Northeast Point. In the back of Mac's pickup, though we could see little through the tiny window squares, we gained an intimate knowledge of the roadbed. Mac's love of speed and refusal to swerve aside from depressions kept the officers bouncing up and down on the hard wooden side benches. I was snugly packed between two companions on the thick leather-cushioned seat behind the driver's cabin. The air grew blue with comments about St. Paul once I assured them that etiquette toward the female sex should not interfere with freedom of expression. The politest remark was the rueful comparison of the dentist: "I never felt waves like this in the —— storm."

After our guests had marveled at the seals and appraised the possible military advantages of St. Paul, we conducted them through the soaking grass to view the beautiful grave of a naval officer. At the head of a tumbled cairn of volcanic rocks the simple granite monument reads, "James Heath, Gunner's Mate, U.S.S. Concord, Born 1860, Died 1894." While the *Concord* was patrolling off the Point in the days of pelagic sealing, Heath died of blood poisoning. Father Rezanoff read the funeral liturgy of the Russian Orthodox Church.[2] Heath was buried on Cross Hill, a tall sand hill near Webster Lake. The next day, for reasons unrecorded, his comrades came ashore and moved his body to Hutchinson Hill at the tip of the Point, putting up a crude wooden marker for the "diseased" seaman, as the recorder of the period described Heath several times. The conventional monument was set up much later. Mac ascribed the inscription to Aleut workmen, a compliment to their craftsmanship if true. The polished granite block is congruous with the stone-heaped grave and a low three-sided wall of basalt blocks. Nearby a slender white Russian cross stands benevolent guard. Inside and outside the plot flowers throng extravagantly. No sailor "home from the sea" could wish a lovelier resting place, infinity above, the roll of the sea at the hill's base, the lone cries of the gull patrol mourning forever.

That blend of the romantic and practical, so characteristically Pribilovian, turned our attention from the solitary beautiful grave to the sealing industry, particularly to the activities administered by the Fouke Fur Company.

First we briefly inspected a wash-house. The Russians air-dried the pelts by stretching them on pegs a few inches above the ground in the open or in huts where slow fires were kept burning. American sealing companies had some blubber removed, dried the skins in salt, and shipped them off in bundles to San Francisco and later to London, which for a time was the world fur center. When the actual killing of seals was removed from private concerns and made a

come out with a book later on and keep going places and becoming an authority. Which I doubt that she could do if she had to worry about starched collars and remember to tell Fedosia to set the table and put tomatoes in the soup a quarter of an hour from now.

. . .

July 31, 1941

And then came the Navy. I heard Mr. McMillin's voice inquiring for the doctor and went out to find him flanked by two men in uniform, the doctor and dentist from the USS *Charleston*. We sat down to chat and M. sent out for Sam whom he located at the Government House. I asked them to lunch, but they thought they had to go to the Company House. The hour came so quickly that they were reluctant to leave and especially to leave me behind. Dr. Leamer asked Sam whether he could not throw a coat around me and take me along. So I dined at the Company House on corned beef and cabbage.

responsibility of the Bureau of Fisheries, a private company obtained the privilege of processing the skins for market and handling the public sale of finished dyed skins. The reforms fought for so bitterly in Congressional halls were but partially accomplished. Under Funsten Brothers and later under Fouke Fur Company, more and more elaborate treatment of the skins was performed on the island. By 1941 the Fouke Fur Company buildings had become an impressively large section of the village. Even to the ordinary onlooker it would seem that it would be cheaper to send off unblubbered skins than to transport equipment and material for buildings and to bring each summer, at government expense, the large number of workers from St. Louis and Seattle and the Aleutian chain. The last benefit from the arrangement. There are few opportunities for Aleutian islanders to earn money. They are enabled to exist the remainder of the year on the savings from their eighty dollars a month wages plus the proceeds of fishing and trapping on their home islands.

Like the killing field routine, the indoor work has a rhythmic tempo that begins when the first truck rolls up to a washhouse window in the morning. The skins are pitched directly through the windows into huge tanks of saltwater piped in from the Bering. We stood in the long dark room between the vats, balancing ourselves on pliant wooden slatted walks that barely kept us above the flowing water. Workmen sheathed in hip boots forked skins from one bath up onto a platform. Others, directing powerful hoses expertly, simultaneously washed and propelled skins across the planking into the next tank of clean solution. I admired the way they extracted pleasure from their job by making pelts dance in the pouring water. The dank, ill-lit shed, the shadowy figures, the hissing torrents of water, the revolting stew of churning skins, the penetrating chill dampness, and the stench of bloody raw pelts created a Hadean atmosphere more befitting sadism than humor. But the Aleuts had the courage to sport in that atmosphere.

Massive slatted frames held the skins beneath the brine in filled tanks. A single fresh skin averages ten pounds. After soaking ten days, the osmotic extraction of oil by the brine had reduced the mean weight to between four and five pounds.

In contrast, the blubbering room exuded light and comfort although it was not much warmer than the washhouse. The air throbbed with the dull scrubbing reverberations of blubber knives erasing seal fat. The blubberers worked on each side of the room back-to-back. Between them, down the center, ran a line of tables. The top of each table was reserved for the limp flensed skins. The sloppy, soggy, blubber-heavy skins were laid on a lower shelf conveniently within reach of the blubberers. Each skin had already been numbered. A foreman kept accurate track of the recipients of the numbers in order to credit the workmen with the correct amount of finished labor and to allot blame for cuts or damage.

The blubberers bent over sturdy rounded wooden beams resembling toy ironing boards set up washboard-wise. These flensing boards were waist high from the floor. Skins were draped blubber side up on the boards. Gripping curved two-handled knives firmly, the men moved up and down like laundresses shoving the knives downward in quick careful movements that took off the fat without penetrating the skin. Each season the new hands, almost invariably college boys, came as skilled laborers after practicing hours on unblubbered skins in the St. Louis factory. As the knives cleaned the skins, the blubberers pulled the pelts upward, keeping them within comfortable reach. The gobs of fat rolled down into a cement trough that extended the length of the room. At night this blubber was swept up and sent to the rendering plant to be made into the number-one oil reserved for processing the furs in the States. With sharp knives the blubberers trimmed the rough edges of the holes where the flippers had been. A quick toss over the shoulder, a deft pull from the lower shelf, and a blubberer was at work on another pelt. As a blubberer paused to clean his greasy knife on the protective canvas apron he wore, he seemed about to commit hara-kiri.

Fortunately this backbreaking work is limited to three or four hours a day. The hardiest human muscles could barely endure more. Blubbering is a steady unrelenting exercise of muscle and mind. If the eyes or fingers forget the knife for a second, the skin is gashed and ruined. Touch must be as delicate as a violinist's. Temptations to relax and work slowly are overcome by the prospect of bonuses for those who accomplish the most. A less kindly economic goad is the requirement that a certain daily minimum of skins be flensed if the workman hopes to return a second summer.

As in a dress factory, small boys busily ran about the room removing piles of blubbered skins and replenishing the waning heaps of fatty skins. Bright orange trucks, attached to overhead cables, ran on rails between the workrooms. They brought in wet skins from the washhouse and carried away the clean ones to a hand-worked mangle. Another conveyer, laden with neatly folded wrung-out skins, crossed the yard to the salt house. Once more the skins were placed in vats, each orderly layer thickly covered with rough salt crystals. After ten days the skins are sufficiently dry to be shipped.

The men in the packing room worked in teams of three. Two men smoothed the last wrinkle from the dried skins, rubbed a handful of boric acid over the surfaces, tossed a little salt on the skins, and folded them deftly into neat rolls. Between them stood the packer. He disposed of the rolls, tucking them in a barrel. When one layer was inserted he hopped into the barrel himself and stamped them tightly in place with his feet as if he were treading grapes.

Staves and hoops arrived in packages and were coopered into shape on the island. As soon as a barrel was packed a workman adjusted the top and tamped the last binding hoop into place. All the barrels were marked for shipment to Seattle. The barrels that contained the fifteen percent of each day's take put aside for Canada were marked with bright orange circles to enable the Seattle longshoremen to separate the barrels more easily. Japan, also entitled to fifteen percent by the same treaty that gave Canada a share, had always taken a cash equivalent.

The Japanese claimed they lacked sufficient knowledge to complete processing the fur. The treaty obligated Japan to give the United States fifteen percent of the seal take from her small Kurile Islands herd. Harry May complained that Japan sent us poor-quality pelts, principally from old scarred bulls and sometimes from females. For years Japan had sent large groups of students to the Pribilofs under the auspices of their Bureau of Fisheries, ostensibly to learn American methods of sealing. Each summer Harry had lectured them about the value of skins. He had concluded they were incapable of learning how to choose good seal skins. It is more natural to believe the Japanese were glad to disguise business sense as stupidity and were delighted to continue palming off worthless skins for the cream of the bachelor crop of the Pribilofs.

Our last call was paid to the by-products plant, bleak in its isolation on the lagoon bank. All summer I had heard the bizarre yarn that the interior smelled less disgusting than the outside. Fortunately, I had been skeptical. The reverse was true from the moment we had to pass the unloading platform where nauseous carcasses were piled high. The gleaming motionless eyes were horrible to encounter. One grisly skinned head leaned out between the boardings, its pop eyes leering at us with malevolent vengeful pleasure. Everyone turned from him quickly.

Our inspection was cursory. The noise of the machines cut down explanations. The sickening sweetish stench clogged our throats and nostrils. Three cookers, fed with carcasses at the top, were busily converting them into meal. We watched the men shovel the shredded substance from the cookers into a pressing machine. It was coarse reddish brown, like the red earth of the killing fields. From the pressing tank a sticky molasses-like oil was piped into a tank. The meal was disgorged, dry and fluffy, through a wide vent beneath which workmen held sacks in place. The number-two oil from the carcasses was purchased by cosmetic factories. Not even Johnston could tell us its ultimate use. I suggested that some of the caustic toilet soap we received on the island must be the seal oil come back for revenge. Some meal was retained on the islands for fox food. Large quantities were shipped to other stations of the Fish and Wildlife Service for fish and animal food. The rendering plant was solely a government activity.

While the rendering plant avoids the waste that went on for years when the carcasses were left to rot in the open, polluting the island air, improvements can still be made. It pained me especially when cod liver oil preparations were becoming scarce, after the invasion of Norway, to know that thousands of pounds of seal liver rich in vitamin D were swallowed up in the cookers. One day, smacking our lips over a tasty homemade appetizer of liver paste, I began to visualize the great industry that could be built up, the manufacture of seal liver paste. As an island industry it would provide winter labor for both men and women and extra money that they need so badly. The cooking and canning process would be simple. I christened my dream child "Pribilof Pâtés." I could see the charming wrapper with gay little seals leaping along the strip of paper. I planned a national advertising campaign stressing the exotic nature of the food and its vitamins content. Sam carried out practical experiments. He weighed seal livers and helped me estimate the amount of meat available each year. When all my data was assembled, we communicated the dream to Johnston who promised with an air of fatherly amusement to suggest our plan to the Washington office. Doc Moore alone shared our enthusiasm. I know my dream is practical. Sometime it will burst the bonds of official lethargy. I shall be able to walk into my grocery and order a dozen cans of delicious savory "Pribilof Pâtés."

When our visitors had finished sightseeing, Commodore Parker invited the official colony to come out to the ship. We trailed up and down the decks of the *Charleston* looking at guns and instruments with solemn faces and little comprehension of the technical explanations we were listening to. Sam and I went off to see the sick bay. I turned green-eyed when I looked at the autoclave of my desires. The smart, trained pharmacist mates were enviable contrasts to our own hospital attendants. Dr. Ellers, the dentist, disappeared at the first opportunity. He murmured something about getting first aid for his "sit-down after that ride."

Coffee and cake were waiting in the commodore's quarters. I was busy browsing through a shelf of Alaskan books, writing down titles I wanted to order. A Filipino mess boy appeared at my side bearing a chocolate soda. Nothing could have surprised me more. Sodas were the only articles I longed for continually. From that moment no one could surpass me as a fervid supporter of our Navy. A Navy that could serve chocolate sodas in the waste of the Bering is a force other nations should leave alone, as the Japanese are beginning to learn. Sam had secured the drink for me. I offered the other women a sip, but they clung to their prosaic coffee and I enjoyed every drop myself.

We watched the *Charleston* disappear in the evening shadows as if dear old friends were departing. The contact with new people had been so refreshing that I was more than evèr depressed by the ensuing

July 31, 1941

Dr. Leamer . . . got some cigarettes for me, two cartons of Chesterfields. I was the only lucky one. He was certainly sweet and charming. He seemed to be so oversolicitous of me that he must have recognized my condition, warning me of slippery spots and projecting rings on the deck . . .

The commodore handed out candy bars. Mess boys brought coffee. I was busy inspecting their Alaskan library and copying titles when suddenly a mess boy arrived with a chocolate soda. I could hardly believe my eyes. Later I found out that the captain had asked Sam if there were anything he would like from the mess and he had asked if it were possible to get a soda. Presto, two of them. What a Navy we have. Prepared for any emergency. Nothing ever tasted better except the first banana I had when I came out of Spain.

When it was time to leave, Doc Moore and Harry May could not be found. Harry came off with a carton of matches in the back of his coat. We were all given two packages apiece, blue and gold wrappers with the ship's name, by the captain.

cont.

conversation among the Service people. I could not sympathize with the guilt they felt at accepting the commodore's invitation without asking the agent's permission. I could not picture Mac even in his worst temper fits trying to forbid the acceptance of such a treat. All during our visit to the boat I kept receiving whispered communications on the subject. By the time we were on land I was so bored with the cringing petty fears that I flared up and asked whether they thought the Nazis had taken over the island. My childish outburst silenced them for the rest of our walk home together. Even Mac suffered from similar apprehensions. I remembered how nervously he had asked Ruth Gruber not to believe all she heard about St. Paul, that it was a nice place and everybody got along together.

> Back on shore, we were walking up with the crowd and I had a chance to thank Harry May for the Camembert cheese he had sent me the night before. He asked if we had crackers and then insisted we come up at once to get a box. Two of them and the crackers are crisp, too. We talked for ages with the Hellbaums and Hoversons and Harry outside the house and then chatted longer inside with Johnston and Harry. Wonderful holiday spirit prevailing. The trip off the island had certainly been refreshing to everyone. And responsible for a great uplift of spirit.

The same chorus began more loudly when the *Spica*, the supply boat loaned to the Service by the Navy, arrived with the principal supplies for the year.[3] She disrupted the sanctity of the Sunday forenoon. The village, somnolent since the departure of the *Penguin* with the majority of the temporary workers, became a lively bustling place. Trucks raced madly through the streets. The men were divided into two work gangs that alternated six-hour shifts of unloading for the duration of the *Spica*'s stay. Only a heavy sea, which the small boats could not breast, could interrupt the work.

Any boat that brought mail was welcome. The minutes we waited at the office for the sacks to be sorted were longer than the weeks we had wished for the letter. We always sat on the living-room floor to tear open the mountains of envelopes, reading aloud to each other, laughing at one bit of news, shedding tears over another. Meals grew cold but we did not care.

As soon as the *Spica*'s gifts to us had been read and answered we spent hours of leisure at West Landing. Swift Navy launches towed our baidars and flat barges back and forth. Our crane never paused, swinging freight from boats to waiting trucks. Before workers in the storehouses could dispose of one load another truck was at the door.

Metrofan enjoyed the *Spica*'s visit. He almost became attached to the window frame as day and night he questioned passersby about the nature of the freight and the conduct of the work. He yearned to parade up and down the dock sporting his naval cap, playing chief of police once more. Sam arranged for a driver to pick him up on the next-to-the-last day. Metrofan dressed early in the morning, crept carefully downstairs, and sat fuming impatiently all afternoon. The driver had forgotten his promise. We found Metrofan grieving, disconsolate and more prejudiced than ever against the younger generation. Sam rushed out to find another driver. Metrofan enjoyed an ecstatic half hour supervising the dock activities from a comfortable seat in the Ford. Some real-life commodores could have envied his jaunty authoritative demeanor. His old heart had to work overtime, but what doctor could have withheld such pleasure for what was apt to be, and actually was, his last supply boat.

Varied cargo kept stimulating our interest. One night we stuffed ourselves with bananas. The next we guzzled slabs of watermelon. Food, lumber, clothing, glass, lead pipe, and coal. Mountains of coal. Fifteen-hundred tons of coal choked the capacious bunkers and were heaped in an enormous mound of sacks along the main road.

Medical supplies were meager. Johnston had warned us that firms had refused to bid on the order. War orders were larger and more vital. Bidding is a device intended to prevent government employees from succumbing to the temptations of graft. It is a clumsy process and sometimes harmful. Since medications could not be ordered by company name, inferior drugs allegedly equivalent to those requisitioned were frequently purchased. Prices listed on the invoices of medications received were shocking. Drugs generally have four price categories, for physicians, for drug stores, for hospitals, and, lowest of all, for federal agencies. Our invoices indicated that the shopping had been done at the drugstore counter.

> August 21, 1941
> The dinner was excellent and the officers were true cavaliers. I was lucky because Captain Granum chanced to sit beside me and we chatted about Annapolis, Greenbelt, and Maryland in general, and I won him over to the idea of cooperative medicine.
> After dinner, there was a delay in showing the movie we had been promised because one of the holds was receiving cargo. Mimeographed song sheets were passed round and a general sing-along went on for about an hour. Then the lights were put out and one of the officers recited "The Shooting of Dan McGrew."

In five complete twenty-four-hour periods the enormous unloading project was completed, the swiftest unloading in island history. The sea had been unusually ladylike and cooperative.

Thursday afternoon Dr. Hill came ashore and invited us to tea. Our neighbors had been accusing Mac of discouraging the officers from visiting ashore and preventing our receiving invitations to go out to the boat. In previous years there had been movies and dinner aboard almost nightly. Of course we went aboard. All the women of Service families except Mrs. Mac had preceded us, accompanying officers who had been distributing gifts to the schoolchildren ashore. We had to believe the captain when he told us Mac had churlishly refused invitations extended through him to the Service families. The employees had had a real basis for their accusations and fears. I remained disgusted at their shamefaced whispering behind his back instead of acting resolutely and concertedly to prevent the continuation of his interference with natural and needed recreation. For the evening the hatchet was buried. The captain asked us to stay to dinner. He sent word ashore to all absent husbands. Even Mrs. Mac joined us. After dinner we went on deck to see a movie.

It was ironical to be sitting out-of-doors in the Bering Sea watching a picture of jungle romance [*Strange Cargo*, with Joan Crawford and Clark Gable]. Just beyond the screen the open maw of a hold yawned. At intervals baidar loads of seal meal arrived and hundreds of sacks were dumped into the hold. Amusing sound effects were added to the story. At tense moments a carrier heaped with sacks would thump against the ship's side or metal would clatter against metal. It was difficult to say good-bye and go ashore. The officers pleaded with us to remain for coffee. We were so contented when no ship touched the island. It took only one new face walking into our living room to make us aware of the world we had left behind.

Stimulated, Sam and I talked late into the night. We paid for our folly. We had to get up at dawn to suture George Rukovishnikoff's smashed finger, the first and last casualty of the unloading. The *Spica* had weighed anchor and was on its way south laden with two million dollars worth of seal furs destined for the fashion parade of the nation. Aboard also were all but one or two of the temporary employees. The social season of St. Paul seemed over.

Chapter 21

Bright August sunshine reminded us one morning that we had never visited Antone Lake except when it lay silvery and somber under a grey sky. The scoria road was a copper red ribbon ahead of us as we drove toward Zapadni. Seaward, green fields slanted unevenly down to the sands of English Bay. Bluish green waters rippled quietly beyond. On our left the flat land gradually climbed to low hill ridges crowned with rocky parapets. The double coronet of Bogoslof brooded high above a bevy of little knolls. Picturesque outcroppings of smoke-grey basalt studding the landscape reminded me of central Spain. There, in similar countryside of copper soil, deep green vegetation, and purple shadowed rocks, stand fragmentary ruins of ancient walls and buildings. There the rocks of a hillside, running jagged, intermittent lines across the earth, may be the remnants of an ancient walled city of the Romans. Here on a northern island that man had known for less than two hundred years, the earth bore the same scarred appearance of lands where men had lived and fought and died for centuries. Here capricious elements had built mock ruins that evoked artificially the same wistful reveries of the transiency of man's works as genuine remnants of the past.

Antone Lake, by bird flight, almost touches the road's end. Our earthbound approach was hindered by breast-high grasses, by sedge hummocks formless under the waving grasses, by small quagmires. Disappointment awaited us when we had struggled through to the lakeshore. The water has shrunk dirtily in toward the center leaving an ugly brown mud rim where clouds of big blue beetles and tiny gnats hovered.

The name Antone had teased our curiosity. Had some breath of France touched this island in remote days? Our suspicions seemed borne out by a study of maps drawn in 1890 by Elliott where he had identified a small building near the lake as "Antoines House."[1] Across the blue of the lake he had written merely "Fresh Water Lake." Again romanticism was dispelled by Dimitri Tetoff's tale handed down by his parents. At some time in the 1890s surveyors asked Anton Melovidov, foreman of the sealing gang, whether the lake had a name.[2] Mischievously, Anton, whose hunting barabara Elliott had placed on his map, informed them that the

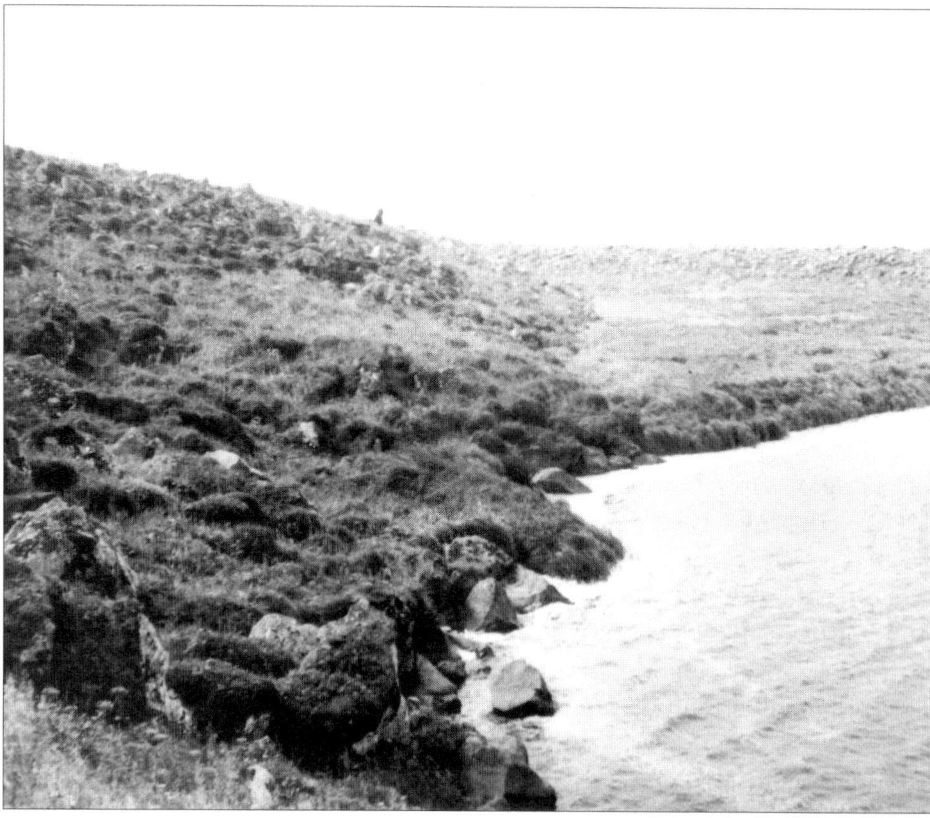

Fredericka Martin at Antone Lake (from the Martin Collection, USUAF210, Archives, Alaska and Polar Regions, Rasmuson Library, University of Alaska Fairbanks).

name was Anton Lake. Anton regaled the village with what he considered a great joke on the surveyors. Many villagers chuckled over the surveyors' willingness to accept misinformation. Actually he probably bestowed a prettier name than the surveyors might have chosen. Anton may have felt that he was annoying his brother-in-law Elliott, for about that time he was signing affidavits for congressional committees that were used to discredit Elliott's more objective scientific testimony. Also the documents afforded an opportunity for obliquely stressing the fact that a sealer was Elliott's brother-in-law. In many of the printed records Anton's name appears as Antoin, Antone, and Antoine. Anton as a foreman was in constant trouble for drinking and other actions that ill accorded with his responsibilities. He was vulnerable to the lessee's pressure for they supported his incumbency when the sealers wanted to oust him. Actually it was quite logical and natural that the lake within his hunting province should bear his name. So few events provided the sealers with inspiration for laughter that his alleged prank was useful.

Many Aleuts recalled their tongue's appellation, *Maanam Amik* [*Maanam Anii*]; the latter word means "lake" but the sense of *Maanam* has been lost.[3] Such informants vaguely remembered that a locality near the lake had first been called

Maanam and the word was later applied to the lake. But *Maanam Amik,* Antone Lake, a mediocre, muddy pond in the bright scenery, repelled us that morning and we hastened to leave it.

Clambering up the steep hillside from the lake to the flat meadow of Zapadni Roadland, we found the beauty we were seeking. The whole slope was a colossal, patternless sprawling rock garden that no human hands could imitate. Great jagged blocks of basalt embroidered with bright lichens and delicate mosses spilled haphazardly when the island was born, provided a bewildering multitude of dramatic backgrounds for flowered patterns. Under springy cushions of *Empetrum nigrum,* the common crowberry, which carpeted flat rock surfaces, or under flowered patches of thin soil between wind-sheltering tilted slabs, we felt the contours of the rock beneath our feet. Angles and arcs, trim rectangular basaltic blocks, and perfect lava spheres composed a harmonious, enchanting geometrical architecture. Under, over, and reaching above the rocks were the flowers. Species bloomed side by side regardless of the season. In the damp mossy grottos it was still early spring. Delicate spring beauties turned pallid faces, unflushed by the sun, upward from shadowy nooks while the shyer sturdier violets nestled confidently against the rocks. Aconite, gentian, several members of the saxifrage family (the rock breakers), arctic chrysanthemums, and the lusty, overgrown northern dandelions flowered neighborly a few feet away from spring's harbingers. The *Empetrum* crept over the rocks in dense, vivid green mantles of fine firlike needles, festooned with jet-black globular berries.

Startling among the delicate colors of spring and summer were the flashes of autumnal red and orange where leaves were already dying. The mere actions of walking were all-engrossing. It was necessary to choose carefully among the profusion of rocks a stable surface for each step, sometimes to swing over a widely gaping crevice, or crawl on all fours up slippery, *Empetrum*-shrouded embankments. Eyes and mind were too occupied with the feet to observe the scenery. So every few yards we sat down to peer into the semiburied flower worlds beneath overhanging nooks or just to absorb the details of the whole beautiful natural garden. I have seen beautiful landscapes in many countries but nowhere else has nature worship welled so vigorously in my heart.

It took us hours at our snail's pace jogging, broken by periods of rest, to reach the sea, probably only a quarter of a mile away. We walked along the wide shingle that formed a natural breakwater to wall the seas from Antone Lake. During storms so much water washes over the bouldered ramparts that frequently the lake is as salty as the ocean that mothered it.

We found a cozy rock shelter from the wind and sat down to examine the flowers I had picked. One of my pet disciplines is to leave wild flowers growing out-of-doors. I have not the same qualms about hothouse blooms, deliberately propagated to brighten homes. But I prefer to visit wildflowers in their own habitat and leave them there to delight other eyes and bring forth seed. There are rewards for such denials. I guarded a small patch of arbutus for years in New York State, where greedy hands have almost despoiled the hills of this fragile beauty. Every April I returned to greet it morning after morning, watching it bud, flower, and die and every April my eye proudly measured the spread and growth of my vine. I do allow myself to pick only specimens for study and my lab was full of treasures that morning. Not only had I gathered species completely new to me such as the arctic chrysanthemum, but I had caught up with the early flowering plants that had finished flowering in other parts of the island before we arrived. Already drooping I was holding a friend I had certainly not expected to meet on St. Paul, Claytonia, whose feminine daintiness ignores the gross fact that she is the namesake of a hearty, masculine, early American botanist, Dr. John Clayton of Virginia. Spring Beauty aptly describes her smooth complexion and wiry grace. What was she doing here among the fire-born rocks, this exquisite lady whom John Clayton had found in the warm Virginian clime? She was my childhood love ever since the first early morning when I surprised her dancing with thousands of her sisters in a stripped woodlot on a windy hilltop in the Catskills. Other familiar plants had equipped themselves for the north by growing fur. Their stems and leaves were glabrous instead of satiny to the touch. But Spring Beauty remained silky and slender limbed, a southern belle who would make no concession to inclement weather.

As I rearranged my booty I speculated on the mystery of the island flowers, how the whole landscape became, even while the last snows clung stubbornly in shadowed hollows, a green canvas spread with colors feverish enough to delight Gauguin and endless variations of blue that Picasso would have ached to capture. Nature had generously offset the lack of bright sunlight by summoning brilliance from the earth. On the greyest days the arctic poppies were a million earthbound

August 13, 1941
We both decided we would like a house made of the stones there at Antone Rocks, facing the lake beneath and the mountains across the lake and fields, and would go to town once in six months. Perfect peace and tranquility. I kept thinking how unfair it was to Tobyanne to be traveling with her across such beautiful scenes and her majesty to be missing it all.

We were utterly confused by the landscape. Made wild guesses about the point of land we could see beyond us, called it Marunich, picked out various mountains and guessed about them. Incorrectly, but at least when I got home and consulted the map in the storybook of *Matka*, I began to get one angle of the island clearly fixed in a corner of my mind, at least. And now that we have *Matka* in the house I can study the outline of this island in quiet moments and gradually get my bearings.

God, but this island is full of beauties. It is impossible to see it in a year. I would have to spend each summer day just hurrying from one spot to another in rotation to keep abreast of changing beauties in each district, before I could feel that I had really seen the heart of St. Paul.

suns to color the smoky air. Before the last poppy fades, the false arnica, *Senecio,* derived from the Latin for "old man," was vigilantly patrolling field and roadside, sand dune and scoria bank, with less graceful but as vividly yellow, broader petaled banners.

In moist spots some hardy flowers drew strength enough from the earth to push their flowering heads above the greedy grasses. That very morning we had measured some high stalks of aconite growing in a dank depression near the lake. They were over two feet high and holding many blossoms above the grass spikes. From the aconite or monkshood Kodiak islanders and possibly the Aleuts distilled poison in which they dipped their arrow points.

In the northern lands, even above the arctic circle, ice-freed earth blooms extravagantly during the brief summers. The plant kingdom of the north contains fewer subjects than in temperate zones but the lesser number of species is more than compensated by lush, tropic-like massing of the intense and vivid floral inhabitants.

Three species of lupine were in bloom on St. Paul. The blue and bluish rose varieties burned like gay candles throughout the island. But here and there, a soft clump of creamy tapers stood gracefully swaying in the wind.

Rose lupine and deeply flushed *Pedicularis* furnished the principal reds in the floral color scheme. The lupine stalks and leaves were heavily haired and looked and felt like wool. In the rain these hirsute clumps turned into silver candelabras, holding up the flower heads. The Aleuts called the lupine "the house of butterflies," but few wandering butterflies reached St. Paul to drift among them.[4]

Flower lovers, recovering from amazement at the incredible profusion of flowers, about two hundred species, might quibble that the majority lacked fragrance. The scented ones, for the most part, emitted disagreeable odors. When I brought some arctic poppies into the house and placed them in water to await pressing in the morning, I woke to a house disgustingly flavored with a fetid odor. I threw the offending poppies into an outside garbage can and threw up the windows at once.

Pootchki, the wild celery, exuded a strong sickening sweet odor that attracted flies to its umbels. I lost my last desire to sample this Aleut vegetable when I saw a vast field of rank plants holding up black flower heads. Each umbel bent under a crowding, squirming busy mass of flies. I liked *pootchki* best in the winter. Then the fields were thronged with stately snow-crowned flowers where the flakes rested lightly on the stiff, dried seedpods.

Chapter 22

Another mid-August morning we were awakened by the unaccustomed feeling of hot sun beating down upon our eyelids. The porch thermometer said sixty-three degrees. A heat wave! Fedosia and I collected a makeshift lunch. Sam coaxed an auto from the island autocrats, unwontedly mellowed by the heat. Stopping long enough to kidnap Vivian Oberg from her housework we were off toward Northeast Point to explore the northern reaches of Naseverni Beach.

The island bloomed in new colors under the sun. Gay ribbons of flowers waved jubilantly in the tender breeze. Birds ploughed the sky excitedly. From the rookeries came the protesting cacophony of the seal sun despisers. The plank road, built like a locomotive track across the unstable sands of the isthmus linking the Point to the main body of the island, was a conspicuous skeleton of bleached silver in the sunlight. From afar the group of buildings at its terminus stood out clear against the sky. On one side of the road were two bungalows, a large building for Aleut work gangs or hunting parties and a small cottage reserved for government employees on outings. Opposite them stood tumbling ruins. An old shack, its roof awry, lay nearly buried in the sand. Here, before the first island road was built, the seal skins were salted and stored.

Beyond the salt house the landscape sprouted beams and planks, the abandoned cribbing and partially sand-blocked shafts of the mines of St. Paul. Ivory mines. Long ago the sand had buried the skeletons of thousands of walrus. Their snowy tusks had been transmitted by earth's metallic influence into many-hued fossilized ivory. Under the rough outer layer of enamel, the tusks were dyed with soft creamy yellows, delicate pink flushing, deep sea–depth greens, warm browns, and, rarely, glassy black. Aleuts and officials have been laboring for seventy years to ferret out the last of the underground treasure.

In Autumn, when the crowding *pootchki* have withered and can be easily downed by the cutting edge of a spade, weekends have become consecrated to the rite of ivory digging, the most arduous mining in the world. The earth is fluid and combative. As soon as one shovelful of sand is lifted two pour into the depression. No man alone can battle the tricky, fast-flowing sand. While some dig breathlessly others insert cribbing as a barrier against the tumbling landslides. Shovel by shovel the sand is tossed away and simultaneously the planks are pushed down into position. The deeper down the harder the toil. The wet half-frozen sand grows heavier. It must be wheeled in a small barrow up sloping planks to be dumped. And at the final layer of bone debris, the diggers may find no ivory lode. Yet so intense has been man's desire for ivory that the earth looks as if gigantic moles had been tunneling for centuries or as if thousands of grave robbers had plied their trade for generations. For many of the mounds beside the pits glisten with more bone fragments than sand.

There are fairly well-defined strata of animal skeletons. Near the surface, seal bones form the thickest layer. Where sea lion killings had occurred, their large frames lie beneath the seal bones. Walrus skeletons are rarely mixed with the others, principally beneath them. Hundreds of skulls, the two long upper canines still firmly embedded in the upper jaw, have been disinterred but the hunt still goes on and prizes are still uncovered. Each year the seekers must dig through the enveloping sands. Of late few tusks have been discovered above twenty or thirty feet below the surface.

The Russians, too, prized the mellow ivory of the north. They seem to have been ignorant of the vastness of the underground trove. They exported principally "green" fresh ivory from slaughtered animals and a few fossil tusks gleaned from the storm-cleaned sand beaches of the Point.

Despite the thousands of skeletons found, the walrus never established rookeries on the island. Pribilof beaches were mere way stations on the spring and fall route of walrus migration. Fifty years ago [i.e., c. 1890] several hundred walrus could be surprised at rest on the level floor of Walrus Island during the traveling season. By 1900 a live walrus was becoming an exciting and rare visitor. The bone deposits corroborate the written record of walrus habits. The large heavy bones of the skeletons and the profusion of "tipi" bones or *ossa peni* among the remains identify the majority of the animals as male.

The puzzle is why so many died at a resting station. Did some disease spread epidemic havoc within a short period? Or are these the remains of valiant old bulls, fighting old age, striving to reach the far north and the icy breeding ground, who crawled ashore for respite and succumbed to age and exhaustion? All we know is that thousands died and their naked bones were covered by the active sand that had not ceased its sexton duties. Present-day diggers hark back wistfully to the good fortune of a group in 1926 who uncovered fifty tusks within an area of fifty square feet only two or three feet under the surface. The deeply honeycombed earth testifies that no one need hope to encounter such good fortune so easily again.

The Aleuts have dug less of late. They seem unable to collect work gangs on holidays. The few remaining Aleut ivory carvers are content to get their material pleasantly strolling the beaches after storms. I salute their common sense. No treasure on earth, it seems to me, is worth the agonizing backbreaking labor that the males from the States exerted for fossil trophies. Ironically most of the officials have acquired the hobby of ivory carving and practice it with electric drills and burrs and with great enthusiasm. I suspect the officials derive greater pleasure from the pastime because no one expects them to carve merely because their ancestors did. The Aleut craftsmen, too, are outfitted with electric carving sets from Sears Roebuck. The officials also like to take enough souvenirs back to the States to keep their memories alive and to shower their friends with mementos of the Seal Islands. The permanent islanders get low prices for their handiwork. With neither need nor commercial gain to prompt them, they prefer to ornament their homes with what is novel and unusual to them, gimcracks from mail-order houses.

The gleam of bones lured us from the car as always, to seek among the debris for teeth, seal, sea lion, or a yellowed walrus molar overlooked by the ivory miners. The chunky walrus teeth are always worn by crunching clam shells almost down to the portion inset in the socket. All three kinds of teeth could be polished and fashioned into jewelry and ornaments. But bones could be sought for in any weather. My heart and feet urged me on to Naseverni sands or "on the north beach." More and more the pleasant old Russian phrase is replaced by "North Beach."

Near Webster Lake we parked the car. Taking turns carrying the basket, we tramped over the hummocks toward the sea. The regiments of lupine rattled their dry pods ominously as we brushed them. Occasionally a pod discharged its ripe seeds toward us, a threat from a child's pistol. Our very passage became important in planting next season's flowers. We routed old bulls from their slumber in the grass. Some scuttled away grumbling. Others were so weary that they posed still as museum pieces although prepared to escaped if we came too close. We had to skirt the most southern fringe of *Vostochnie* or Eastern Rookery until we could find access to the shore without disturbing crowded seal beaches.

Emerging among scattered rocks we gasped at the gleaming scintillating carpeting of shell fragments between the boulders. Nowhere else had I found such abundance. Excitedly I dug into each miniature shell heap and collected a few dozen perfect or only slightly chipped oyster shells, worn to exquisite golden and opalescent tints. Graceful rose Oregon tritons denuded of their protective brownish green bristles, like abandoned fairy craft, lay here and there among the oyster chips. Had not the ugly jagged teeth of the underwater reefs lain in wait for such fragile jetsam, there would have been treasure on the shore to satisfy the greediest collector.

With a lunch basket grown triply heavy with its cargo of shells we reluctantly left the rocks behind us and set off down the sleek sands of Naseverni. As far as we could see southward extended a line of solitary bulls, sentinels guarding nothing but their own privacy. One by one as we neared they slipped off into the sea and swam lazily about watching us. As soon as we had passed each returned to his post to bask.

It was wonderful to walk straight toward the sun, even to have our eyes blinded by the brilliance. Nowhere could our eyes find rest. The sand beneath our feet danced, sending the sun's light stabbing up at us. The smooth blue waters shone like the lustrous face of a southern sea. By keeping my eyes closed for a few minutes I could open them and see the rude land swell that was Marunich six miles away. Beyond, the old volcanoes, wholly unwrapped from mist and rain veilings, towered in the luminous air falsely assuming a stature and majesty they did not possess.

We sprawled back against the warm sides of a barrier dune to eat our lunch, grateful for the tossing shade of the grass fringe on the dune's summit. Not until we had each devoured a ham sandwich, well spread with mustard and accompanied by a sour pickle, did we realize that I had forgotten to include a beverage. We ate fewer pickles and nibbled on apples to assuage our thirst. Otherwise the meal was a perfect picnic. No ants browsed contentedly over our food. The sand was quiet instead of invading our sandwiches. We were mindful of our fortune, savoring a day that St. Paul may not know again for years.

One visitor almost called. A bull came out of the sea. Immersed in his own thought he loped directly up the beach toward us snorting and shaking his head from side to side. We held our breaths while Sam fumbled for his camera. A few yards from us the old fellow paused and saw us. With an outraged bellow that made our hearts quake though we knew better he wheeled about and rushed for the sea. There his courage returned. Cautiously he crept back and lay down to sleep not far away from us. He wallowed in the sand and complained to the heavens about the interlopers. At last we took pity on him, roused from our pleasant after-lunch lethargy, and left his neighborhood. Had he not troubled us with his discomfort, we might have loafed the afternoon away, lulled by the soothing seal ballads from Vostochnie. The sea was mute. Gulls spoke occasionally over our heads. Then a new sound, a faint steady hum, swelled louder in the air. The seal plaint was drowned by its rough crescendo. Incredulously we stared into the sky. It was a plane. First a silvery dot no larger than a seagull. Then the great silvery wings were sweeping toward us coming lower and lower. We could see the insignia of our own Army, a dark shadow that must be the pilot. We waved frantically. It passed over us and then we saw, far below us near Marunich, its fellow patrol bomber.[1]

We watched the empty sky. A few minutes later both of them winged back over Marunich. Although they had been but wings passing we had been quickened by a poignant realization of life beyond our lonely sun-drenched beach, of affairs and men who guided the destinies of the world. A faint pang of homesickness, of longing for daily papers, crowded streets, for bustle, haste, and noise, swept over me. Then I relaxed. The world the planes came from would be mine, probably too soon. It was good to sink back into the beauty of the landscape, to taste the sun, to feel the soft sand dragging my footsteps.

When we reached the village in the later afternoon, the vibrations of excitement had not died down. Playfully the aviators had swept so low over the houses that people who had seen planes only in the movies had flung themselves on the earth expecting a swift rain of bombs. A few bold souls boasted they had seen the faces of the aviators clearly. I could imagine the pilots chuckling at the thrill they had given a lonely village. They forgot that in the most isolated byways of the earth the radio accounts of war in Europe had educated people to fear. Their exploits of skimming over the roofs, lifting their planes from one terrace level to another, left a memory that burned dreadful after the seventh of December.

Naturally no one wanted to hear about the really important event of the day, our picnic in the sun. The next day I had the painful pleasure of exhibiting a souvenir of our outing, a two-inch bracelet of sunburn on my ankles. Wary from sad experiences, I usually protected my fair skin from too prolonged sunning. My ankles unwittingly exposed while we lunched were a burnt offering of which I was proud, the one and only sunburn of which I shall ever boast. Never before had a physician of St. Paul had the opportunity to enter in his log the phrase "treated for sunburn." The next mail carried testimonial snapshots of our outing to friends who had worried lest in the far north I miss my perpetual picnicking.

Chapter 23

After I had trampled several beaches, peered into rock crevices, searched industriously the length and breadth of each sandy sea rim, I rechristened St. Paul the Island of Broken Shells. A few handfuls of shells, most of them chipped and battered, were slender gleaning for diligent hunting. Had I not fared north with the fixed notion that seashores and tide-abandoned mollusks inevitably go together I might have learned from books or people that regions touched by floe ice harbor few mollusks and that few shells were apt to withstand the buffeting against Pribilof rocky sea edges. Occasionally a perfect specimen of the less than two hundred known species of the region rewarded my unceasing vigilance. Ironically this bivalve is more attractive to the nonscientific collector when its shell has been divested of its chestnut-colored cloak and polished by the friction of wave and rock and sand to glowing nacre, purple, and delicate rose brilliance.

The lure of the happy accident of coming upon an unmarred specimen imbued the briefest seaside stroll with excitement. Had we been able to fill our pockets on our first outing, shell stalking might have grown a dull pursuit at once. Instead the next-to-the-last day I spent on St. Paul I was hunting a tiny striped snail on the slippery kelp-entwined rocks off Marunich with so much gusto that my mind was utterly free from anxiety or even the remembrance that Japanese foes were not many miles away.

Two beaches near the village were daily goals, easily accessible when cars were not available for distant journeys or when time was limited by medical duties. Less than half a mile apart, these beaches belonged to different worlds. Black Bluffs turned its somber naked face seaward and guarded a short range of shingle. Zolotoi Sands was as familiar as the strand of an Atlantic pleasure resort, for that unmistakable trace of civilization, garbage, littered the soft shore.

Black Bluffs must have been named at storm time for I have seen its burned brownish red face darkened when the sky turned black and the sea boiled among the beach boulders. The village slope of Black Bluffs is such a gentle hill that it is startling to reach the abrupt brim and look down a hundred and ten feet to the rocks at its base and the dock at East Landing. It is nothing but a large ash pile,

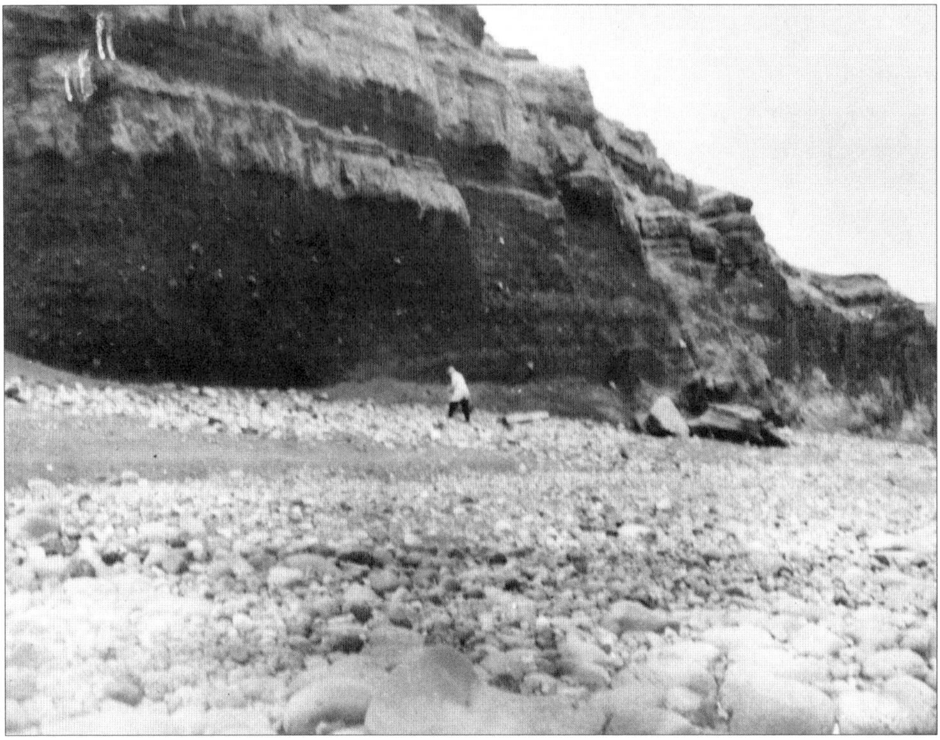

Fredericka Martin at Black Bluffs (from the Martin Collection, USUAF210, Archives, Alaska and Polar Regions, Rasmuson Library, University of Alaska Fairbanks).

grass grown and flower decked on its inland incline, bald brown along its crumbling brink. Not a thread of vegetation clings to its seaward-scape where the rough, irregular cinders are packed together with various matrices in strata of diverse blending and conflicting colors.

Red and orange-brown strata of cinders are banded one upon another with an occasional vein of chocolate clay or broad grey sticky cement streaks. Rocks and boulders, reddish shale-crumbling slabs, spherical pebbles dot the surface wartily. Rarely did we traverse the shingle without seeing a few protruding rocks break off and slip stridently down, sometimes too close for comfort. The lower quarter of the cliff had a smoother surface from long washing by waves during high seas. Early spring, when frost is loosening the breccia, or just after storms was a time for wary walking as far as possible from the foot of the cliff. During the thaw period, Black Bluffs became almost animate, waiting to hurl one or more of its gargoyle boulders or unloose a formidable landslide when a human being approached. Yet just at such times do the curious want most to linger at the cliff's foot.

Buried in the walls of Black Bluffs are the only clues to the age of the Pribilofs or, more truly, of St. Paul. When the sea floor cracked under the pressure of volcanic action thousands of living sea creatures were trapped and encased in molding rock that preserved their form, imprint, or actual shell. Nowhere else in the island group has a shred of fossil remains been found.[1] Although Black Bluffs has suffered more dramatic wind- and sea-wrought erosion and has shrunken far back from the sea its veins still bear a host of fossils. The winter waves cut away so much of its bases that huge masses of breccia deprived of support crash to the beach splitting into thousands of chunks exposing conglomerate masses of grey rock decorated with fossil imprints or fracturing smaller global fragments so that the actual fossilized mollusks protrude like petrified birds from a sculptured nest.

By the summer's close I had collected a few rocks marked with the faint indentations of shells. During my winter readings I came across photographs that revealed the enormous loss of bulk the cliff had suffered. As winter proceeded I watched the bluff being battered, broken, and changed into a new piece of scenery. By spring a new cliff face greeted us. We had fresh, raw-edged slabs of breccia to climb over or skirt on our walks. The upper edge was scarred with unfamiliar scallops from the recent landslides. Vertical fissures had breached the sea wall. Familiar earth cracks had been filled in by breccia debris. The lower sea-washed portion was a smoother curved indentation. Our footsteps crunched in the unsettled layer of lately fallen cinders. We wore high boots to avoid filling our shoes with irritating sharp particles as we sank deeply into the loose debris.

The fossil clues have not yet settled definitely the geologic birth date of St. Paul. Just before 1850 Il'ia Voznesenskii of the Imperial Academy of Sciences of St. Petersburg examined Black Bluffs and gathered specimens.[2] Dall's investigation in 1868 will be remembered because at least one fossilized species bears his name. Elliott, Brown, Palmer, and Townsend collected many specimens for our Natural History Museum. The specimens of American scientists are not very old. Although there is disagreement as to whether certain forms found belong to the Tertiary period or to the post-Pliocene era, the specimens have living counterparts in the Bering Sea today and could be dredged from the seabed not far from Black Bluffs. Whether living forms were caught up from the sea waters and imprisoned in the breccia or whether fossil beds on the sea floor were disrupted and the fragments incorporated in the body of the cliff is another matter for speculation. Perhaps both processes contributed to the accumulation. As all the fossils have descendants alive in the neighboring sea, St. Paul is geologically brand new. That conclusion would be accepted without question if the Russian collector's list of specimens did not contain names that belong to an older geological period. Possibly these names result from errors in identification and classifications. If not, the collection may contain fossil forms from the sea sediment tossed carelessly by the seismic action into company with living forms that had been flitting about their calcareous tombs. The chance that they too were living during the island's birth casts just enough doubt to keep scientists interested in every new specimen uncovered and seeking further confirmation of St. Paul's natal date.

In March we braved bouncing pebbles, the suddenly personified boulder that jumped down at us, and gathered splendid specimens. I found a few cardia embedded in crumbling rock, the brittle shells intact until the gentlest touch shattered them. Some shells were as brightly colored as the fresh young specimens I found in the sea wrack on the same afternoon. Others were ghostly white with a prison pallor befitting their age and situation. When the shells of the cardia fell apart the fossil of the once living animal was polished so highly that it seemed a brown or grey glass reproduction of a mollusk, soft to the touch like sculptured marble.

Not all life on or near Black Bluffs was entombed and mummified. The kelp beds at its foot were alive with marine snails and limpets. Sandpipers and turnstones loved the flat kelp-festooned rocks exposed at low tide. On its upper shelves in tiny recesses the rosy finches nested. These most companionable of the island birds lingered all winter about the village, haunting the houses for stray crumbs and suet.

At the northern end of the beach a formation of rocks, once aptly labeled the "Round Tower" on the maps but nameless today, terminated the cliff arc. A high platform of convoluted lava abutted seaward in front of the tower. Peering around the tower from the slippery rim of this balcony I caught sight of a picturesque arch built of gleaming lava blocks. Shadows darkened the opening and my imagination ran away with me while I waited for a day when low tide and sun-dried rocks enabled a clumsy pregnant woman to find safe footholds. I approached the entrance, stepped into the shadows, and found myself staring at oozing muddy walls a few feet from me. My fairy castle was only an ugly dank shaft. I was comforted when I climbed its broken side and found a natural seat sheltered on three sides from the wind. Sam and I loafed there frequently watching the theater in and on the sea.

From Kitovi Point, the next land projection to the north, troops of young seals came swimming in orderly single file and broke into dolphin leaps one after another as if at a trainer's command. Alternating ordinary swimming with breaching, as the graceful arching leap is termed, the procession would proceed until the leader deemed it too close to the man-haunted dock of East Landing. He swerved abruptly and started back to Kitovi, his followers whipping in his wake as in a game of follow-the-leader.

The first time we explored the rim of Black Bluffs we reached the top by climbing a steep point near Tower Rock. On a narrow ledge, which we could sit on without straddling only by extending our legs carefully in front of us, we dropped down to catch our breath. Sam behind and above me complained that he was sinking into a hole. When we started off, I climbed to his resting place and realized he had been reposing on the entrance of an obviously inhabited fox burrow. If the occupants were at home they missed a rare opportunity to attack one of their enemies in a vulnerable area. It taught us to part the thick vegetation warily when we sat down in grassy spots. The foxes that resided along Black Bluffs attempted to feed on our friends the rosy finches. I always wished them ill hunting when I saw them prowling in the neighborhood.

My first pets on St. Paul came from the beach at Black Bluffs. I started an aquarium with a few dozen of the small purplish brown sea snails in a Pyrex baking dish. The experiment was brief. Daily we brought them fresh seawater. The labor did not discourage us but the inability to provide them with the merest slit of air space without their escaping did. It is very unpleasant to cross waxed floor space and hear the crunch of a shattering shell as a fugitive snail met with a fatal traffic accident. We found them crawling everywhere on the floor and the furniture. Unless I gave them frequent ventilation the creatures turned bottoms up in a few hours. I repopulated the aquarium a few times from the millions that lived at East Landing and then decided to use my casserole for more practical and normal purposes.

Homeward from Black Bluffs we never came empty handed, if laden with no more than a bird feather or a curious-shaped cinder. We found a knotted club of driftwood, a more fiendish and brutal weapon than any caveman's club of fact or fiction. It gave our living room a grotesque air. Sam found a piece of whalebone, rubbed by rock and wave out of all semblance to known anatomical structure. It seemed ideal for a wall shelf. Being weighed down with fossils, Sam carefully wrote, "Please deliver to the Doctor's house" and parked it on a sturdy breccia ledge that seemed high above the waterline. A storm delayed our return for a couple of days. When we sought our new house furnishing, the breccia shelf was gone and our bone fragment with it. Weeks later the slab of bone washed back. It eventually reached our front porch but never our wall.

I found an interestingly hollowed stone that I thought might be a primitive Aleut lamp. Since oldtimers scoffed, I restrained my hopes although I was sure I could trace the tool marks in the hollowed space. Dr. Hrdlička's definite decision that it was a man-worked vessel gave me untold joy. To think that back in civilization I can look at that lump of rock, at a reminder of those harried, beaten Aleut hunters who camped out near Black Bluffs obedient to their Russian master's will. It is a reminder both of the tragedy of a people and a spot of earth where I was very, very happy.

Zolotoi Pesok, the Golden Sand, conjures up a sunlit glittering beach. I rashly assumed one of those fur-mad Russian hunters nursed a poetic but inaccurate spark. Zolotoi sands were sleekly soft and grey darkening to purplish black when wet. Veniaminov disillusioned me about the name's origin.[3] When the Russians arrived the floor of the cove was hidden under the crowds of sea otter. Their soft silky pelt was the beach's gold. The Chinese market paid a fabulous price for perfect skins. The ugly murderous mass slaughter to fulfill the dream of gold to be garnered in oriental bazaars inspired the island's most romantic place name.

The first hunters had specific quotas or definite hours for securing furs for their employers. Like the Fouke Fur boys of 1941, they spent many leisure hours gambling. They played for higher stakes than the low ones permitted by island agents during recent years to prevent the men from losing their carfare home. Dice as well as cards amused the Russians. They had the right of peltry, of procuring and sealing as many furs as they wished for their personal enrichment. Their gambling counters were always at hand, either drying on a frame outside their huts or still alive on a nearby shore. It was customary for the winner to step to the threshold, point out a fine sleek animal, the fur of which he deemed sufficient recompense for his winnings. The loser would immediately creep upon the luckless animal, club him, and bring back the warm oozing pelt to settle his debt. Reckless slaughter to satisfy the company's orders and gambling debts despoiled the sea otter herd. Six years after the Pribilofs were discovered only an occasional otter appeared. After 1811 none ventured back. The refugees had found lonelier kelp beds far from man's neighborhood.

The garbage that cluttered the beach often prevented our loitering. I credited it at first to passing ships. I soon realized that no such armadas plied the Bering. I stumbled across a bottle from the dispensary. Local garbage, I found, was dumped from two points along the cliff behind the house. From both, the currents carried all floatable material to mar the lovely beach.

I found fragile rose limpets on *Zolotoi Pesok,* so minute that I gathered one only by sliding my fingernail beneath it. Occasionally the sea tossed up perfect sand dollars, so lovely a shell when bleached that I would not trade one for the silver dollar it resembles. The delicate filigree on the upper half of the shell is one of nature's daintiest designs. Dried specimens I kept in thick cotton. They dissolved into grey chalky powder at the slightest pressure.

Zolotoi in early autumn was the playground of Reef pups. Swimming clumsily the pups sought the cove because the rougher waves they could not swim under or through tumbled them on soft sand instead of bold rocks. We spent long afternoons in rocky nooks close to the sand watching thousands of pups romping. Frequently our own offspring lay swaddled in blankets in a rock niche, sleeping unaware of the other young Pribilovians so near her.

The oldest swam well and were practicing breaching. At first they leaped above the water and fell back lumpishly, to be picked up by an incoming wave and tossed carelessly ashore like driftwood. Squealing and shaking their heads vehemently they snapped angrily at the water, tried to bite the waves, and waddled about the beach sputtering and bumping into one another. Then off to charge the wave once more determined to conquer. Back they came more indignant but never too discouraged to try again immediately. Their antics were always fascinating. Ashore they mocked their elders' behavior, lunging at one another like fighting bulls. They worried strands of kelp like puppies enjoying bedroom slippers. They sat fanning and scratching with the sophisticated nonchalance of their parents. No gesture belonged to their youth alone.

Lonely was Zolotoi in November when the pups had gone south, sturdy tireless swimmers fit to life in the ocean until the next morning. Then the shore became an animate actor that we came frequently to see perform. The wide sandy swathe of beach was submerged. Water and sand writhed and seethed where we had walked all summer. The invading water propelled by violent winter tides and winds clawed at the tall grass-topped dunes that had stood so proudly beyond the reach of summer seas, leaving massive indented wounds in their smooth sides, biting enormous chunks of sand from their flanks. Snow fell along the edges of the caldron. The waves paved the drifts with sand. The mixture froze into a cement highway that we raced quickly across to reach Reef. The familiar way was bleak and fierce and frequently remodeled.

Gradually the sea withdrew. Our friendly summer beach was partially restored to us. Former rocky resting places were lost in the sand. Dunes sprawled drunkenly from the waves' lashing. New dunes stood up where a sand flat had lain smoothly. The ground gave unexpectedly beneath our feet where buried snow was melting. We had watched the elements at work remaking the island's face. In the spring sunshine we knelt on the new clean sands to gather rose limpets and, on an ecstatic afternoon, six perfect sand dollars.

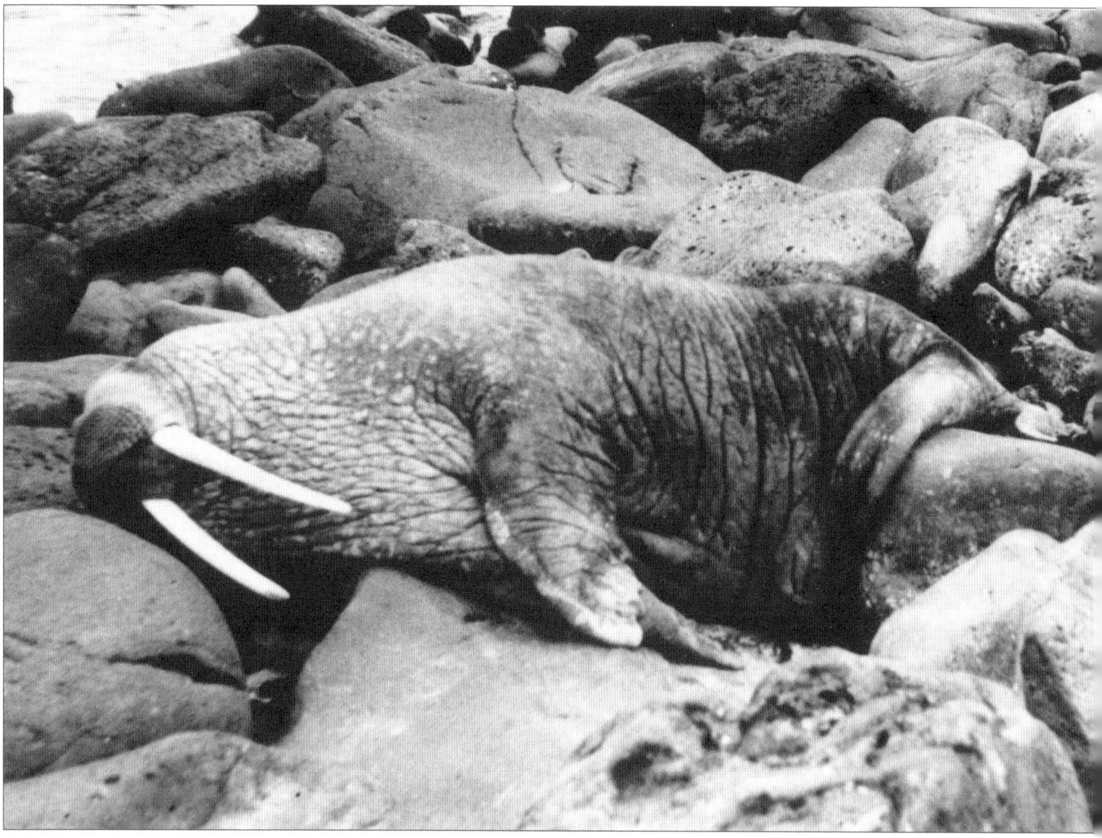

The walrus at Northeast Point (from the Martin Collection, USUAF210, Archives, Alaska and Polar Regions, Rasmuson Library, University of Alaska Fairbanks).

Chapter 24

Sunday the twenty-fourth of August was an ordinary day. As we drove toward Northeast Point in the afternoon, the sky was brightened by the sun, which never quite shone through the clouds. Fine rain bombarded the windshield spasmodically. Jack Eggis, Lowell Livingood, Ford Wilke, one of the two young biologists who had arrived on the *Spica* to study seal life, Sam, and I strolled leisurely along the borders of the rookeries watching the seals enjoy their freedom from harem bondage. Far back in the grass the seals were sprawled in lazy sleeping groups, males and females, young and old intermingling. Pods of pups gamboled near them, careful not to disturb their tranquil elders too often. Lone pups wandered up and down between the water's edge and the green fields bawling hungrily for their mothers.

At the shore we sat quite close to the kingdom of the sea lions. Some basked on the rocks. Others sported in the sea mingling sociably with hundreds of seals. Comfortably ensconced in rock nooks we were content to loaf and be entertained. We chuckled over impish pups. We admired the regal poses, the sleek majesty of sea lion bulls or the graceful breaching of swimming seals. Mother sea lions hovered around their young, supervising their swimming efforts. One leonine male was spread out over the beach shapeless as a collapsed circus tent. Only his magnificent massive head set back in carven dignity identified him. A whim to bathe in the sea set him in sudden motion. His enormous body moved agilely seaward. At the brink, indifferent to other bathers, he threw himself from a ledge and unloosed a tidal wave that sprouted upward, tangled full of squirming astonished animals. One squealing pup was lifted skyward and then tumbled back into the safety of the sea. With the characteristic resilience of youth, the pup resumed paddling as if nothing had happened as soon as he felt the comforting natural embrace of the waves.

The afternoon ebbed quickly away. Sam, Ford, and Lowell prowled back and forth snapping pictures whenever the light seemed graciously favorable. I sat lazily talking with Jack. Jack chewed snoose and spat at curious pups. The kelp-stained brownish yellow teeth of the pups made them seem his companions in the

August 25, 1941
Saturday [August 23] we continued our dawdling. I completed volume 4 of the investigation of 1896 and read and inserted markers for finding interesting bits for the book in reports, almost continuous from 1920 until 1935. Sam spent some time with John Yatchmeneff, developing pictures. Mr. Hellbaum was with them both for a time.

Sunday we slept latish. At seven when I was awake for an interval, the front windows were veiled in white fog. But when we rose a couple of hours later, the weather was clear and the sun came out to warm us. We discovered that Heretina had arrived and was busy cleaning up the office. I decided not to discourage her. But had her do the most important tasks of the day and sent her off after lunch to go on a picnic with her family.

The combination of sun and ripe berries on the island seemed to have stimulated the wanderlust in every heart on the island.

Sam went reconnoitering about the chance of a drive and came back to announce that we could go out to Northeast Point with Jack Eggis and a few of the boys. We had lunch. The Yatchmeneffs dropped by for a little visit. They seem very nice people indeed. They also were on the lookout for a drive. Several trucks just jammed with people had already left the village. When the car stopped for us there was still a crowd standing at the machine shop awaiting their turn.

vice of tobacco chewing. The pups could not leave us alone. They sniffed at our boot tips and hissed disapproval. They retreated still facing us, snorting frenziedly. They baaed like lambs with sore throats. One chap fleeing from us looked back over his shoulder and went sprawling over a rock. The racket he made showed he blamed us for his loss of dignity. He was physically unhurt, protected by his wadding of blubber. No one could ever call a seal pup pretty. Most of their charm I think comes from their constant activity despite their ball-like figures and the ironical combination of chattering exhortations and the comic popping eyes streaming endless chains of tears.

Half dreaming, absorbed by the animal theater, I thought how insatiable human beings were. A few weeks before I had been overjoyed and full of awe to approach the rocky ledges of the sea lion. Now I neighbored with them companionably, accepting them as part of my ordinary life and dreamed of walrus and hoped the winter ice floe would carry a polar bear within my vision. Almost impossible dreams. No living bear had been ashore since 1870. Almost a quarter of a century had passed without anyone meeting a stray walrus guest. To leave the islands without a glimpse of a walrus seemed worse than visiting Manhattan and failing to look at the Statue of Liberty.

Jack, Sam, and I walked back to the car to await the others. I felt chilly. We had taken a direct path through knee-high *pootchki.* The wet embracing leaves had finally soaked through my heavy corduroy slacks. I was anxious to return to town and steam heat. When the boys caught up to us, Ford, whose drawling manner of speech persists when he is most excited, was insistently interested in the laws concerning walrus hunting. I explained the regulations, renewed almost automatically every three years. Only Alaskan Natives were permitted to kill them for food. An occasional scientist could obtain a permit to collect one or two specimens.

My wet legs were turning to ice but his questioning continued. How often were walrus seen on St. Paul? When was the last visitor there? Finally he smiled broadly and pointed toward the beach, "There's a walrus down there asleep." We stared at him. It could not be true. A miracle had happened.[1] Could we reach the spot again before the walrus finished his nap?

I forgot cold damp slacks and numb legs as we dashed heedlessly through the same wet thickets of vegetation. When we reached the stones we slowed our pace, picking our footholds cautiously to avoid dislodging a loose chunk of lava. Then we saw him, still asleep on his rocky couch. Only one tusk was visible as he lay stretched full length on his side. My heart thumped wildly. How quickly my dream had come true. Had I been touching a wishing stone when my thoughts had turned to walrus? There he was, almost a phantom beast, legendary, a true symbol of the past grandeur of the great beasts of the sea.

We crept closer. Only Sam had unused film, just part of a roll. Sam usually consulted a Kodak instruction book before he essayed pictures. Forgetting at the moment to seek details about light, perspective, focus, he was advancing straight toward the sleeping beast with his camera glued to his eye. Ford and Lowell crept closer until the walrus was almost encircled. Sam began to snap photographs. The walrus opened his small eyes lazily. He lifted his head, turning a surprisingly amiable face toward us. Instantly we were as rigid as the rocks we stood on. The yellowish brown hairs on his rounded

August 25, 1941
Wilke told us yesterday that he and his companion had been instructed to survey and take soundings in the lagoon to see whether it were capable of landing a seaplane. Now they intend to do the same at Big Lake. If the results are good, Dr. Scheffer hopes to take a census of the seal rookeries by air photographs next year. Serious doubt about the rate of annual increase being eight percent evidently exists. Too bad Johnston is not engaged in this angle of the work but is a bureau functionary for all more commonplace details. He is a born naturalist and probably no one could excel him in power of observation and in judgment.

Andy Holland, the Company House cook, is a sketch. He calls the scientists "bug hunters" in such a tone. He told us that a couple of years ago a scientist from Ann Arbor was here, among other places, studying the work of the Bureau. And when he got back to Seattle, he had an interview with reporters and was quoted as saying, "After the whites and the Fouke Fur Company get through, there is very little left for the poor Natives. They come right up and steal the seals off their doorsteps." And, of course, he lost his job, ended Andy. He said the name was Hub or Hubbard.

"The seals," said Andy, shaking his head sagely, "have been coming here for thousands of generations without political or financial advice from anyone." He alludes to Dr. Scheffer as the "Flying Dutchman."

nose stuck straight out, reminding me of a withering cactus. I caught a glint of ivory. When he lifted his head from the ground I saw that one tusk was broken. The beasts use their backward-slanting tusks to dig clams and other shellfish from the sand. They either wear away a portion of the tusk gradually or accidentally break off a piece against a rock. Mac had told us men often killed walrus merely to open the body and extract a few quarts of freshly swallowed clams, which they rinsed and cooked. A roundabout and cruel way to get a seafood dinner if true. In all likelihood, this is one of the tall tales of the north.

As our guest was about to settle to napping again, Lowell's foot slipped. Never had the clatter of rock against rock been so thunderous to my ears. Without unseemly haste the walrus raised his head, stared once in our direction, and swerved toward the sea. It was the hour for the movie camera. Sam's pictures were a perfect running sequence of the beast's movements. Heartbroken at his desertion, we watched him plunge into the sea. Without a backward glance at his admirers, he swam steadily down the coast out of sight.

Had Lowell's balance been steadier, we intended to race villageward to rouse everyone to inspect the visitor as soon as the pictures were taken. Instead, we had to face the envious eyes of every inhabitant. We gave dozens of sets of photographs away as consolation. Searching parties haunted the eastern beaches for two days before it was definitely concluded that the walrus had sought a quieter refuge to finish his nap.

The walrus is a member of the *Odobenidae* family whose most striking characteristic is the elongations of the upper canine teeth. His yellowish brown rugose coat is almost hairless. His tail and the nails on his flippers are vestigial. His haunts are arctic waters whether above the Atlantic or Pacific. The Pacific species has longer, heavier tusks. The male grows to between ten and eleven feet long and weighs between two and three thousand pounds. Our guest was a full-grown male.

When Sam developed his pictures and realized how near he had been to that huge body he was astounded. Intently viewing the animal through the viewfinder he had been unaware of the diminishing space between them. Fortunately the walrus had no desire to tangle with a camera fiend.

Chapter 25

Five days after we encountered the walrus, Tobyanne was born a little after eight in the morning. All day Thursday I was impatient at the tiny premonitory pain that foretold her coming. While I fretted at nature's dilatory methods I supervised the installation of hospital furniture in our bedroom and its vigorous cleaning. I never realized that Heretina, who had started to work for us just a week before and now wielded her disinfectant-tainted washcloth, was very puzzled at the transfer of delivery-room fixtures to our own sleeping room.

Fortunately we had many callers during the day to divert Sam. He was most anxious about the progress of her successful arrival. I was complacently, smugly wrapped in the certainty that this delivery was to be the most successful I had ever witnessed or assisted. I was not able to imbue Sam with my own assurance. He was longing for civilization where he might pace a corridor in the ordinary expectant-father role, trusting in the skill of a specialist. While he sat tense and miserable, I curled up on the couch, impatient but delighted that the nine-month vigil was so soon to be ended, eager to meet my daughter.

August 12, 1941
I don't think Sam is sleeping well and I hope it is not too much due to worry over the ordeal of delivering the baby. I am getting very anxious to have the baby arrive, not because I am worried but the time is so close and I am anxious to see what my little companion looks like. Awfully excited about it. And now that Sam is more at ease and relaxed he is very sweet about the baby, despite his worries.

At the last moment a little nagging doubt assailed me. Perhaps not a daughter. Hastily I ran over all the names of boys I could think of and decided Christopher would do if my daughter failed to arrive.

By midnight I was weary of being the center of curious eyes who watched my every breath for a sign of greater pain. Besides, I was anxious for solitude to finish "Mountain Meadow," one of Lord Tweedsmuir's engrossing adventure tales. Rudely, I ordered out the kindly visitors and sent Sam to lie down, although I knew he could not sleep. At two thirty I had just turned the last page of my story when I received the sharp signal I had been waiting for. Actual labor

August 17, 1941
We really had a pleasant social chat but this social life is killing us. Every evening either out or at home. But I suppose we should really be thankful that the people are as nice as they are and that they like us, instead of being completely isolated.

But every night.

Mrs. Elliott just dropped in to say that the little Hellbaum youngster is having a birthday today and she wanted a medicine box to wrap the ivory cross Mr. Elliott had made her. I am trying to think what I can dig up to give her.

Mrs. E. also volunteered her assistance when Tobyanne arrives. That may be a ticklish situation for I hate to have people's feeling hurt because they aren't allowed to hold my hand. But the fewer people around, the better it suits me. I'd rather be alone, even without Sam, until I absolutely need his help. I realize more and more how swell he is to be willing to deliver me all by himself.

For the first time Fedosia abandoned the scorched-earth policy in baking, and the oatmeal cookies she made were soft and edible without dunking.

Sam's shirts are surely going to the devil up here. I had hoped that there would be some on board the boat, but so far the only package put ashore has been the botany book from mother.

It is noon now and the ham is ready for lunch when Sam comes. And I must turn to something else. I think I will try another version of our being tempted to come here.

pains at last. I waited a quarter of an hour before rousing Sam, until I was sure of my symptoms.

It was at last time for me to go to work and prepare my delivery room. As if I were preparing for a patient, I scrubbed my hands, donned sterile gown, mask, and gloves, and began to unwrap packages of sterile goods. Pausing to rest between the pains, I worked as quickly as I could. Double participation in such an event had advantages. Instead of succumbing to pain, my attention was centered on preparing every detail of equipment so carefully that Sam could work efficiently without nursing assistance. I poured out sterile solutions in bowls on one table, Merthiolate, green soap, glycerin, and covered them with a sterile sheet. My linen and instrument tables stood ready, also covered with heavy sterilized sheeting. One table, pushed to the side, I grimaced at defiantly. Here I had laid out obstetrical forceps, tubes of suture material, and instruments in case surgical repair was necessary. They were there as sensible precautions and for Sam's peace of mind. I was too egotistically set on doing a good job of bringing a child into the world to regard them as my assistants.

At last every detail was in readiness, as perfectly arranged as in the best hospital delivery room. Even the hypodermic of pituitrin, to be administered after birth, was ready, the needle protected in a pledget of alcohol-soaked cotton.

It was after four o'clock. I was glad to climb into my own bed and relax between the waves of pain. During the next four hours Sam urged me to take a little lemon-yellow capsule, a dainty pellet that promised respite and escape from reality. When I continued to refuse, he left several on the bedside table to haunt me. Sometimes the capsules swelled into grotesque sulphurous giants, with thick derisive lips ridiculing my human weakness, daring me to take them. I would grin back at the imagined specter and vow mutely, "I am not going to take you and lie here quiescent, prolonging my muscles' efforts. I am in haste to meet my Tobyanne. I want us both to be wide awake when we meet." And then it would be necessary to clench my hands lest they disobey my will and grasp the alluring medication.

As the night bore steadily toward dawn, I whispered often to Tobyanne, to encourage us both, "This is just one more steep cliff to ascend. We've been running up cliffs together all summer. Just a little longer climb and we'll stand on the headland and see the ocean streaming by and feel the wind ruffling our hair."

I have seen hundreds of babies born. I know, as well as any onlooker can, the agony of childbirth. Even after I had been nursing for years, I've choked up and wiped away tears while I cursed the cruel natural laws of birth. Yet as the life-bringer, I, a woman of thirty-six having her first child, put away my hatred of birth processes and played a game with my aborning child. "We've been running up and down so many hillsides all summer. A little higher and we'll reach the summit," over and over I whispered and, then, Tobyanne was crying out the reply I had been waiting for. Her fresh voice was caroling our successful journey through the shadows of pain to the heights of joy.

The bright light of day was streaming in through the windows. Tobyanne, bright-eyed, vibrant, a light wisp of delicate flesh, lay in my arms and Sam's tired and beautifully happy face leaned protectingly above us. We three had reached the hilltop together and could rejoice in the new day, the new life that had begun for the three of us on that island in the endless space that men call the world.

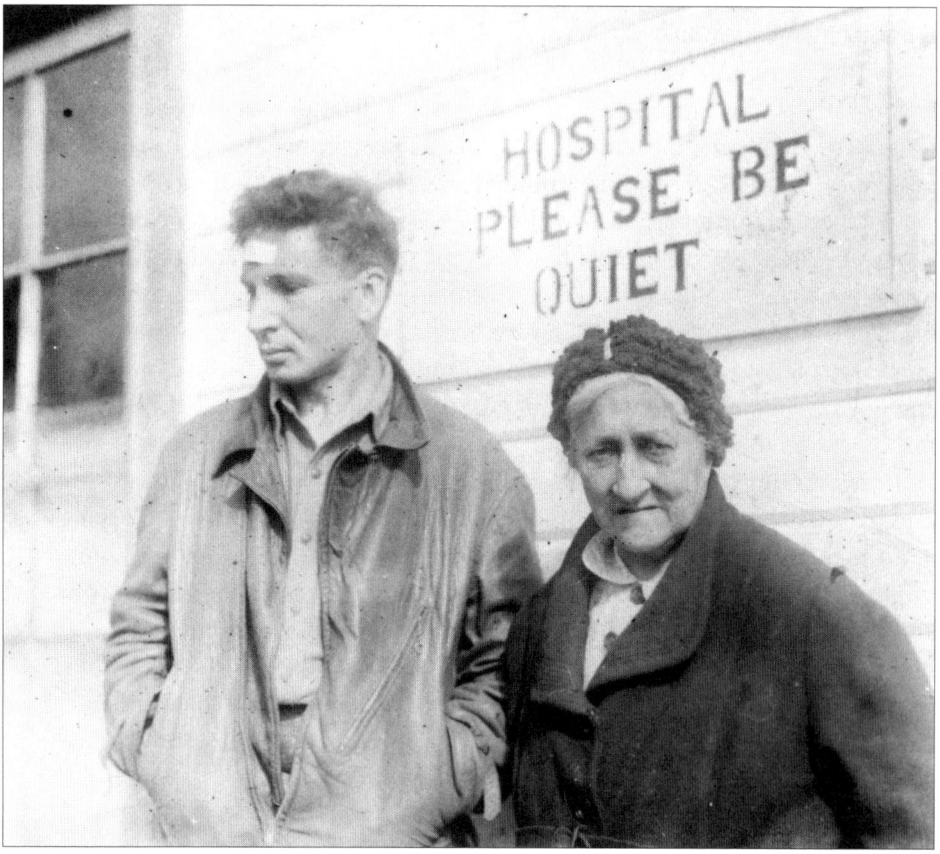

Samuel Berenberg and Anna Stepetin (from the Martin Collection, USUAF210, Archives, Alaska and Polar Regions, Rasmuson Library, University of Alaska Fairbanks).

Chapter 26

Comedy entered my bedroom at nine o'clock. Heretina came large-eyed and incredulous to meet the lively new member of the family. Having failed to recognize the portents from my appearance, she had been utterly baffled by the introduction of hospital furnishings into our home. Her elation dulled a little when she realized daily diaper washing had been added to her household duties. She became attached to the baby and proud of her proximity to "Snow White," as the village youngsters christened Tobyanne. Heretina could see the baby have a bath any day she liked. Other girls who wanted to attend the rite had to come ask for the privilege.

Postnatal confinement to bed differed little from such an experience in the allegedly more comfortable atmosphere of the States. The wives of other employees came to help. For most of them it meant mainly supervision of Heretina who patiently bore with a succession of bosses. Inez Elliott, frail wife of the radio operator, was a trained nurse. For a couple of weeks despite her own poor health, she came in, trim and professional in her starched white uniform, to give me the necessary professional nursing care. She took my place as Sam's assistant when Andre Melovidov was born in September. Dainty foods, books, magazines, and precious flowers raised in the greenhouse by Service wives flowed in an unending stream from the members of official families.

There were many Aleut callers, too, coming with gifts. Almost first to arrive was old Anna Stepetin, wheezing after her climb up our front steps and laughing joyously as she rocked Tobyanne in her arms and crooning Russian endearments. She procured a fluffy cap from her pocket, apologizing for the lavender ribbon laced through the brim. For weeks small paper parcels arrived containing knitted or crocheted gifts tossed off by Anna's busy fingers. She had all the pride and interest of a real grandmother.

Five-year-old Lubova Stepetin called Friday afternoon. Although she had been motherless for two years, she was still searching for an ideal mother to replace the loving one that tuberculosis had stolen. Her foster mother, John Hanson's wife, was kind but too old and reserved of manner to fill the void in

> October 27, 1941
> After nearly two months I shall begin to pick up the thread of our lives for our memory book. A vast variety of details and slight anecdotes may never be recorded but the general tenor of the past weeks has been baby care and resting in bed trying to get completely well from the complications of childbirth. It has been a trying period for Sammie but washing diapers and holding bottles is not so nerve-wracking for him as waiting for the delivery.
> . . .
> Friday afternoon [October 24] Sam and I went up to Government House to see the starving pup that they were trying to nurse by forced feedings of milk. . . . I took the opportunity while there to look over some of the books in the library and brought down an armload to work with. Sunday Sam and I enjoyed reading part of the 1913 hearings when Elliott was presenting his case about the dishonesty practiced on the islands and covered up by scientists, including David Starr Jordan, against whom he was most bitter, and government and previous company agents. So far in our reading, I am inclined to believe him. While we were reading, Mrs. McMillin arrived with an armload of magazines for our perusal and informed us that the island had once possessed a copy of Elliott's monograph on the seals (1882) but that it had disappeared from the doctor's house during 1926 or 1927. So there seems no hope of finding it among the jumble of books in the lab as I had faintly hoped.

Lubova's aching heart. We played our usual game. Lubova turned the pages of a magazine until she found a picture of the true triangle of life: man, woman, and child. Then we began our ritual, Lubova identifying the figures to her satisfaction and I confirming her statements. "That's the doctor. He's my father. That's a lady. That's you. She's my mother. The little girl is me," she said. "Where is Tobyanne?" I queried tactlessly as a trio representing us prepared to get on a train. Lubova's lovely deep brown eyes filled with tears. "She isn't here," she cried fiercely. A few minutes later Lubova said good-bye and departed with a handful of cookies as consolation. From that evil day forward, Lubova's visits were infrequent. She never evinced interest in the old magazine game. Had Tobyanne's arrival shattered an intense optimistic dream? I fear that it did.

Old Metrofan, temporarily out of the hospital, came in huffing and puffing to inspect the baby and received a stern reprimand from Sam for walking so far. Unabashed, he sipped tea and gave me advice about bringing up children.

Convalescence was brightened by new arrivals. Father Makary Baranoff returned to resume charge of the village church after a year's absence. The ringing sound of his resonant voice when he opened the door evoked pleasure. Ford Wilke and his fellow scientist, Hank Banner, dropped in more and more frequently as our acquaintance deepened into friendship. Dr. John P. Harrington, of the Smithsonian's Bureau of American Ethnology, arrived on the same boat with Father Baranoff to begin a thorough study of the Aleut language. He was accompanied by two assistants. Almost immediately he was lending me books and coming in frequently to share interesting bits of knowledge with us.

At last Sam, strict about long bed rest after childbirth, began to relax his regulations. I ventured out of doors on wobbly legs, walking a little farther each day. Life had a new rhythm dictated by Tobyanne's needs. Her simple wants imposed on us regularly, inflexible but not confining. She woke, ate, and slept in perfect accord with her schedule. Her presence gently disciplined us to adhere to a routine of work and play and helped protect us from succumbing to temptations to idle free hours away. For the time had come to stop dallying and begin a systematic study of the history of the island, of the Aleuts, and to uncover the *via dolorosa* that the Aleuts had followed to their debased present that troubled my heart and conscience.

Armed with notebook and pencil I began to spend more of each day poring over the pertinent books in the island library, winning the confidence of the Aleuts I knew best, and recording the facts they chose to disclose. Simultaneously with my detective work I prepared mail for all my friends and acquaintances for the last outgoing boat of the autumn to carry south. When the enormous mass of correspondence was ready, the personal letters padded with copies of daily journal notes, we estimated that I was sending out more than a hundred thousand words. Just in letters. The figure astounded me so that I sat back to work at the past more determinedly than before. Instead of distributing random bits of the story to my friends, I ought to be writing that story for a wider public, for Americans such as I had been a few months before, to whom the name Pribilof Islands was strange and alien. I vowed to record the story of one small island mothered by Alaska, a realm of birds and flowers, a refuge for sea animals, and a cruel prison to the dreams and aspirations of a people whose past was forgotten and whose present was a sea-bound secret.

Saturday [October 25]
Sam decided not to go digging for ivory. But we spent a very quiet day. And began to try to teach her majesty to have her last bottle at ten. It proved quite difficult so we did not get to bed until eleven thirty. She did not call us until a little after seven but we were still groggy and went back to bed until her next summons, after eleven. Heretina did not show up for work after church. When I was dressed I asked one of the boys to go get her and was informed that she had gone riding with a truckload of kids. Her father sent her in at five thirty and she did the washing for the day and one or two other jobs, getting done just in time to make the movies. Sullen of course at being sent here. But it is comforting to our hope of a regular life of work, study, and writing to see that Peter has some influence over her . . .

Chapter 27

I don't know how those teachers could say they earned their salaries," Elary said. "They didn't have reading books beyond the fifth grade. They didn't teach us grammar."

Elary Gromoff sat in our living room pouring out his heart. Psalm reader in his church, manager of the Native Canteen, and exempt from sealing, Elary might be counted as one of the few Native white-collar workers. A thin, tense man with fine Russian features, he sat nervously on the edge of the rocker, twisting his cap in trembling hands as he spoke of his lack of education, of his weak, unguided attempts at self-education. When he referred to knowledge hidden from him in books, his voice quivered. His spoken English was clearer, more grammatical and fluent than most of the islanders. As a child he had longed to become a priest, but his foster mother, Iuliana Gromoff, had frustrated his desire to attend a Russian seminary, because of the expense, or even to go outside to an industrial school lest he be overcome by temptations in the States. Elary was still suffering from the denial of opportunities for himself and the same frustration for his two older children, Alice (baptized Alexandra) and Smiles. Smile, as his name appeared on the island census, had been baptized Ishmael and was called Smiles by everyone but Father Baranoff.

Too often Elary expressed his craving for recognition by emphasizing the Russian side of his ancestry. But on St. Paul he was an Aleut among Aleuts despite his Russian heritage. Once, under stress of personal sorrow on the death of an infant son, he had wandered out across the island, talking wildly to himself until a searching party found him and brought him back to warmth and human society, away from the tempting oblivion the sea promised. The confused victim of social caste, a naive soul scorched with a thousand ardent desires, for knowledge, for equal participation in American citizenship with his American overseers, for escape to the States, he was sometimes an enigma to both the unambitious Aleut and the contemptuous non-Aleut.

"Those teachers," he continued, "they wanted me to go outside to school. But the agent said no and Mrs. Gromoff was strict. She wouldn't help me. So I stayed here and went to work. She was old-fashioned. In the States everybody can go to school. Isn't that right?"

His bitter accusations against his teachers were unjust for Mr. and Mrs. Alvin G. Whitney were exceptional champions of the people they had come to educate.[1] In both 1912 and 1913 they composed voluminous detailed reports of the shortcomings of the island educational system. In one report the Whitneys recommended that one of their brighter pupils, a lad more Russian than Aleut in physical appearance, should go outside for further studies to be trained as a teacher for his own people. That boy was Elary, who, bitter because he had been cheated of one of the basic American rights, railed at their memory thirty years later, without realizing why textbooks were limited and classes circumscribed or that those teachers had appealed to Washington to make his dream of education come true.

Endeavoring to delineate so realistic a picture of the unwholesome social conditions and the failures of the school system that the hearts of Washington officials might be moved to order reforms, the Whitneys outlined carefully the history of educational efforts from the onset of American guardianship to their arrival. Fearlessly they ascribed blame where it was due, whether to the deliberate limited interpretation of contractual obligations by the lessees and their agents, to the indifference and callousness of government officials sworn to supervise the companies' fulfillment of their contracts, or to the conscious desire of either type of employee to keep the Aleuts ignorant and amenable.[2]

The Whitneys were not the first to expose the defective nature of Pribilof schooling. Nor the last. Again and again in the more meager reports of agents of both islands since 1870, the indictment "the school is a farce" was repeated. Twenty years of American government and "it seems incredible, but it is true, that young men and women who have been to school here for seven years do not know how to speak or read a sentence of the English language," assistant Agent Murray wailed in his official report of the year's events on St. George in 1890.[3] A decade later the charge was repeated. A decade later the Whitneys presented their facts. In 1941 the teachers were still begging for more books, for visual aids to teaching English and bewailing their students' lack of knowledge. Seventy years after the Americans took over the islands most of the report compiled by the Whitneys could have been applied word-for-word to the classroom of 1941.

The contract between the Treasury Department and the two commercial companies simply stated that the lessee was to maintain a school and provide a teacher on both islands. No specific standards of education were demanded by the government or rules concerning the qualifications of the instructors issued. The first school on St. Paul, a class of twenty-nine students from five to eighteen, was held for two hours in the afternoon in the dining room of the Company House. Attendance, though voluntary, was ninety-five percent, a fine showing. In 1871 the ancient Russian storehouse, apparently useless for commercial purposes, was patched up for a schoolhouse. A longer school day was instituted.

November 1, 1941
Saturday afternoon, lunch over, the baby bathed and sleeping and both of us in the study while the rain is coming down in oceans outside. The wind is blowing furiously and the rain is coming down the windows of the living room almost as hard as on the outside.

Thursday afternoon, after I had done a little typing, Sammie and I walked down to West Landing and up on top of Spilki. The ground was lit up with silvery patches of reindeer moss, which dominates the earth now that the high vegetation is sere and yellow. The rocks are still gay with green mosses and some of the yellow-orange lichens. The view from the top of the hill was especially magnificent. So clear was the air that it seemed as if we might stretch out a hand and touch the sides of Reef. Otter Island sailed close to us in the blue waters with purplish shadows claiming the water around her rocky sides. Her center ground glowed dimly with yellowing vegetation. Off toward Zapadni, the landscape was soft with yellow, grey, and purple tones.

Coming down to the village we stopped in at Gov. House and chatted with Joe White a few minutes and then with Harrington. The latter seemed so pleased that we had come to see him. He has a wonderful book on Aleut archaeology that is filled with markers and therefore not in a lendable state. I am dying to read it. I brought down Hultén and yesterday and today I have been copying all the material that I want from it.[4]

Then the attendance began to wane. The novelty wore off. When the classes were almost empty, officials charged that the Russian Church stirred up the parents of the children against learning English lest it wean them from their religion. A lone contradictory voice explained the Russian clergy discouraged female attendance because of the debauching proclivities of the schoolteacher and the government agent. The wife of Charles Fish of the signal corps, stationed on the island to make meteorological observations, opened a school in 1872 and was later accepted by the company as the accredited teacher at sixty dollars a month. In 1873 Agent Bryant visited the class for Christmas exercises and discovered that a dozen children could read and reckon, a few could write, and the remainder were diligently struggling with the alphabet. But the success of the teacher was brief. Mrs. Fish bitterly accused the company of breaking up her efforts by withholding coal issues for heating the room during the second year of school, just because her students were making enormous strides in learning. There is little doubt that many company officials and government agents who strove to please the company shared the opinion that the less the Aleuts knew of English the more contented sealers and sealers' wives they would be. Basically they regarded the Aleuts as inferior and incapable of progress. At the same time they feared lest education contrast their contempt.

James Buterin, son of Kirik Buterin, St. Paul chief, was one of the few Aleuts who received extensive education in the States. He was educated either by the Alaska Commercial Company or its general agent, Dr. H. H. McIntyre, in Vermont. Gossip said his opportunity came because the company desired to win the loyal gratitude of the chief and have one exhibit of their philanthropy. From 1878 when James was twenty-one he taught the village school until [ill health] forced [him] to resign a short time before he died of tuberculosis in 1883.

It was in 1875, three years before James became the instructor, that government agents began to rail most bitterly against the Orthodox Church. Father [Paul] Shayashnikoff, first resident priest, fiercely proud of his Russian birthright, championed the retention of Russian and Slavonic (church language) classes.[5] He did not intend to attack the English language but merely to preserve the languages the islanders already knew and to preserve, especially, the language of their religious services. But the Aleuts' confused dissatisfaction with their new governors and new working conditions became focused against English education. The militant priest bolstered the islanders' timidity. Mothers who had kept their children home from school to help with housework found a new, potent excuse for pandering to their indolence. Casual truancy became an almost community-wide campaign of rebellion. Father Shayashnikoff requested the part-time use of the school building for Russian classes and lessons in Slavonic liturgy. Not satisfied with permission to use the building on Saturdays, he demanded the privilege of entering the school at any hour of any day to discourse to the pupils on religious themes. Refused by local authorities, his grievance against them grew more intense.

The Treasury Department had finally defined the school year as the eight-month period from September until May, for five days a week, and had ordered all children between six and sixteen to attend school. Now new regulations began to issue from Washington. However, the conscious or unconscious feeling of superiority among the majority of employees from the States further weakened the dicta from Washington and counteracted the earnest labors of good teachers and humane scientific-minded physicians. English was the sole language to be taught on the Pribilofs. The intent of the communications was excellent although there were better means of making English acceptable than coercion. The Aleuts came within that group mentioned specifically in the treaty of transfer from Russia as the civilized tribes, entitled to the rights, privileges, and responsibilities of American citizenship. How could they assume their responsibilities or appreciate their rights and privileges unless they made the language of their new country their own? But the regulations, translated into Russian and posted or read to the community by an interpreter, did not put an end to truancy. Agents blustered and raged, sent foremen to round up delinquents, to no avail. Finally a fine of fifty cents for every absence not excused by the physician, a serious financial drain on the slender cash income of the sealers, broke up overt resistance to English education. It was replaced by a subtler passive resistance to English education. Led to school forcibly, the children could close their minds to the precepts of the teachers, could not be compelled to absorb knowledge. They conformed. They sat at their desks, their minds safely blocked off by lack of interest, by annoyance at discipline, by an unawareness of the fruits of application.

Simeon Melovidov, another Aleut, educated in California, taught the St. Paul school for two decades.[6] Conscientious, he worked loyally to educate his people. The lists of books he ordered for his pupils contain excellent texts and storybooks. But as an Aleut, no matter his personal feeling about school progress, he was handicapped in struggling for more benefits. Aleut schoolteachers were economical for the lessees. At first they received only the first-class man's share of sealing proceeds. Later Simeon was paid a regular salary of fifty dollars a month.[7]

October 30, 1941
Monday noon while Heretina was eating her lunch I sat down and had a long talk with her. I seasoned my mild scolding with all sorts of pleas and reasons for better behavior, and I think a few little seeds were planted. I have beautiful smiles from her every time I look at her now. And although lots of things slide by her attention or are not well done, I can see some evidence of her trying to be better.

I mentioned among other things that I wanted this to be a second home to her, that I wanted her to bring her friends here, etc. She went racing off after lunch to sew on her Girl Scout uniform and came back at three with Elizabeth Titoff, who sat about stiffly with her coat on for some time. I was typing when Heretina returned. Soon she came in and asked a question about making cocoa. I told

cont.

In 1911 after the Bureau of Fisheries had been assigned to manage the Pribilofs, Dr. Walter L. Hahn, naturalist and storekeeper, prepared a thorough and painstaking social analysis at the request of his Washington superiors.[8] Most of the blemishes in the social structure he traced back to the failure of education. He exposed the vicious circle by which the low social status of the Aleut deadened his ambition for himself and his children and how the defective educational system built a barless prison within which the Aleuts vegetated, neither hoping, knowing, or caring for escape, for physical or mental betterment. He assailed the unregulated choice of teachers whose main qualification was a speaking knowledge of English, the meager school equipment; one teacher to carry the burden of imparting knowledge to fifty pupils. He pointed out the absurdity of making government agents, devoid of experience as teachers, responsible for educational matters. Hired and retained for their ability to manage the sealing gang, they were unable to judge merits of teachers or teaching methods or the kind and quantity of the requisite material. Because of his own experience in teaching in grade schools and a university, Hahn criticized the problem constructively. Undoubtedly his plea brought the employment of two teachers, Mr. and Mrs. Whitney, in 1912.

The instructions to Mr. M. C. Marsh, the next naturalist sent to St. Paul, stressed first the necessity of studying the fur seal herd and secondly directed him to supervise all educational matters and all matters relating to public health and the well-being of the Natives. The very next paragraph began, "Your first and most important duty lies, of course, with the seal herd." Quite unconscious of damning its own program, the Washington administration laid bare the fatal flaw in its approach to Pribilof society, the attitude that has weakened all local and federal attempts at reform. There was no villainous plot to keep in subjugation the people reputed to be, by heredity and nature, the best sealers; not even cold disinterest in the human beings whom the past had stranded on the Seal Islands. The Bureau of Fisheries was organized to deal with animal life. Food and shelter were factual problems to be solved in neat accounts and estimates. The souls and the minds of the sealers were subtler problems, and mechanical rules could not regulate their activities. It was not enough to order schools into existence without taking into consideration the special problems of overcoming language barriers, of presenting novel ideas of a world and life beyond the students' ken, of providing social outlets where the new knowledge could be utilized, and of proving to the Aleuts that study would advance their social and economic position and widen their horizons in a thousand ways.

The Whitneys certainly found their task heartbreaking. On every side they were beset by difficulties, petty trifles and major problems, too. The school building was in need of repair, of cleaning and painting when they arrived. The week necessary for renovation was clipped summarily from the school year by the agent, from a school year already curtailed by numerous religious holidays and sometimes by inclement weather. The single room was crowded, impossible to ventilate and heat at the same time. The children's damp outer clothes steamed unsavorily on a rack on the wall. Their muddy footgear cluttered the floor space. Whatever minor improvements of any kind the Whitneys suggested locally were blocked immediately by tradition, by the agent's curt rejoinder, "not customary." Their requisitions for teaching aids were disallowed by the agent though, as they pointed out, he ordered plenty of liquor for the island stock with no thought of economy.

her and presently through the study door I saw them sitting in the dinette sipping cocoa and eating some of the English Huntly and Palmer cookies that Aunt Sybil had sent us. At suppertime I thought perhaps I better ask her to invite her friend to stay before she just kept her. She seemed thrilled and after we had eaten, she prepared, with Elizabeth's help, bacon and omelets, cake and raspberries. They seemed to be having more fun. Elizabeth was not so frightened and was of assistance to Heretina in many ways. I rather expected there would be a run on the house after that but she brought no one home from sewing yesterday.

Monday night we were late going to bed because of vain endeavors to have her majesty eat. But Tuesday I was still able to grit my teeth and type and I did eight pages of stuff about village events.

The tone of their second year's report, illustrated with a large number of photographs showing the squalid school building, the unkempt appearance of the village was more discouraged than the first. Since it seemed impossible to institute reforms on the islands, the Whitneys advocated the removal of the entire population from the island before the Aleuts became more pauperized, more debased, and more incapable of citizenship. Sealing, they averred, could be carried on by laborers imported for the summer period. Sealing was nothing esoteric, a rite for which the Aleuts were especially evolved by nature to carry out, but a job that an ordinary laborer from the States could handle as deftly and efficiently, if not more so. They proposed that a large boarding school be erected at Unalaska for all Aleut children under the U.S. flag, where, removed from the influence of casual overseers and families subverted by the evils of civilization, the children would live in an atmosphere where English would be their main means of communication and expression of thought. In such surroundings they might catch a glimpse of a broader life and find an impetus for studying.[9]

From St. George Island in the years of 1912 and 1913 came the same indictment: The people know no English and their social environment is at fault.

After the Whitneys, a long procession of teachers, most of them sympathetic to their pupils, others mechanically carrying on the motions of teaching for the salaries' sake, attempted to cope with the teaching problem. From the best of these teachers came always the same appeals for aid from distant Washington. Irregularly but monotonously the reports that reached there were noted and filed away.

Chapter 28

In 1941 the roll of St. Paul's school included eighty names. The two-storied schoolhouse, from its eminence on the brow of Village Hill overlooking the other buildings, was imposing despite its drab painted exterior. Photographs make it even more impressive. In the wide hall of the main floor the children's garments hung neatly on hooks along both walls. The two large classrooms were furnished with conventional desks and benches. The walls were decorated with the children's colorful crayon drawings. On the lower floor were a manual training shop, a domestic science room, and the shower rooms. Outwardly the appearance of the classrooms had improved. It was vastly different from the crowded sitting-dining room of the Company House, from the cramped patched-up old Russian storehouse, and the small one-roomed building erected by the first American lessee.

Only the processes of imparting and absorbing knowledge failed to keep pace with external development. In 1942, sixteen-year-old Alice Gromoff, officially that rare Pribilof creature, an eighth-grade pupil, could not write a small paragraph in complete sentences. In after-school classes with us, she struggled to get a concept of a sentence with heartbreaking intensity. Mr. Hellbaum tried to find spare time to prepare special studies for her eager, hungry mind. He had, after a long search among yellowed books, found a dull prosey American history book for her to read in the classroom

February 2, 1942
I omitted one fact that Gabe [Stepetin] told us yesterday that was very interesting. He said that an older brother of his, Nicholas, had finished high school and was starting college. This brother's dream had been to educate himself so that he could come back to help his people. He had promised to take Gabe "outside" with him that fall. During the summer, he had been working on a ship and was lost overboard. How it happened, no one knows or at least never told his family. When Gabe told us, I said I had seen an item in the log that mentioned that the body had never been recovered. "That is true," said Gabe, "but we never told Mother the truth. We told her the body was found and buried somewhere." Which I thought was very sweet.

cont.

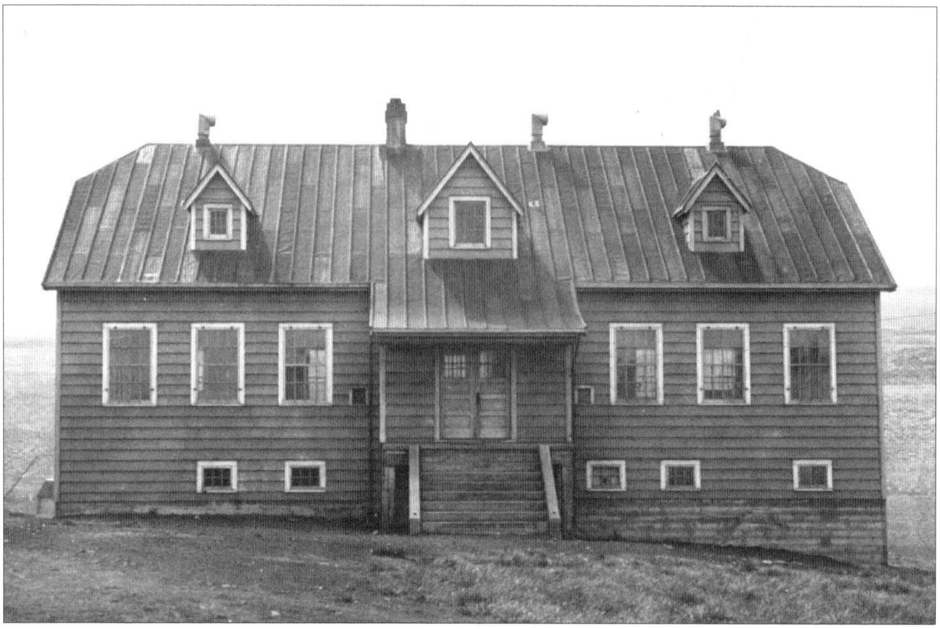

The school building on St. Paul Island, June 1938 (courtesy of NOAA National Marine Fisheries Service, Department of Commerce).

This morning I went inside the schoolhouse for the first time. I think it is quite a pleasant building inside although a more cheerful paint scheme would not be amiss. But it smelled and looked clean. We put TB patch tests on each kid in the senior class. It took but a very few minutes.

Walking up was certainly an adventure. Fortunately, there were thin streaks where ice had frozen in rough irregularities and to these spots it is necessary to cling to get up the hill. Otherwise just sheets of sheer thin ice.

while the others recited their fourth- and fifth-grade exercises. With great effort Alice was learning to converse in halting labored sentences of badly pronounced English. The other children spoke in broken phrases, with a hugger-mugger of words that garbled the meaning into a jumble of anagrams. Scarcely one could pronounce an English vowel sound correctly. Teachers had come to believe that an anatomical defect prevented the enunciation of "sh." Conversational clarity was befogged by the universal inability to differentiate between *he* and *she*. In the course of a brief story the characters revolved dizzily back and forth from masculine to feminine.

There could no longer be the excuse that education was hampered because the students lacked the desire to learn. Alice was exceptional because she was innately very intelligent and had been brought up by a father whose obsession was to have his children well educated. For three years of her childhood she had been hospitalized in the States for a tubercular hip and she longed to return and become like other American girls. When she was eight years old and returned to the island, she had forgotten Aleut. Relearning the Native tongue, whatever correct pronunciation she had possessed in the hospital had been butchered. But her ambitions differed from those of many girls her age only in intensity.

The autumn before we came to the island a group of sixteen-year-old girls, automatically debarred by their age from further schooling, had petitioned Mac for permission to continue their studies. He refused because there were not enough desks, chairs, and books for them and certainly no teachers.

Qualifications for teachers are either not clearly defined or very peculiar. A main consideration seems to be the marital status of the applicant. Illegitimate babies fathered by lonely bachelor schoolteachers led to a preference for a married couple. Perhaps the most severe indictment of the caliber of single, male schoolteachers who have been here is the fact that no teacher has ever married and taken outside the girl whom he chose for his island companion. Men so heedless of maintaining the respect of their scholars and their families and so callous about the ultimate fate of the abandoned girls and their own children could not inspire much reverence for learning in the community.

Married couples, each of whom are well-trained teachers, are not exactly commonplace. Too often for the rapid progress of education, the wife of a teacher, long sequestered as housewife and mother, had dusted off her normal-school diploma, hurriedly boned up on some rudiments of teaching methods, and taken over the lower grade room. Nor are there many really good teachers willing to accept a position that includes six weeks of labor on the killing fields in summer for the man, while his wife is responsible for various sewing tasks in the village such as making curtains for public buildings. The low salaries are sufficient to deter the best teachers.

Curious disparities in educational status occur. On St. George in the autumn of 1941 a domestic upheaval left the male teacher, who had not completed his normal-school training, in sole charge of the

December 12, 1941
Sam got involved in a religious discussion with Alice Gromoff—tried to implant in her mind that she should always ask for proof of anything before she accepts it as truth. That made supper late. We were just going to eat when Smiles came in. He is still sitting in the living room reading away at a *N. Y. Times*. We have discussed a course of study and Hellbaum has some eighth-grade books for him to use. I am to start him typing tomorrow evening. I do not think he is really so interested but he is a quiet youngster so perhaps it is more than his father's dream that is bringing him here. We will see how he sticks to his studies. He wants to learn shorthand and typing—the latter of which I can help him with. But he wants to be a mechanic, he says, and I do not see what all this study is leading up to, if that is the case. But let us give him a chance. Alice has such a fine mind and Smiles is probably very intelligent and bright, too. But he certainly had a wonderful experience in the Russian school in Pennsylvania. He learned Russian last year and was learning Russian grammar this year. Nothing else. Some education.

school for several months. His wife was finally replaced in December by a young man who possessed a master's degree.

The Hellbaums were just rounding out their first year on St. Paul when we arrived. Mr. Hellbaum, a former high-school teacher in California, presided over forty-five pupils from ten to sixteen years of age, assigned to groups from the second grade to and including the eighth. His wife, a secretary before her marriage, had been a busy wife and mother of her two daughters from her wedding until her arrival on St. Paul. Despite her inexperience, guided by her husband she was attempting miracles in the primary room. Her thirty-four pupils divided into pre-primer, primary class, and the first grade, included youngsters from six to eleven years of age.

Picture Mrs. Hellbaum at the commencement of the school year in September. Confronting her is a group of tiny newcomers, five years old and ready for school—with either not one word of English in their vocabularies or else such poor language aids as "hello," "OK," "yeah," "naw" to start them off. Very little of their teacher's time can be devoted to helping them untangle the mystery of new sounds. The majority of the youngsters in that room are lively, squirming imps who can apply themselves to their primers and reckoning only when a vigilant eye supervises them. Scarcely more than beginners themselves, the victims of the teacher's limited time and the absence of visual aids to make the English sound intelligible, they have memorized the appearance of words and can repeat sections of their primers by rote. They mouth the English phrases badly because the words are meaningless. They lack practice in pronunciation and they have had scant opportunity to hear English spoken. The fragments of their lessons that are assimilated are retained in a mental compartment labeled school; the written or spoken word remains foreign to their thoughts. Show the class a picture of a cat and ask the English name. A chorus answers promptly "cat." Chattering among themselves, even within the classroom, they say "*kuska*" [*kuuskax̂*], a mutilated Russian word long ago adopted into Aleut.

Could the tongue-tied newcomers spend their first school term in a kindergarten routine of songs, games, and play in which the English words became meaningful pleasantly and the correct pronunciation unwittingly picked up, the pre-primer class would soon become an average American classroom. As it is, the children, no matter their potential intellectual powers, limp badly from grade to grade and are graduated because of their age, not for the successful completion of studies, still unable to speak the language of their country. Mrs. Hellbaum's request for a piano, by which she might make English palatable and delightful to her young pupils, was peremptorily turned down as a needless luxury. Her plea for more drawing materials met a similar fate. This lack she partially overcame by collecting magazines from officials on the island and relatives in the States. Actually, we became rival collectors, as we sought pictorial magazines for our tubercular patients. Cutting out colored pictures and making scrapbooks made a slight impression on the children. It at least entertained them and kept one group happily out of mischief while she heard another recite.

But, except by pictorial lessons, how were her pupils to understand "dog" without a picture? No dogs had been on the Pribilofs during their lifetime. A horse? An elephant? These were pictures simple to find in advertisements. Other nouns were not so easy to define. How explain the nature of a brook on a streamless island without a photograph of a rural countryside to clarify the word?

Lacking modern or even a sufficient number of outmoded textbooks, Mr. Hellbaum procured prepared lessons of the true-false variety from the States. He and his wife mimeographed copies during their supposed evening leisure. They stressed, throughout all their teachings, the necessity of becoming like other American children and emphasized and tried to make attractive the rewards of learning English. Their words fell upon the ears of children who knew only too well that they could never leave the island to get more schooling or escape their destiny of becoming sealers and the mothers of sealers.

Some of the ironies of teaching were in the textbooks themselves. I borrowed the hygiene text the children have to read. Every page recounted the healthy habits of Bobby and his friends. The book described how he obediently drank his glass of fresh milk after each meal, ate fruit daily, and, of course, bathed and took meticulous care of his person. How far from the little Aleuts was Bobby! What use to teach drinking milk when the cow's milk went to government families and to the hospital and the canned milk of the government issue was just sufficient for cooling coffee and tea and moistening oatmeal. How puzzling to learn that fresh fruit each day is vital to growth and health and yet receive only a sack of fresh oranges twice a year from the Fouke Fur Company, supplemented by a few expensive pounds of fruit from the Native Canteen. Nor is there much use to preach daily baths to people whose household water must be carried in by hand.

If the Aleut children had not known that the Service people had fresh milk daily and fresh fruit most of the year, what grandiose ideas they might have acquired of life in the States. They would have pictured a land, not paved with gold as European immigrants were once told, but a holiday land where a more munificent, more doting Fouke Fur Company transformed every day into a Fourth of July or a Christmas for the lucky Bobbies of the country.

School days devoted to instruction from 9:00 a.m. to 3:00 p.m. throughout the term, guided by stimulating teachers, might assist the Aleut youngsters to pick up a few more crumbs of knowledge. But the unfortunate teachers had many duties besides imparting book lessons. The more-to-be-pitied students had very little time under the school roof to devote to actual studying. The school morning had other interruptions besides the quarter-hour recess. Daily tooth-brushing drills and the administration of cod liver oil three times a week stole away a few precious minutes. Children took turns at various janitor tasks, dusting, sweeping, mopping, and cleansing the washrooms. Mr. Hellbaum himself and some of the older boys had to tend the furnace, neglected by an irresponsible adult janitor.

Three afternoons a week the lower class was dismissed to roam the streets footloose and lesson free. While Mrs. Hellbaum devoted those periods to domestic science for the older girls, the upper-class boys learned manual training from her husband. On Tuesday and Friday afternoons all the children carried little packages of clean clothes to school instead of books. "Shower days," as the children called them. No one escaped the biweekly scrubbing. The big girls helped the little girls. The big boys kept an eye on the smaller lads. The teachers inspected the results and sent back for reshowering those who had skipped some vital bit of anatomy.

Everything but lessons to usher the native Pribilof children into the fold of Americanism.

The girl students aroused my pity most. During the winter Mrs. Hoverson, formerly a schoolteacher, asked me to give her newly organized Girl Scout troop some talks and simple nursing lessons. Making a bed with a person in it was one project I selected. Then I thought in dismay, "More housework. I am becoming a part of the conspiracy." From cradle to the grave the Aleut girls are pursued by household drudgery. Generally, as soon as they can toddle, they are helping their mothers already beset with a younger infant to tend. During school years their household tasks increase in scope and finally are supplemented with domestic science classes three afternoons a week. At sixteen, they face the unpleasant alternative, housework at home or employment, either as maids in homes of Service employees or in the hospital where inadequate porter service limits nursing to scrubbing and dusting and sweeping. Household duties until the crowning date of their lives, their wedding day, takes them to new homes where the whole burden of home responsibility becomes theirs, where they will raise children in accordance with the traditional pattern of their mothers. Housework of the most demanding kind, handicapped and primitive, enveloped

December 22, 1941
Smile Gromoff came down to arrange about lessons and we started him off typing Thursday night. He has been practicing about two hours more some nights since then until yesterday when he had to go foxing at Zapadni for this whole week. But on Saturday he arrived with books that Mr. Hellbaum lent him, for eighth-grade work, and Sam went over some grammar lessons for him to study out there and assigned some stories in a reading book. When he comes back he will begin his arithmetic. He is to write down all the words he does not understand.

Poor Smiles. He seems very bright but I cannot find out whether he has any definite ambitions beside wanting to be a mechanic. But he seems willing to put forth some effort and his typing manuscript has been uniformly excellent. I doubt whether there have been ten mistakes in the whole business. Much better than I did in the beginning and than I do now.

them forever. Whichever way an Aleut girl faces, the dishpan, the broom, the mop, and the water bucket confront her.

And there was I, the feminist, desirous of seeing those bright girls escape their limited horizon, become teachers, secretaries, nurses, whatever they wished, actually weaving another strand about them. But how, because of language difficulties, because of their immaturity in meeting quite ordinary problems, could I teach them more complicated and interesting nursing projects? I was restricted by circumstances to imparting the most elemental rites of a career that of all womanly professions is the most varied, demanding not only mechanical aptitude for household tasks but scientific, spiritual, psychological knowledge. The Girl Scout ranks held such diversely equipped girls as Marie Melovidov, whose English was nonexistent, Alice Gromoff, and Elinor Hellbaum, the teacher's own daughter. Apt and deft in their handiness, remembering from week to week the whys and wherefores of their procedures, the girls concealed their boredom very politely. Slim balm to my conscience, troubled by inflicting such exercises on their recreational hours, was the slender hope that since hospital housekeeping is streamlined to prevent all useless expenditure of energy one or two of the next generation of sealers' wives might avoid a little backache and fatigue from making up the family beds.

There are few Elarys with a bitter, burning dream of finding means of equality in books or tasting frustration for their children's lack of opportunities. Another unusual person was Heretina Kochutin, a brisk lively woman in her middle thirties, who chatted volubly in poor English. When Sam asked the reason for her fluency, she retorted vigorously that she was an American, too. But, she added, she had learned her vocabulary from a former teacher who had administered generous portions of castor oil to children who used Aleut during school hours. Others of her age seem not to have acquired so large a vocabulary by this harsh method.

For a number of years after the leasing system was discontinued, a few adolescents were sent to the Indian Industrial School of Chemawa in Oregon. The custom died out at least a decade ago.[1] One official excuse was that the children could not endure the warmer climate. To which I would like to retort derisively that there were probably no red-hot kitchen ranges around which to huddle in equatorial temperatures. Such a tropic atmosphere caused me to cut short many a visit to an Aleut home. In sober fact, there are enough hale and healthy people who have moved from the islands and adapted themselves to life in the States to disprove the idea. The former teacher, Simeon Melovidov, and his sister, Alexandra, widow of Henry W. Elliott, are enjoying vigorous old age in California. The official excuse is based on very flimsy support. Many children did become ill at school. Most of them, bewildered by the sudden transposition to a daily regime of strict discipline, were homesick for their fond families and frightened out of their wits by their new supervisors. The tales of former Chemawa boys and girls are woefully unhappy. It is not unusual for mental agitation to find expression disguised as physical illness.

There was Peter Kochergin's story, for instance. For weeks after he arrived at Chemawa, he wept for hours daily and nightly cried himself to sleep. He was terribly frightened. Everything was strange and alien. No supervisor spoke or acted in a kindly or affectionate way. Because of his feeble understanding of English he misunderstood instructions and then was punished severely for his blundering attempts to comply, as severely as if he were guilty of outright deliberate disobedience. He was too terrified to try to explain his apparent noncompliance. Penalties for misdemeanors were not light. Long hours of guard duty were usual sentences. A martinet matron who inspected the children's sleeping quarters copiously doused ill-made beds, dust on furniture or floor, and ill-arranged articles with water. Then she stood watch over the culprit as he cleaned up the mess. Such strict discipline, accounts of which brought pages of Dickens to mind, was a startling contrast to the home life the children had known. There were other factors that made school life unbearable so that children fretted and became prey for passing germs.

"Gee," said Peter, "I was hungry. I was always hungry. They just had everyday food on the table." It took several tellings of the story before I ferreted out his definition of "everyday." It meant insufficient. Just a little. Not enough for the appetite of a growing boy. Sadly enough, it meant just like on the Pribilofs.

One day he confided to a chum that he was always hungry. The other lad was an Indian and a Catholic. He invited Peter, who had been classified as a Protestant, to accompany him to the Catholic church the next Sunday and share the meat and bread refreshments at the conclusion of the service. Peter could hardly believe his ears. What kind of a religion gave food away? All the rest of the week he looked forward to Sunday. On the great day he slipped away from the groups preparing to attend Protestant services and joined his friend. He knew he would be punished if he were found out but his protesting stomach urged him on. He found the ceremony unduly long. All during prayers he fretted and doubted and annoyed his pal by asking when, when, when? At last everyone stood up. Church was over. Everyone marched into an adjoining room. As soon as the door was open, Peter breathed in the wondrous odor of hot dogs and bologna. Peter wolfed down as much as he liked.

He recalled, "Gee, that preacher man was nice. When I went out he shook my hand and thanked me for coming. But I never got no chance to go again. I got caught and went on guard duty for a long time. But I never forget that day so long as I live. And I didn't mind the guard duty, cause the eats sure was good and filled my belly."

We teased Peter and Dan Shabolin, the dairyman, about their Indian accent. They both had a curious way of smothering their words that made them less intelligible than many Aleuts who knew less English. To my surprise Peter took my fun in earnest. Since few of the Chemawa pupils spoke English outside the classroom, they had even picked up phrases of Indian dialects.

"Very hard," Peter said and Dan confirmed it. "Very hard to learn English good there. Just like here."

At Chemawa the Aleuts could learn trades and farming. Peter had learned a little about dairy work and harness making. He always regretted that he had not been in the right class to learn tailoring. I never met a student who had remained long enough to master a trade and find work in the States. One St. Paul woman and her daughter found work at the school itself, in the laundry, and shook off the scoria dust of the island permanently. Those who returned were indistinguishable, save for slightly more facile English, from those who had never been outside. Old students were always talking of their experiences as if to assure us that they were sophisticated about the world and could talk to us man-to-man. I listened and I asked questions. I never encountered a hint that their school stay had been other than a harsh, disillusioning experience from which they returned as ignorant as they left and more confused than before about America and Americans.

Peter unconsciously summed up the quality of the industrial school. "Them farmers around the school liked it. They got five dollars for every runaway kid they found. By golly, they make plenty of money."[2]

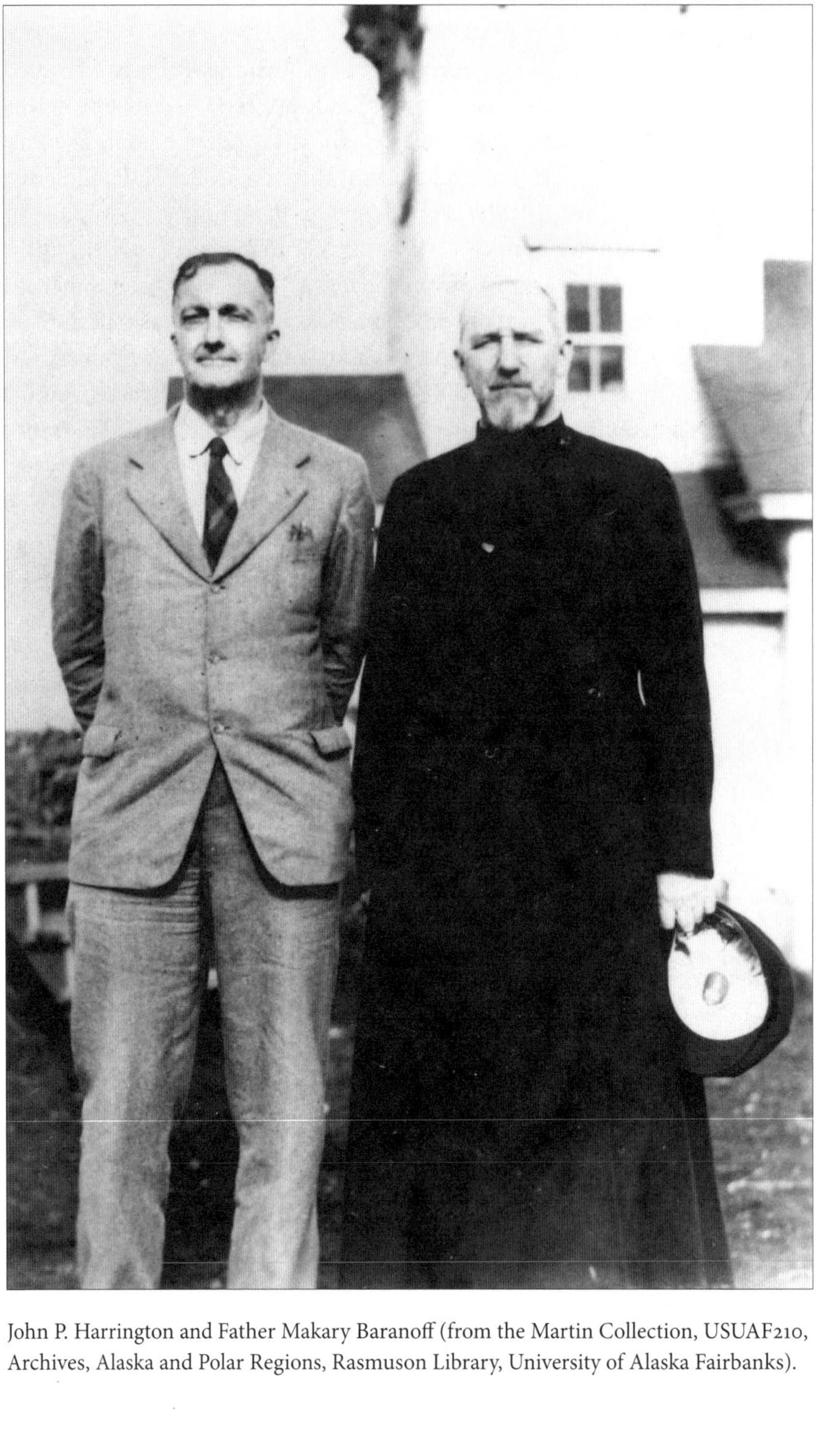

John P. Harrington and Father Makary Baranoff (from the Martin Collection, USUAF210, Archives, Alaska and Polar Regions, Rasmuson Library, University of Alaska Fairbanks).

Chapter 29

Before I left Greenbelt I was making enthusiastic plans to study Aleut. I thrilled at the prospect of learning enough of the language to enable me to understand, in gross patterns, the modes of expression of a different people. The fascination of grammatical construction was outweighed by the hope the Aleuts would be easier to know if I were able to understand and speak a few words of their tongue. I rang up a dozen individuals and institutions to ask, "Where can I get an English-Aleut dictionary?" Invariably the answer was, "I haven't the slightest idea." One person knew that a Russian-Aleut dictionary existed but thought it must be out of print. Again I had the sensation of going toward a completely unexplored area. There on my map, flung across the wide Pacific, lay the island chain where these people lived and above those islands the important industrial islands of the Pribilofs with nearly five hundred Aleut inhabitants. Yet the scholars and museums to whom I applied could not help me.

But one man did not fail. Just half an hour before the *Penguin* sailed from Seattle, a special-delivery letter arrived from Vilhjalmur Stefansson containing the addresses of two people who might direct me to Russian sources of information, and I wrote them as soon as I reached St. Paul.

I was lax about undertaking studies on my own. The days were full of varied tasks and interests and studies of other kinds. Local officials warned me that the Aleuts resented any attempts by whites to become too familiar with their personal privacy, the greatest safeguard of which was their own speech. I had had no intention of asking for information and appearing idly curious until I had established friendly relations with the villagers. During office hours I overheard the chatter of waiting patients. I recognized words and phrases, sometimes enough to gather the drift of the entire conversation. There were Russian words, some so distorted either by actual syllabic change or mispronunciation that I would sense a familiar note but be unable without much mental effort to recognize them. Cautiously, I commenced to admit my awareness of words. Always the reaction was pleasure, a flashing smile. Apparently, as in so many other conventional official beliefs, the warnings I had heard had been very much exaggerated. If I requested

November 1, 1941
Heretina, the general, has Anna helping her scrub and clean in the kitchen and the gales of laughter are continuous. Who said these kids are sullen? They were trying to teach me Aleut this noon. Heretina actually made a joke by telling Anna that I understood Aleut and meanwhile was winking at me to agree with her.

After noon had fled rainily away, the kids were busy cleaning up the kitchen and I tactfully reminded Heretina of her duties in the office.

November 4, 1941
Yesterday morning I broke off typing and Sam and I went up to Gov. House to see Harrington (who was out) and to try to locate as many books containing the Elliott/Jordan controversy as possible. We found none of the early stuff, the 1890 beginnings. But we did find the complete set of volumes of the hearings from 1911 to 1914. So I have several months of reading ahead of me. And the testimony still holds me entranced. Sam read aloud to me for an hour last night while I rolled cigarettes. And laughed.

In the afternoon we went back up, after stopping off at the Canteen to buy tobacco. On the way to the Canteen we saw a workman skinning a white fox at the machine shop. It had been found dead. Small portions of the inner surface of the pelt were greenish and they were not sure whether it could be salvaged or not, but they were trying. The fur is glorious. I do not see why it is not popular.

cont.

interpretations, the response was prompt, willing, and colored with expressions of delight at my interest.

Such dabbling merely proved how thoroughly Russian had been woven into their speech to endure for seventy years in an English-speaking community. I vowed to study seriously in the (I hoped) less cluttered days of winter. Then, as if in response to my heart's wish, John P. Harrington arrived to study and record Aleut before it should decay still further and follow their folkways into oblivion.[1] His ultimate goal was to establish a body of material to be compared with Siberian tongues in hopes of uncovering a clue to the route of man's migration from Asia to the Americas. Basic likenesses or differences might aid in solving the riddles of the early migration.

Until early December we lived on the fringe of his interesting work. Most of the aids we gave him were, naturally, nonlinguistic. Sam hunted out the most intelligent, fluent informants. I rallied two of the amateur botanists of the Service colony to arrange a flower collection he had purchased from Father Baranoff so that the correct Aleut names could be affixed to the specimens. My own delving in the library enabled me to provide him with the almost-forgotten place names recorded on early maps or used in early accounts of island life.

Dr. Harrington worked as only a zealous enthusiast can toil. He lived, ate, slept words. He withstood our intense coaxing to waste a few hours in seeing the island and watching the seals. He had no time for such folly. He had come to snare words and the last autumn boat would remove him from his hunting purview too soon. He had no time for social calls. Human beings he viewed from a cosmic angle that permitted sympathetic toleration for those unfortunates who did not appreciate the drama, the magic, the power, and the glory of the Word. Up at five thirty, he ceased work only for the half-hour respites of mealtimes and fretted through the brief delays forced upon him by unpunctual informants.

Almost nightly he dropped in after his dinner to chat with us while he waited for a laggard informant to return from the evening meal. Armed with a sheaf of papers he would send me flying for paper and pencil, either to note some interesting fact he had unearthed that day for my own journal or to take down instructions for some minor bit of detecting he was assigning me. While he fussed uneasily because his Aleut helpers were catching their breaths at home he either regaled us with entrancing Indian legends, comic experiences he had encountered on his research trips, or he analyzed the origin and development of words. Sam's philological hobby was given an outlet. Strange sounds winged through the room. Sanskrit, Greek, Latin, Arabic, Old Slavonic, Gaelic, and Welsh words, not to mention such mere striplings as German, French, Spanish, and Russian terms, were bandied about like juggled coins. All too soon for the Berenbergs a timid knock would announce the informant's arrival. Dr. John would depart in a bustle of crackling papers hastily gathered, a scurrying for wraps, a search for his hat, frequently found abandoned on the floor and serving as a comfortable couch for one or both of our kittens.

Harrington's choice of word-gathering station had accidentally been most fortuitous because the temporary summer Aleut workmen came from almost every archipelagic settlement. Despite the thinned ranks of the Aleut people, there are still people who speak

We found Harrington taking a bath and were instructed to go into Jack's room and see what was going on. Jack Marr is the man who takes the recordings for him. He played back a record for us, which contained a few giggles and murmurs from Mrs. Elliott and a nice clear statement in Mr. Elliott's voice and then some Aleut with Irish Stepetin speaking. Irish was not very fluent. Jack was reading some simple lines to him and Irish was fumbling in his answers. Jack's bedroom was littered with little piles of papers, sorting out the various kinds of information gathered. I picked up the one on the Pribilof Islands and copied down a few facts.

Harrington rushed in still dripping and explained the Russian alphabet to us. Very interesting. He took us off to his room to chat and regaled us with his problems and yarns until we were late for office hours as usual.

He dropped in after supper and Sam and I tried to interest him in an account of Elliott's doings but we rather failed. But we did give him some leads about reports that will send him searching for new words. And introduced him to the story of "Matka." He told us that Jordan was a smooth politician and that much of his work on fishes is rumored to be bolstered up by Edelman.[2]

I have asked him down to have dinner with us Sunday. I hope he enjoys it as much as he does the others he talks about. We heard about his preparations for coming up here yesterday. They had no

cont.

idea where they were going to stay. They brought provisions. They have had to give away their cheese and bacon because it is beginning to spoil. They would have bought a tent but Harrington had no chance to get one until he arrived at Ketchikan. He had the money in his hand and the clerk said they would have to send to the warehouse for it. Just then the *Penguin's* whistle blew and H. had to rush. Just in time, for the gangplank was already drawn up when he got to the dock. But this is another instance of the lack of courtesy or something worse that the Washington office is guilty of.

John Yatchmeneff was telling us stories about the Unalaska trees today so I have learned that Hultén has made a few errors, too. He says no seedlings came up. Yatch says there are a few, three or four feet high, and that one man transplanted some to his yard and has a nice yard as a result. Expedition Island is the Treasure Island of today. Yet Hultén says that the picture in the Harrington [*sic*, Harriman Alaska Expedition (1902)] book is of the clump of trees on Amaknak Island.[3] So the authorities are rarely as authoritative as they would have us think. I will write Hultén about this some day when the war has ebbed enough to permit mail to go to Sweden.

the three main dialects into which their language had been divided, the Unalaskan, Atkan, and that of Attu. The speech of the Pribilovians, stemming almost directly from the Unalaskan tongue, had been influenced by immigrants from Atka and Attu and had undergone changes due to the geographical and social isolation of the people. There were even differences in speech between the residents of St. Paul and St. George, principally in the adoption of Russian words and in changes in pronunciation due to careless inflection handed down from one generation to the next.

However, representatives of St. George were few on our island during the summer although some St. Paul people were familiar with the idioms of the other island. So Harrington sat at the hub of the Aleut world and could collect and compare samples of all varieties of Aleut without stirring from Government House.

Whoever turns to Aleut must go first to the old Russian sources, still almost wholly imprisoned in the untranslated publications of Veniaminov and the minor fragments in other Russian writings, or to word lists, usually compiled from Russian sources, in other European languages.

Harrington set to work translating into English the photostatic copies of Veniaminov's grammar and dictionary, which he had brought with him. His good fortune extended to his discovery of valuable assistants, Father Baranoff and John Yatchmeneff.[4] John's father, Alexei, had been the living source of information for all types of scientific investigators during his lifetime. Upon John's shoulders his father's mantle had fallen. He had become the chief spokesman for and interpreter of his people.[5]

John was good looking and very non-Aleut in appearance. Well poised and slightly conceited, he knew more about the world than most of the Aleuts. He was an excellent conversationalist and pleasant companion. He spoke, read, and wrote, with equal facility, Aleut, Russian, and English. Because of the social disadvantages of being Aleut, his really brilliant mind was often a detriment to him. There was no other outlet for his frustrated dreams except the forgetfulness of a drinking bout. Jobs of court interpreting and general interpreting, assisting visiting scholars, and filling various lay church positions were spasmodic and provided no regular livelihood. Jobs, menial and socially looked down upon, such as hospital porter or janitor, were his lot in Unalaska. As a blubberer on St. Paul he was an exemplary workman and rarely joined in local kvass drinking parties. And for a few weeks he was tasting the headier intellectual wine of being the authority on Aleutology. Next to Father Baranoff he was the Russian expert.

Harrington appraised John's potential weaknesses: the probability that John could not permit himself to confess ignorance and was capable of credible invention. Consequently all information was checked and rechecked against the testimony of others before acceptances.

With such helpers the work went quickly. One by one other informants were interviewed and squeezed dry of knowledge. How they reveled in their contributions! Until, toward the end of the project, the village grapevine spread the rumor that the island authorities, always contemptuous of intellectuals, were unusually disdainful of the eccentric word gatherer. Fearful of official disapproval, villagers flocked less readily to his rooms. But they still retained the inner pride that their language was going into a book for people far away to learn about. It seemed odd to me that the local nabobs were so careless as to ridicule publicly one whom the Aleuts would classify as another "white." All successful imperialists know that those who strive to impress supposed inferiors should maintain at least a public appearance of unity.

> November 8, 1941
> We stopped in at Gov. House and wasted some time discussing alcoholism, how much a person can drink and remain healthy, and the cure for hangovers. Then upstairs to see Harrington who showed us a delightful tale of the Aleuts about the volcanoes. He found it in an old report and copied it out for John Yatchmeneff to translate.
>
> November 10, 1941
> Dr. Harrington arrived a little after five, a bit gashed around the chin from rapid shaving and bearing his copy of Yatch's translation of the volcano story. I will be able to get the story later from the government report he is using.
>
> We had a pleasant meal, illuminated by Harrington's charming stories. And the stories and conversation lasted until he tore himself away at eight thirty. He should have gone up at eight for Yatch was supposed to be there working. Vivian came in just when he was telling us an interesting yarn about government graft, slight scandals of the Indian Bureau before Collier. So we did not hear the end of it.

Tracking down the origin of place names fascinated me. A flavor of early times clings to old names. A hint of the personality of the name bestower makes

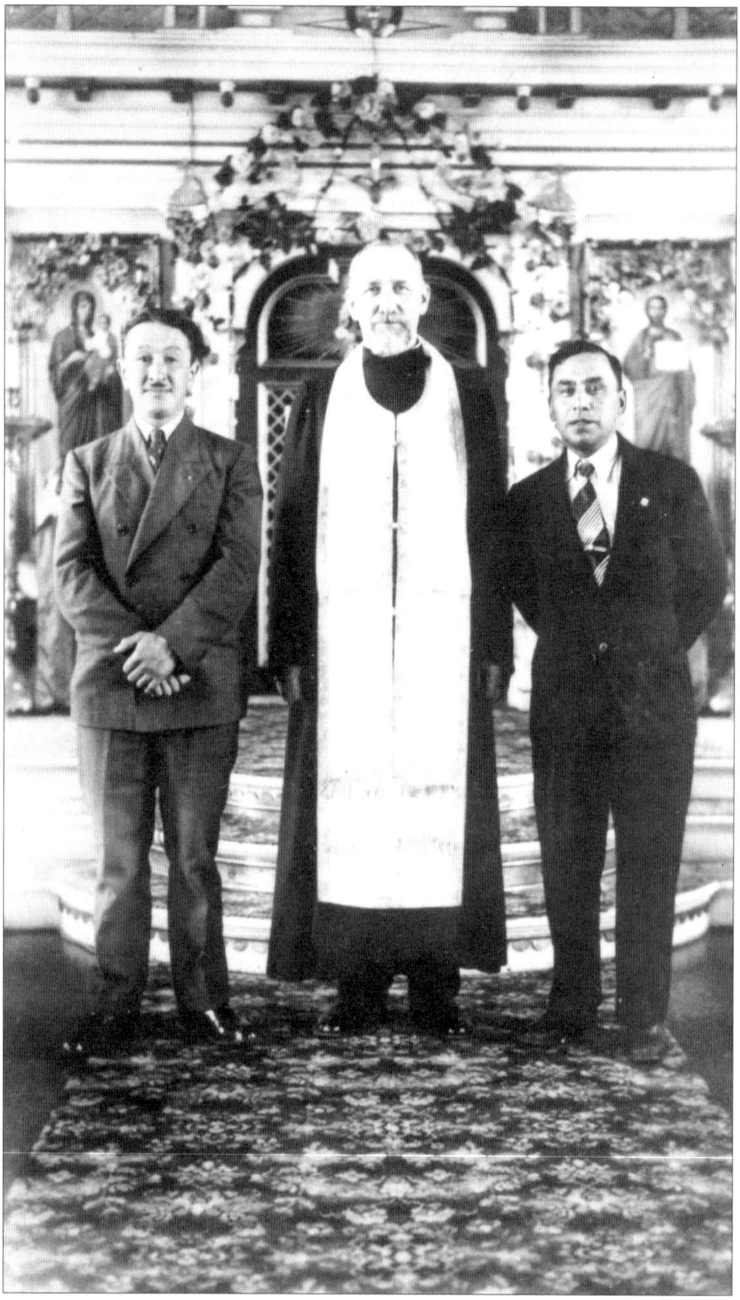

John Yatchmenev, Father Makary Baranoff, and John Hanson inside the St. Paul church (from the Martin Collection, USUAF210, Archives, Alaska and Polar Regions, Rasmuson Library, University of Alaska Fairbanks).

dry history more alive. Two names especially gave us good hunting. The Jordan Sealing Commission of 1896 had christened a small rookery on the Zolotoi side of Reef *Ardiguen,* defined as the Aleut word for a heap of stones.[6] The word seemed non-Aleut because the language had no *r* sound. No contemporary villager could decipher the mutilation. We pounced on every luckless patient who came into our office: "What is the correct meaning of *ardiguen?* How do you say `heap of stones' in Aleut?" At last everyone in the village was asking his neighbor about the name. The village concluded that the word was foreign. But still we hunted and delved. Jordan, in the text and accompanying map of his charming seal story "Matka," designated the killing field as *Asascardano,* a pleasing word to roll on the tongue but again extremely non-Aleut in spelling. Once more the alien *r* intruded.

One Sunday morning I woke with a romantic idea bubbling on the rim of my conscious mind, as if left behind by a dream. Perhaps the word had been SS *Cardano.* Had a ship of that name ever been anchored in Village Bay near the killing field or run aground in that neighborhood? Eagerly I confided my romantic notion to Dr. John who kindly refrained from squelching me immediately.

That afternoon John Yatchmeneff was playing hooky from his word games at a local name's day party. Harrington, compelled into inactivity, dropped in while Alice Gromoff and Peter Kochergin were calling on us. Our visitors found themselves on the witness stand, interrogated by three fairly gentle but very persistent bullies. We tried out the many possible variants of *ardiguen, arthiguen, arditheun, athuen;* no success. "Where was that place?" asked Peter. I told him once more. I showed him the map. Peter's look of mystification continued. Just when we were about to give up, Peter asked, "Do you know what we used to call them rocks in front of the Lagoon?" He uttered an Aleut word. It exploded in our ears.

[This entry describes Martin's first meeting with John Yatchmeneff. His father was an Aleut from Morzhovoi and was chief of Unalaska from 1902 until his death in 1937. The "church seminary" referred to was the Russian school operated by the Orthodox church.]

July 9, 1941
We were a bit late getting up because I had such a bad night topping off with an evil dream that aided in exhausting me. So Sam was in the tub at eight thirty when a very nice-looking patient arrived. He is a blubberer from Unalaska and looks more like a New York Jewish intellectual. Sam learned that he is a free citizen with voting powers and acts as court interpreter. His father was a Russian Jew, his mother an Aleut. He is here with his wife and child. And will stay until November. [The log for December 11 noted that he, his wife, and child Florence returned to Unalaska with Lilly and Myrtle Hope, who had been visiting.] Maybe when the rush season is over, we can learn some Russian from him. He once studied at a church seminary at Unalaska that then was closed after the Russian Revolution for lack of funds. Such ramifications.

"What? Say it again. And again." And Alice chimed in to repeat it. *Adgun* would be the English spelling but tongues would say something more literally close to *athguen*. *Adgun*, a heap of rocks.[7] The mystery of that slope of lava boulders on Reef's flank was solved. The American ears that listened in 1896 had caught a nonexistent *r* and made it official. They had taken an Aleut name from one locality and bestowed it on another.

> November 11, 1941
> It gets dark so early that it was already quite dusky as we approached the village about four thirty. Because of afternoon baths we don't have much time to hike in the afternoon. Next time there seems the promise of a nice day, I think we will bathe her in the A.M. and park her with her bottle with Vivian. But the difficulty is that perfect weather at nine thirty, the time for a morning bath, may be replaced by a blizzard before noon.
>
> When we got back, Heretina was busy cleaning the office and had a helper, Dunya Kochutin. With much prodding I managed to get the housework finished and supper started. But once supper was ready we were delayed listening to *Information Please*. And then the cook came from the Company House, in for infrared treatment, and Banner dropped in to discuss seal pediatrics. I dragged him into the kitchen with us. When we were through and back in the living room, two more Kochutin kids arrived. After that there was an enormous outburst of activity in the kitchen. And dishes were soon done.
>
> Vivian dropped in with a pound cake and sat about chatting until nine. We had tea and some of her cake. As soon as she was gone, I dashed to this machine and tossed off a letter to Bayla. One more ready for the boat.

After another quarter of an hour, stimulated by success, Peter stumbled over a word and Alice caught it and turned it over on her tongue and there was *asa*—a point of rocks sticking up above the water. And *cardano* was a mutilated version of the Aleut phrase for "long ago." Long ago, offshore from the old killing grounds, rocks had lifted their peaks above the washing tides, rocks that now lay concealed beneath the water. And a fact of physical geography, a hint of the changing contours of the island, lay concealed behind the name bestowed by some oldster who recalled the protruding reef. No shame to the ears who heard the *r*, for the guttural *a* too often suggests that sound to beginners.

Those Aleut vowels, just three of them, plague the beginning student. How many shades of tone can be given to *a, i, u*. Variations that an Anglican-trained ear would bank his reputation on as *e* or *o* transform phoneticians into frustrated delirium and reduce an amateur to a state of gibbering idiocy. Somehow the Aleuts, whose pronunciation actually is not standardized, achieve an intelligible communication that the noninitiate must sweat to imitate. Consonants affect the vowel sounds. For instance the *a* that seemingly had an *r* in tow preceded the *th* sound and the combination deceived carefully attentive ears.

The consonants, more easily transliterated by the Russian alphabet than the Roman without using such combinations as *ng* and *ch*, are further complicated in living speech by aspirated variations. The Aleut alphabet is easily expressed by sixteen Russian letters. One American authority, Geoghegan, used sixteen Roman letters, a combined *ng*, and a diacritic sign.

Knowing the grammar of modern European languages is no help. Aleut, while definitely a strongly differentiated branch of Eskimo, so different as to be almost a distinct tongue with a subskeletal eskimoid structure, lacks the harsher and more difficult sounds of the regular Eskimo and the languages of the Indians of southeastern Alaska. Like the Eskimo dialects, the existence of the verb is a question over which linguists fight fierce duels. Luckily with pens. An Eskimo does not trifle with an actual expression for "being," a condition that is self-evident. What we consider verbs, action words, Aleut and Eskimo brethren express via nouns in a state of existence. *He runs* is therefore in the Aleut mind *his running*. But it is possible for the non-Aleut to handle this unusual thought pattern in terms more familiar to his own background.

The rich web of inflection is a labyrinth for the uninitiated. Veniaminov found about seventy terminal endings for nouns and four hundred for his so-called verbs, squeezed and manipulated into the conventional conjugations and declinations of the classic languages.

Demonstrative pronouns are bewildering obstacles to the student's progress because so many special words identify the position of the speaker or his posture. As examples, *wan* means the one nearest to the speaker; *ingan'*, second from the speaker; *ikun'*, third; and *akan* means one far off. Other words denote whether the person alluded to is sitting or standing.[8]

November 17, 1941
Sam spent all Saturday developing and printing pictures with uneven success because, among other factors, the power is low on Saturday and the current fluctuates badly. We have an excellent view of the village that Wilke took from the radio tower and accidentally took two of the main part of the village that match perfectly.

Monday night we were up talking with Hank and he found the portion of Elliott's monograph on seals that was published among the documents of the tenth census. So we lugged down two colossal tomes that have portions in them. His sketches, which are unique and comical, are in the other two volumes. I shall chuckle over them on my visits there. I am chuckling over his writings here at odd minutes when I can sit where such a big volume can be read. I've tried reading them in bed, but the effort required to handle these awkward outsized books is too much for comfort.

The Aleut, of course, had no grammatical problems himself until the Russian Church required a means of communication with their new converts. He had no written literature of his own except the few fragments picked up by Veniaminov and recorded in the imposed Slavic symbols. The bishop's labors led eventually to the publication of nine books in Aleut, all religious in character. A few other scattered religious manuscripts, mainly sermons, exist.[9]

December 3, 1941
Harrington's financial troubles gave us a very unflattering picture of research via the Smithsonian. He and most of the other men pay their own fieldwork expenses from their salary. I doubt if H. gets more than twenty-six thousand dollars. He mentions a fifteen-percent wage cut that came from the last world war and not until Roosevelt came in was ten percent restored. Now new economies are in the wind.

Harrington is a glutton for punishment in his search of words. He came across the continent in a Greyhound bus, pays Jack Marr a salary and expenses as well as his own, and pays his informants—all from his meager salary. No wonder he has no family or is so out of touch with the world or so naively thankful for dinners people have given him. He always throws in such details in every account of his work. Pathetic. Scholarship in the U.S.A.–Bah . . .

In the course of our conversations when we were expressing our disgust with such a system, Harrington told us we had not heard the worst yet. He had learned the facts just a couple of years ago. For years he had dreamed that when he retired he could go to some foreign country where he could live better and more cheaply while he enjoyed some other language, but there is a regulation or law that the annual medical examination of people on pensions must be performed in the United States. He said many people went to Europe and hoarded

cont.

However effective these books might have been in stimulating Aleut culture, the cultivation of written Aleut was completely stifled by the American acquisition of their homeland. The Russian Church continued until 1919 to print editions of the religious texts for their most active mission field. Individuals here and there in the Aleut settlements nourished their borrowed writing medium and handed it on to their children, but in each generation the will to pass on their heritage weakens.

For the scholar, the review of Aleut is complicated by the necessity of both studying the records of the Russians and investigating the contemporary speech. For the amateur like myself, more anxious to establish contact with our Aleut associates, it was simpler to strive to absorb the sound range and pick up homely phrases and learn them parrot-wise for usage. Thus Sam learned to say, "Breathe in, breathe out," and similar directives to his patients that made office calls more pleasant.

If I had expended much effort in learning Veniaminov's grammar before reaching St. Paul what a muddle I would have been in trying to formulate conversation on my own. For the Aleut tongue, the research disclosed, had been and was still deteriorating, wasting from the blight with which civilization had sapped tribal vitality. Not alone had it ceased to grow and expand, except by the artificial means of borrowing first Russian and later a few English words, but it had actually shrunk, diminished in volume as far as the vocabulary of daily conversation was concerned.

To me this discovery was the most pitiful I had made about my Aleut friends. First I had been shocked at their lack of English after seventy years of American guardianship. Then I had been disillusioned about the average Aleut's fluency in Russian. Only a few old people could express themselves in defective Russian. The churchgoers knew by heart the sound but not the meaning of Old Slavonic prayers and hymns. At least I thought they possessed their own tongue completely. Then I learned that their thought range was circumscribed by an ever-shrinking vocabulary.

Father Baranoff's carefully gathered statistics revealed that the old men over fifty and a few younger men of St. George spoke Russian passably, while on St. Paul only the old women spoke and read Russian. The reason for the sexual division of devotion to Russian is a mystery. The exact figures of those who could read and write their own tongue were six on St. Paul and four on the sister island. The truth is even less pleasant than the numbers indicate. The totals include those who struggle with the intricacies of the curlicues of the Slavonic alphabet as well as the more expert.

In retrospect, I became wise to circumstances that forethought should have predicted. Their living language of the past had been limited to the conditions and attendant thought processes of a simple mode of life. Two foreign cultures had imposed new conditions and the terms in which to express those conditions. Alien pronunciation affected the Aleut sounds. Imperfect, sloppy habits in new media of communication led to carelessness in speaking their native tongue.

Daily I saw examples of the difficulties of transference of thought around me. I heard Heretina try to impart my instructions to Paul, our janitor, in Aleut and merely confuse him. Sometimes in despair, she herself

pennies so as to make a steerage trip back to the States in summer just for the examination and sometimes are forced to stay as much as six weeks before all the red tape is cut. This seems definitely a problem for the United Federal Workers. So many of such cruelties are so completely unnecessary that one wonders what type of sadistic mind proposed them.

Even to spend one's money on fieldwork, the powers that be at the Smithsonian must consider plan of work and grant permission. Harrington, who seems to have been there since 1916, had been caged in Washington for nine months and hated the office routine. He outlined the following reasons for studying Aleut.

Hrdlička had been at work so long, trying to dig up some traces of past men in these northern areas, to try to locate some indication that man came to the American continent from Asia, via a northern route. Harrington explained to them why the artifacts that excavations disclosed could never supply the missing link. Harrington mentioned Henry Bascom Collins as a follower of Hrdlička and credited him with excavations on St. Lawrence Island.

(Incidentally, since I have heard there are no funds for carrying on research except from stray angles, I do not judge Hrdlička so much for his unsavory practice of luring college students to dig for him and making them pay their own expenses. Another dishonesty necessary in a dishonest society.)

cont.

Harrington pointed out to his superiors that language alone might hope to reveal a link between the continents. Words and perhaps the melodies of songs might disclose the relationships of tribes and throw more light on the mystery. So that is his aim and I hope he comes to some final conclusion. If he does not get Aleut wholly recorded now no one else will be able to. Old people are few and far between. I should say people over fifty, for they are the old people here. An old blind woman, mother of Nekifer Mandregan, is eighty-five, the oldest one alive here. And her memory is none too good.

December 5, 1941
Yatchmeneff has told Harrington that at Kashega, a small village at the westward end of Unalaska Island, on the north side, lives an old Native who remembers the days of otter hunting. Harrington longs to visit him for the occupation of otter hunting carries with it a tremendous vocabulary of particular terms, for equipment, for hunting techniques, etc.

resorted to crude English, ending rudely, "You dummy, you."

Carl Hoverson described Nekifer Mandregan's attempts to interpret simple orders. Nekifer would address the work gang for a few minutes volubly. No response. He would pause and start off on another tack. Failure again. A couple of simple English sentences would develop into a long, obviously clumsy Aleut harangue. It was actually often easier for the officials to explain in broken English, illustrated by signs, than to prompt and reprompt an interpreter. It seems incredible that distorted English phrases, uncomplicated by grammatical constructions, articles, prepositions, adjectives, or adverbs, the barest skeleton of English, should be more intelligible than their own language. But the facts were to be faced and could not be denied.

I came to believe that the average Aleut had an English vocabulary almost as large as his Aleut one. The English words simply needed dusting off and made useful by being spoken and heard constantly for a while. The Aleuts had a reason for lack of practice. The few who were articulate in English were conspicuous. Able to talk man-to-man in the agent's tongue, they looked directly, without shyness, into his eyes, unconsciously less dependent in demeanor. The reward of fluency is peculiar, particularly in the face of constant criticism of the villagers' inability to learn and speak English. Troublemakers, wise guys, soreheads, even Nazis and Communists, are only some of the labels. It matters not how well behaved the speaker is. Once he talks like a "white," bureaucratic minds recoil, recognizing the potential strength and independence of English-speaking sealers. Happier is the Aleut who keeps his mouth shut and conforms to the almost kindly intoned epithet of "stupid native."

Keeping their English vocabulary locked up in their minds is an instinctive safety device that had deleterious effects the sealers did not recognize. A sense of values, human, personal, familial, and social, depends upon thought and the exchange of thought with others. The exchange of ideas, so vital to an integrated human group, had for nearly two hundred years been shrinking. Floundering in a transitional stage for generations, never welcomed into American, English-speaking circles, never stimulated to open-hearted acceptance of the new language nor admitted to opportunities for full usage of it, the Pribilof sealers are actually an encouraging reminder of the toughness of the human spirit. Their present is heartbreaking to individuals among them and shameful to Americans who have to accept responsibility for their plight, but their own future, and certainly the future of their children, is not hopeless.

The increasing changes to the Pribilof Aleut dialect came vividly to light in comparing local informants with individuals from the Chain where bureaucracy had not consistently dominated the way of life for seventy years. The languages of men from Atka, Attu, and Belkofsky were not so sterile or arid. The difference was one of degree, but the pressure of the worst of the twentieth century lay most heavily upon the people of Unalaska and the Pribilof Islands.

Nightmares were not my only reaction to the revelation. My waking hours were invaded by unhappy thoughts. I found myself in a prison whose bars were compounded of shame and disinterest. Could I turn to no aspect of the islanders' lives without being confronted by the warped results of racial discrimination, symptoms of social ills, and the wounds of injustice? If grammar and word lists were not free from social distemper, the inspiration of the island, its flora and fauna, could but be a mockery of man's eternal indifference to man, or at most but a temporary solace of a wounded spirit.

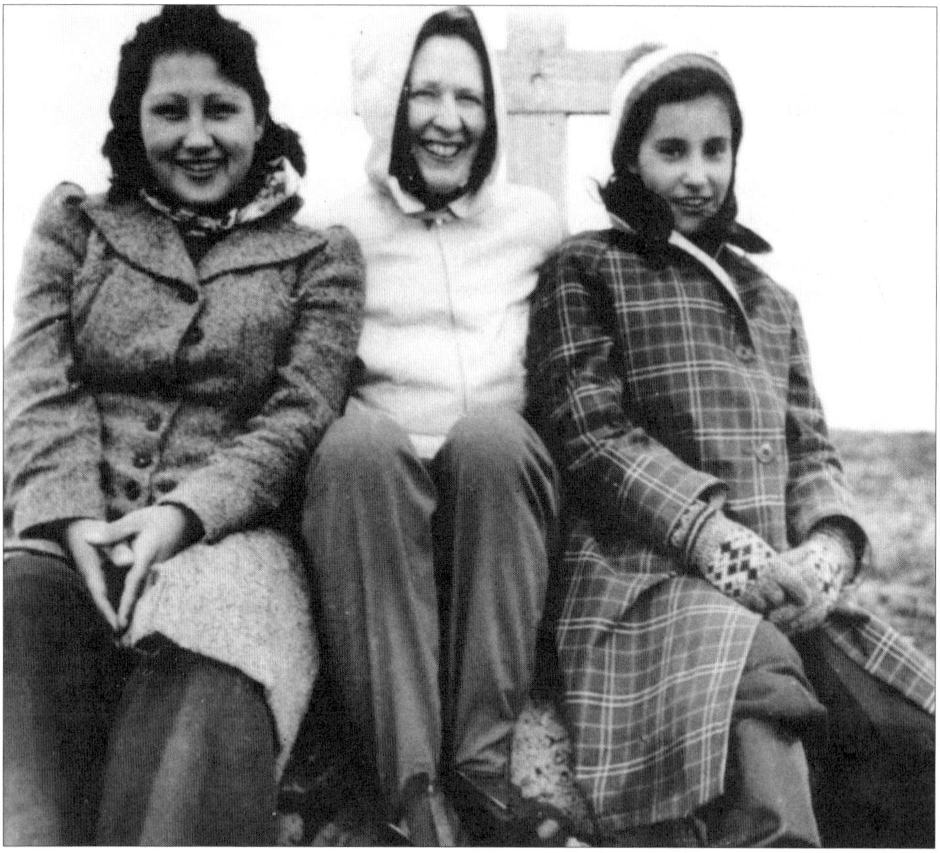

Heretina Kochergin, Fredericka Martin, and Alice Gromoff (from the Martin Collection, USUAF210, Archives, Alaska and Polar Regions, Rasmuson Library, University of Alaska Fairbanks).

Chapter 30

When mankind's ill-wrought schemes threaten to suffocate the mind and heart, contact with a generous, whole human being refreshes and renews the atmosphere and inspires the lagging will. My reminder arrived in the mail sacks of the *Penguin,* late in November, in the innocent form of three bursting envelopes bearing the return address of R. H. Geoghegan, Orientalist, Fairbanks, Alaska. One of Stefansson's suggestions was coming to life. The overstuffed appearance of the envelopes was imposing. The contents overwhelmed us. In answer to an obscure stranger, one not even an academic linguistic student, R.H.G. (we used this alphabetical appellation until he wrote us that the Gaelic syllables of his surname could best be slurred together by the non-Irisher into the sound of the German verbal form *gegen;* by that time the initial habit was strong and cannot yet be broken) had toiled laboriously, not merely to give us a bibliography, as we had asked. Since what we needed most was buried in old Russian books that he possessed, he had provided us with word lists and a condensation of large sections of the grammar wonderfully simplified by his explanatory comments.

The size of Geoghegan's contribution to us proved his warm generosity. It expressed a spirit met rarely in the normal walks of life. It marked a scholar of great heart who said, "I have knowledge not in books. Let me give it to others." Just to look at the many closely

December 3, 1941
The difficulties of the *Penguin* on this trip would make a romantic tale. Poor Captain Knudsen must be inventorying all marine superstitions endeavoring to find what jinx is hovering over the ship. He has never encountered so many varieties of obstructions, delays, and misfortunes on one journey before. We who scoffed at the tales of ships standing offshore for long periods have been humbled as we watched, day after day, the *Penguin* at anchor far out from land while heavy seas battered away at our landing places.

Misfortunes began in Seattle. Just what damages necessitated the *Penguin* being put in dry dock, I have not learned. But into dry dock she went and weeks dragged by while repairs were going on. Three times, Mr. Johnston wrote us, the perishable stores

cont.

were ordered. Three times the orders had to be countermanded. At last, November 8, the *Penguin* up-anchored and steamed through the locks into Puget Sound. There was a long stop at Ketchikan. Julia Merculieff, whom Sam had sent to Seattle to procure an artificial arm, had been extremely seasick. She began to vomit blood. The captain was alarmed and radioed an account of her symptoms to Juneau. He was advised to put into the nearest port where a doctor would be available. So the ship stopped off at Kodiak.

Captain Knudsen had reason to be worried. He feared that if he were forced to leave the girl there, with her father and without instructions from the Service, he might be held liable for her bill. So he radioed here and to Seattle to secure promises of financial backing if it were necessary to leave her. But Kodiak doctors pronounced her well enough to proceed and apparently ruled out the feared diagnosis of appendicitis.

Storms were blowing up around Kodiak. There were too heavy winds to make good enough time to assure entry into some of the more dangerous bays where stops were necessary to let off weathermen and other government personnel. Between stops, while anxious hearers on St. Paul listened to the radio conversations between Sparks and our Mr. Elliott, the nightly report would come: "Anchored for the night." The personnel here, straining at the leash to get away on leave in time to celebrate Thanksgiving in

cont.

typed pages, with barely a suggestion of margin left clear, imparted salutary humbleness of spirit. As we pored over the pages we found personal notes inserted at intervals that made our unseen teacher more alive to us. He penned an apology for a scratched out phrase because at seventy-six his right hand was partially paralyzed and hindered his efficiency. Life became more spacious, more invigorating, because an elderly scholar, handicapped by a physical disability, had so wholeheartedly poured out his knowledge for unknown people at the cost of long hours of painful exertion. It was nearly a year before our loving admiration for him was increased by the knowledge that the stroke that impaired his muscles had also dimmed his eyesight and dulled his hearing.

There were no dull shadows in his mind. His driest grammatical explanations scintillated. The letters sparkled with whimsical quips and roguish wit. His saucy observations about knotty grammatical points etched the means of applying the rule in our memories as no factual explanations could have. So sure were we of his humorous instinctive understanding that when the February mail boat did not arrive to take out letters for him we dared to wire, "With assistance of your lessons now teaching Aleuts their language." And R.H.G. reading it in Fairbanks a few hours later chuckled as heartily as we had expected.

The crowning gift of all was in the third envelope, a translation of the portion of the journal of Bishop Veniaminov that described the Pribilofs. Something I had expected to have only by obtaining photostats of that old, unobtainable volume from some library copy and toiling slowly over the Russian sentences with a dictionary in my hand for months and months. And there it was in my hand as a casual gift. Because translating and typing had gone on simultaneously, in order to get the last autumn mail boat, R.H.G. defended any crudities of English, crudities that close carping inspection could not reveal. We persuaded the agent's secretary, John Stacy, to type copies for the two island libraries, for the Seattle office, and Father Baranoff's historical files. Nine months later my conscience smote me when R.H.G. admitted he had kept no personal copy.

Carbon copies seemed alien to his nature. Once he had presented the complete translation of the Veniaminov dictionary to the Smithsonian. Then he requested that the manuscript be transferred to the fledgling Territorial Museum at Juneau, where it vanished into nothingness. Because that valuable translation found no safe niche accessible to scholars, a Smithsonian ethnologist had just been forced to repeat the labor of translation as a basis for further studies.

At other times R.H.G. had translated large sections of Veniaminov's works for interested individuals, keeping no record for himself. Each time he assumed that he was finished with what was for him a minor linguistic interest, a pleasant interlude away from the Oriental studies he enjoyed so much more thoroughly. He never foresaw that someone else would continue to spring into view to ask to borrow the English key to Aleut. Public interest, academic interest, the two faces that might have crowned his studies with pleasurable satisfaction of seeing his efforts in print, were lacking. Only here and there, in Copenhagen, in Paris, in an American college, individual scholars knew the value of retaining a complete record of Aleut. Not even the foster country of the Aleuts had realized the vital stimulus such

the States, would sit back and sigh. Another night wasted.

Sand Point, King Cove, and finally Unalaska. The day of the 1941 official Thanksgiving the *Penguin* came to rest in the harbor at Unalaska and settled down to wait word from the islands that the weather would permit unloading. Day after day McMillin raced around the island, from one cove to another, seeking a landing place. Day after day the winds swept in contrary directions and the shores remained inaccessible. Big swells rolled firmly toward the land against which the baidars could make no progress or furious seas threw themselves menacingly against other sections of the shore. Sunday came. McMillin spoke the magic words but the *Penguin* reported her position that night at Unalaska. Great anger and chagrin were expressed by the impatient passengers waiting here, for the captain did not explain the reasons for his delay. He had been forced to take on a new hand at Unalaska because one of his men had left. He had started out for the islands. The new hand went crazy. The *Penguin* was forced to turn back and take the man to a hospital and secure a substitute. Finally, on Monday the *Penguin* made a fresh start.

At St. George she was supposed to pick up the radioman there to relieve Mr. Elliott for the winter. The weatherman was cautious. He refused to go out to the ship. "You're crazy if you think you are going to get me out in those seas in a small boat," he is supposed

cont.

to have said. They cannot call him fool or coward for the baidar made the trip safely to the boat, received the mail, and, on the way back to shore, overturned. The poor Aleuts had a cold ducking. Some of the parcels floated away. The contents of others were ruined. The mailbags are supposed to be waterproof, but I do not think they are tied correctly to face such experiences. We have heard no other details about the consequences of this sudden bath, but Herd was exonerated from the charge of sissiness . . .

The *Penguin* came directly here, arriving off West Landing about five o'clock. At six the baidar brought in passengers and the mail. Mrs. Wilke was here at last. On two occasions she had spoken to her husband over the radio and had been most frank in her expressions of disgust at the delay. But for her delays were over and she and her husband could settle down to a pleasant winter of work and companionship. For the outgoing passengers, there was no milder joy. They felt that it might be a few days before they could get started for home, but after the long wait, the sight of the *Penguin* at anchor was tantalizing but just suppose—and "just suppose" came true. The next day, long before light, a little before six, the workmen were called to man the baidars. Unloading went on as quickly as possible. All day long the trucks roared past the windows and stopped often to give us precious parcels.

a guidebook between Aleuts and her other citizens would be.

Consequently, whenever a call came, dear R.H.G. propped up his Russian texts, pulled the lid from his typewriter, and patiently repeated his previous work, always improving his material and enriching it with his own observations of the spoken language.

Armed with R.H.G.'s texts (more came to us in January), we were able to penetrate a few grammatical mysteries, acquire a skeleton vocabulary, and continue our studies in the winter after Harrington's departure. Then we met fresh difficulties. Patient Aleut listeners we had aplenty. Our bookish grammar fitted us to tackle the religious Aleut texts Father Baranoff had given us, but was unwieldy, unintelligible to our island listeners. Evening after evening or during afternoon calls, our Aleut acquaintances pored over the typed word lists with us. Some words had acquired a different connotation since Veniaminov's time. Mainly the insidious vowel pronunciation tripped all of us up. A typed word spelled with a Roman *a* that was pronounced locally with a *u* or *e* sound evoked no recognition among our friends. Given two more years on St. Paul, with faithful daily practice, we might have acquired fluent conversational ability.

Not that our brief studies were futile. I retain an appreciation of thought patterns to be earned in no other way. I have warm memories of the liveliest hours spent companionably with many Aleuts I may never see again, hours of laughing contact to be won in no other manner in the island social atmosphere of suspicious timidity and resentment against the "whites." And if Harrington's studies are resumed and completed after the war and are finally published, the Smithsonian has at least one customer ready for a book that will definitely not be a best-seller.

Best of all, our intent to learn Aleut gave us R.H.G., whose fat letters follow us wherever we go, filled not with Aleut now but brimful of the awesome intricacies of Gaelic, the language of his childhood and of my father's ancestors. Still unacquainted physically but only *correspondentially*, as he writes, our mutual affection had grown and grown until he is among our dearest friends, as close as real blood kin.[1] Specialists in Alaskana will know of him as the editor of the valuable Russian section of Judge Wickersham's monumental "Bibliography of Alaskan Literature." How tragic for a generation of youth who might have been stimulated by his instructions, by the witty inspiring textbooks he might have published, that the currents of life bore him into the secluded heart of Alaska, to be known only by the greatest linguistic savants of the entire world, by a few fortunate people like ourselves, and the very lucky little Ten'a damsel whom he entertains. Describing his frivolous pastime, he wrote, "I play 'shop' and cut out salmon strips and money and blueberry pies and candy and snowshoes and heaven knows what else from old paper by the hour for a husky Ten'a damsel of seven summers who lives across the street from me and between whiles we solemnly criticize the adventures of Rumpelstiltskin, and the Green Dwarf, and Faithful John, and the Frog King and other heroes of faery lore. It had always been a great hobby of mine to consort and condole with the small fry."

November 19, 1941
Office filled with waiting patients who were soon dispatched. Dinner. Then a bath and supper for her majesty who was delighted to see us and not very interested in food. Dr. Harrington arrived during her feeding while we were listening to a news broadcast from the States. He was in search of my references for certain statements I had made about old Russian maps of St. Paul. So I had to lug out those huge tenth census volumes and others and read the excerpts to him. He flopped down on his knees and began to write. His pen ran dry. He dived into his pocket and brought out his pet bottle of ink, which I suspect he sleeps with, and filled his pen. He kept appearing about to lean on the wooden radiator cover where he had put his ink. I read breathlessly, waiting until he should dislodge the cover that does not fit well and be baptized, not only with his own ink, but with the sand of my miniature garden in a baking tray and a dish of seashells. I was glad when he was finished and had gone back to an easy chair.

Some Aleuts are consciously aware of the progressive desuetude of their language. Adults frankly berated their language limitations and regretted the limited opportunities for acquiring more English and using it. Others feel like Agnes Melovidov's aunt. Since four-year-old Agnes was motherless and pathetically shy, she was dragged limply into our preschool clinic for a physical examination by her elderly aunt. Finished with height and weight, heart and chest, and other data,

Agnes was being pushed into her coat when her aunt idly observed, "Agnes don't talk." But Agnes knew her name and her age in English when Sam asked her. "I can't find anything wrong," he told the aunt. "She seems to be speaking all right."

"Yes, she speak English," said the aunt. "But she don't talk."

Communication difficulties too often limited our social conversational attempts to weather and other banal topics. That we could not share very intimately the islanders' social life was unimportant to either the Aleuts or ourselves. Really serious was the lack of accuracy in discussions of health and disease with patients.

"Are you giving your baby strained vegetables?" Sam would ask a young mother. Since the regulation government-issued food provided no food of any kind for children under two and nothing but oatmeal for youngsters from two to four, it was necessary for parents to purchase canned supplies from the Native Canteen. The expense deterred many mothers anxious to nourish their children. Consequently it was necessary to check and recheck the child's diet.

The mother's reply "I get some" was a puzzle that had to be deciphered by further questions. It might indicate she had been buying it and was still faithfully using it daily for her child. On the other hand she might have purchased a few cans once or twice and no more. It might be a promise that she intended to go straight from the office to the Canteen to buy some and would introduce the new food to the child that very afternoon. This battle of the tenses went on over practically every instruction given a patient.

"Breathe in and out with your mouth open," Sam ordered the patient, who continued to stare at him uncomprehendingly. "Like this," said Sam, panting. The patient's face would light with understanding as he or she began to imitate Sam. How many minutes were saved when Sam had the Aleut phrase at his tongue's tip. And how relaxed and free from embarrassment were the patients at hearing their own tongue.

I told Heretina how to identify a pie plate reserved for the cat's milk only. "Take a little piece of adhesive tape and stick it on the edge of the pan," I enunciated clearly. I saw her carrying some long loops of adhesive from the doctor's office and warned her gently against wasting medical supplies. Hours later I happened to glance under the stove. The pie plate was taped securely to the floor by two long pieces of adhesive. No wonder she had required so much tape! My English had been at fault in some way. How puzzled she must have been by my motive in fastening the pie plate to the floor. Probably scornful, too.

It was not so amusing the nights she misread the directions for the griddle cakes and baked all the dough in cake tins or boiled the lettuce like Swiss chard. Pribilof housekeeping would have been less of a strain to both of us had we been able to understand each other.

We tried to be so friendly, Heretina and I. But every time she started to chatter to me, her mixed-up personal pronouns and tenses would force me to ask clarification. If I did not question her, I often failed to respond to her tale as she expected me to. Either way, the story was speckled and she lapsed back into monosyllabic comments, the animation subsiding, to leave her face a smooth mask.

Sam had English classes. I taught typing. Smiles and Alice Gromoff were my pupils and they learned their mechanical tasks rapidly. The perfect deft coordination of their fingers in the touch system was balked by their slowness to read English text quickly. Their reading tagged way behind and the copying from sight was a complete failure. Neither of them could compose their own thoughts in English swiftly enough to keep up with their mobile fingers.

Smiles started reading *Treasure Island* for his reading assignment. The words he handled fairly smoothly, but there was scarcely a sentence that he really understood. He had no background to prepare him to enjoy that boy's classic. I had never realized the potentially immoral influence of the opening pages with the scene laid in a tavern and full of songs about rum and grog drinking. Smiles seemed confused by it. The story certainly clashed with oft-heard precepts against drinking.

When Julia Merculieff joined the class she asked immediately, "Can I learn fast?" "As fast as you can learn," Sam encouraged. Julia took home a multigraphed copy of fourth-year grammar lessons, borrowed from the school, with an assignment to study certain rules and fill in blanks on two or three pages. Three days later she was back with the entire booklet filled in. Everything was wrong. Punctuation, spelling, grammar, everything. She had seemed so much more fluent than the average young person that her handiwork, or mental work, was extremely disappointing. It took sev-

November 19, 1941
The hospital improves gradually. Peter Kochergin has finished the walls of the green patient room and the yellow and white waiting room. He has begun to clean the floor of the green room. I am anxious for him to finish one floor for I have my doubts about this grey floor paint we are forced to use for lack of better. I'm afraid it will be so dark it can conceal dirt and it may detract from the dainty aspect of the rest of each room.

The village lake froze over hard enough to support about forty youngsters skating this afternoon. The children skate well, swooping and gliding like the gulls that usually frequent the spot. I learned from Harrington last night that some old informant stated that the Aleuts used to make sled runners and skates of the walrus tusks. How long ago he did not know for his informant was vague as to years passing–only, "when he was a boy." Since dear old Metrofan died I have lost my best check against rumors and tales. He can worry no longer over the Japanese invasion and the news these past few days would have worried him a great deal.

I met his wife Sunday coming back from the cemetery. Few people seem to visit the graves and I was surprised.

Now to supper–to be continued?–depending upon the professor and Aleut words.

eral weeks to dampen her ardor long enough to impress the fact that she must sit down and study the rules at the tops of each page and apply them to the exercises.

May 11, 1941
Alexandra reported proudly that she had been in charge of the schoolroom for a short period in the morning and had reported twelve pupils for talking in Aleut. The Hellbaums have suddenly become very strict about this and movie privileges are forfeited once for one remark in Aleut-for longer periods if the offense is repeated. Some kids have already lost several movies, which means that the street outside our house is noisy on movie nights when at least in the past we had two quiet evenings with no hoodlums running and shouting around the hospital.

Father Baranoff has been trying to locate the site of the old village and has this much information. On the site of the present radio station there were once barabaras. When John Hanson was a boy he used to play in those depressions and remembers the whalebone timbers.

But Dimitri, the pump man, has introduced a new puzzle. He insists there were once barabaras and a small village behind Lukanon, between it and Diamond Hill. He has promised to show the depressions in the ground to Father one of these days. I am anxious to see them. I wish I could find those around Polovina Lake and the site of the old graveyard there.

Some people expected the radio to stimulate interest in understanding English, force an awareness of English words and American sentiments upon unstirred minds. They overlooked the average American family's indifference to a blasting radio and that special radio deafness that is a new social phenomenon until in thousands of households all conversations and activities are carried on comfortably only over the constant drone of music and voice. Only the turn of the dial that brings silence startles. The same process happened even faster on the Pribilofs. During the absence of sound in the hours of daylight when static interfered with radio reception, the villagers supplied their own programs. A few small broadcasting appliances from Sears Roebuck, a dozen hillbilly records, and a few families took turns supplying the whole community with radio entertainment, with background music.

The men, most of them, hung over their radios at news time. They heard some peculiar facts, sometimes they complained bitterly of the announcer's too-rapid speech. It was not unusual for their radios to blast on and on in Japanese, Spanish, Russian. A good comfortable sound. And almost as intelligible. How often the village quivered with excitement because the words *Alaska* or *Aleutian Islands* had been caught in the hurly-burly of talk. "What was it?" they asked each other. The question raced round the village. It was sure to reach the hospital. Peter Kochergin would run in apologetically, "Did you hear the news? Something about Aleutians. So-and-so just came to the hospital to ask but the boys (meaning the tuberculous patients, practically chained to their radios) they didn't hear so good either."

I joined the optimists by putting faith in the talking movies. Out of the proceeds of their own Canteen, the villagers began, not long before our arrival, to rent movies. I didn't know there were so many bad movies until I went to the Pribilofs. The Cisco Kid was the healthiest regular feature and became the boys' hero.

The movement, the action, requires the accompanying conversational concentration so the people strained their ears. Since they saw most films two or three times, they began to memorize snatches of conversation. I overheard the children who came to play with Heretina repeating whole scenes. Often they asked Sam or me to explain a word. A few words must have been absorbed from the radio; many more became real to them on the screen. But as long as the "whites" of the island sit in the small gallery without paying admission, leaning back against plush seats, enjoying the movies paid for by the Aleuts who sit below on hard, backless benches, how can English become their own beloved natural language? Not until their American associates open the gates and admit the Aleuts to mingle in their society and converse with them can English be the natural speech of the Pribilofs.

> July 21, 1941
> I learned that the movies attract the St. Georgians. They have never visited here in such large numbers before. Helena Mandregan's mother was returning home. She came up and shook hands with us and said thank you. One of those evidences of a natural courtesy that I am sure they did not learn from the so-called "whites." Mrs. East commented on the same fact being proven because so many were taking back bunches of dried straw flowers, which do not grow on St. G. And contrasting it with her daughter's roommate having to be reminded by her mother to give Mrs. East flowers when she was a guest in her home.

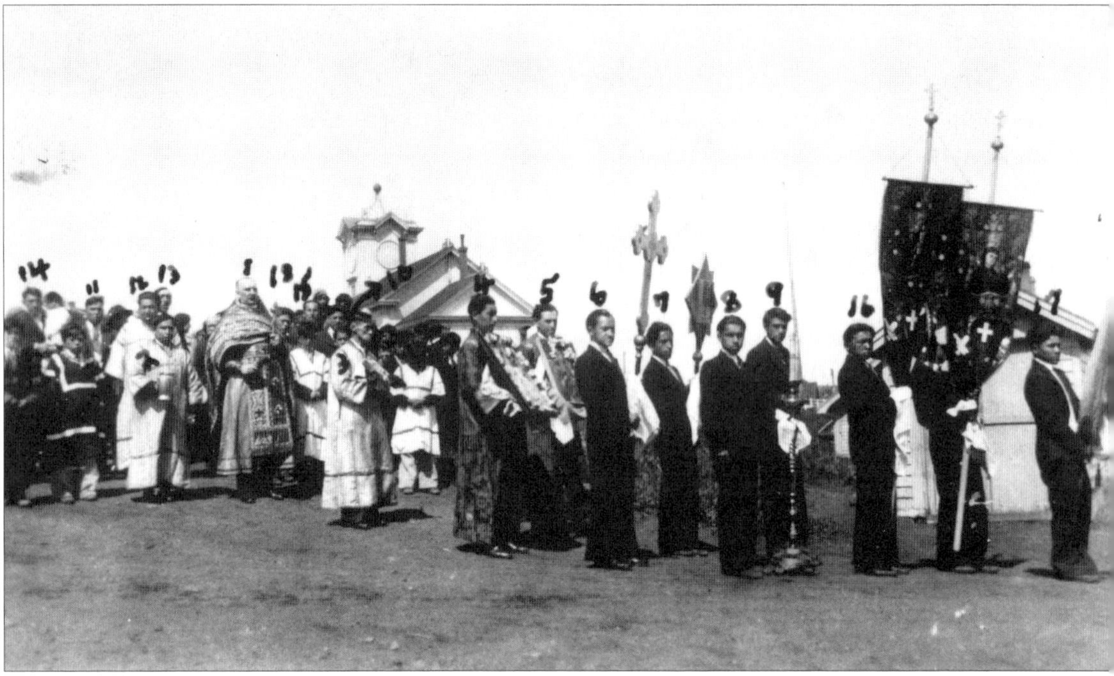

Church procession on St. Paul (from the Martin Collection, USUAF210, Archives, Alaska and Polar Regions, Rasmuson Library, University of Alaska Fairbanks).

Chapter 31

As I began to understand the shortcomings of the educational system, the tight circles of persons, institutions, commercial practices, and business aims that had encircled and molded the Aleut, I wondered what the Greek Russian Orthodox Church had given him, since the first mission monks landed on Kodiak Island in 1794, that it had retained his fealty. What had this faith contributed to his development? How forceful was the local church as a spiritual and moral influence in the community?

I remember Ward T. Bower in Washington saying the only punishment that really touched the hearts of the sealers was exclusion from church services for a short period. When we arrived no priest was in residence. Nekifer Mandregan, one of the two foremen and an ordained deacon, was conducting services. Because of his success in retaining the job of foreman, he did not have the complete confidence of his people. He loved gambling and, to me, Nekifer, whom I liked very much and whose ever-smiling wife I loved, seemed hardly the perfect representation of holiness and sanctity.

When the church bells began to toll at six thirty every Saturday night, I liked to stand at the window watching people stream from their homes. The men wore ill-fitting Sears Roebuck suits. The women and girls were gay in colorful modish dresses, hats, and coats from the same mail-order house. Usually all the girls and many little boys, no matter the weather, pattered along in white shoes. Everyone walked with an animation and purposefulness rarely observed at other times. I wanted to see into their hearts and analyze the urge that took them out of their normal passivity, dressed them in their best, and sent them stepping proudly forth toward the bulbous-domed, cross-decked building.

The first priests had need of courage and faith and patience. The trader Shelikov, canny enough to realize his efforts to secure the fur monopoly of Russian America would win more support if sugar-coated with benevolent aims of uplifting the peoples, had asked for missionaries. Much to the chagrin of company directors and colonial officers, his request was successful.

Naturally the first group of priests, having given up their placid monastic life and endured the vicissitudes of the long sea voyage, expected the company that summoned them to welcome and assist them to begin their religious duties. Instead they were met with lukewarmness, indifference, or hostility. Russian hunters chafed at priestly rebukes for promiscuous relations with Aleut women and grumblingly permitted themselves to be joined in holy wedlock to the mothers of their children. They resented most the presumption that the livelihood of the priests should be provided by their labors, from their shares of the season's furs. The priests complained they were forced to work for their living like the ordinary hunters, to build their own shelters, to procure their own food, and to construct their own houses of worship. Rezanov's report of colonial life in 1805 critically assailed the priests as lazy, fault-finding troublemakers.[1]

The rights and injustices of each side are more apparent today as well as the almost inescapable sources of friction. The merchant stay-at-home who headed the company actually had no interest in Christianizing the Natives until, as Veniaminov sadly admitted, baptized Aleuts proved more loyal and obedient. The priests whose expectation of a warm welcome from their countrymen, of less primitive settlements and houses, of a high status in a colonial social hierarchy that did not exist, were too accustomed to civilized living to withstand the shock of reality and adapt themselves to a simple, rigorous way of life. Not even a dugout set aside for church services was prepared for them. It could not have been, since no one knew they were on the way. But they were informed that if they wanted a church or a room for a school they must build it, as each man fashioned his own shelter. There were no excess workmen to be spared for such labor. The difficult native tongues entailed years of study before the monks could truly communicate with their potential parishioners and gather them into their fold.

Not until Veniaminov arrived in 1824 to labor and earn the title of Apostle to the Aleuts was there a new spirit in missionary activities and better relations between church and commercial governors. Veniaminov was born in the Siberian province of Irkutsk and ordained a priest in 1818. Five years later the Holy Synod sent him to Russian America. He and his family arrived in Unalaska June 29, 1824, and had the summer to rebuild the old church, which had begun to collapse. The young priest began immediately to master the native language. He formulated an alphabet so that the tongue could be written, and he worked on translations of several religious texts as well as composing a dictionary and a grammar.[2] Ten years later he was transferred to Sitka, where he studied the Kolosh tongue and wrote a study of it. Recalled to Russia in 1838 he traveled home the long way around the globe while his family returned directly across the Pacific to Irkutsk. His wife died before he could rejoin his family and he decided to become a monk. Taking the new religious name of Innokentii, he retired to the monastery but not for long. As a result of his own efforts, Russian America was becoming an important mission field and needed the supervision of one familiar with religious problems. The synod called him from his quiet cell to meet the tzar, who approved him as a bishop for the newly created diocese of Alaska. In 1841 Veniaminov revisited Sitka, inspected the mission activities, and on his way back to Russia visited all of his previous parishes. He settled down in Yakutsk where, between attending to the duties of his diocese, he studied the Yakut language. In 1862 he was living on the Amur River and feeling too old for further responsibility. When he requested leave to retire, the Holy Synod was unwilling and five years later he was selected to become the metropolitan or chief prelate of the Russian Church. In 1879 he died, a great religious leader and a great human being. Among those who mourned him, few could have grieved as much as his old Aleut parishioners to whom he had ministered with love and tenderness for so many years.

The Aleuts should have remembered him always as the first champion of their rights, but too many of them today have never heard of him. The world owes him gratitude for the most accurate history of the Russian colony and for rescuing the few fragments of pre-Russian Aleut culture.

The Aleuts received their greatest gifts from the Russian conquerors through the church that, though it helped to erase their previous culture, gave them a recorded history, a written language, and some education, even in secular matters, in trades and crafts, in agriculture, and even in literature. The church demanded and obtained legal marriage for the Aleut woman and legitimacy for her partially Russian children. Before the Aleut could lose the last vestige of self-respect, he found himself caught up in a spiritual equality with his masters, confessing and receiving absolution side by side with them. Pious Aleuts and Russians were the equally beloved children of God. Into the drab dugout came the bright holy picture, the gilded icon, color and brightness restored to their dolorous lives. Not as innately beautiful as the intricately patterned dyed baskets, decorated vessels and weapons, the feather-decked garments, and other artworks of the islanders, the garish religious articles were only partial substitutes but better than no ornamentation at all in the huts.

Between 1795 and 1797, a decade after the Seal Islands were discovered, a driftwood chapel was built somewhere on St. Paul. Its site has been forgotten but it was either at Zapadni or Polovina.[3] Veniaminov described a wooden oratory erected in 1821 in the environs of the present village. He praised the collection of icons and religious ornaments and vestments, all purchased by the sealers from their miserable earnings. Later the Russian-American Company built a larger chapel, halfway up our Village Hill, in the area now fenced off as Government House lawn.[4] In that building hung a *lustra,* an elaborate candelabra, wrought of whalebone and walrus ivory by the islanders. For years walrus blubber burned in many light cups. Then the spirit of progress invaded the church. An ordinary brass candelabra was purchased and the homemade one was pushed out of sight. Just a year before Father Baranoff first came to St. Paul,[5] someone, infected with housecleaning fever, had condemned it to the rubbish heap. Over the cliff it went with the garbage. The few who remembered its beauty and history spoke of it with tear-filled eyes. This chapel on the hill was roofed with walrus hide. Next to it stood the parochial school, the only building with a shingled roof in the village.

In 1877 a wooden church was erected, supposedly with the aid of the Alaska Commercial Company, less actual than reputed. The credit they received for purchasing and freighting the bells from Philadelphia to St. Paul was unearned. The nine bells cost the sealers three thousand dollars. One third of the amount was the shipping charge although the bells came all the way from Philadelphia aboard the schooner *St. Paul.* Not even a reduction in shipping rate was given the Aleuts.

When that church was torn down to be replaced with a larger structure in 1906, its principal cross was set up on the crest of Telegraph Hill to guard the village. In the Company House library we examined the large model of a new and finer church the sealers were saving money to erect. The fund was nearly ample to fulfill their wishes.[6]

According to the Treaty of Transfer the land on which the church stands belongs to the parishioners. Consequently the only portion of St. Paul to which the Aleuts have a legal abiding property right is the churchyard and the graveyard where their ancestors lie.

During the Russian period, the Pribilofs were one of the most remote missions within the immense area of the Unalaska parish, a realm that included the entire archipelago.[7] The priest came, if transportation were available, every two years to bless and baptize, to hear confession and give communion, to marry and read burial services, and to untangle the spiritual problems of his isolated communicants. Deacons and lay preachers served faithfully in the interim.

When Father [Paul] Shayashnikoff, son of the Aleut foreman whose journals have been destroyed, arrived to be the first resident priest he brought not peace to his flock but a sword. Energetic and a natural leader, his resentment of American practices and regulations kept his people alert to the inroads of Americanism and sullenly resistant to American injustices until his death in 1893. He was a great man who loved his people but he was fighting historical changes with the wrong weapons and unwittingly he harmed his congregation. Three other priests who followed him were Aleuts. Sometimes there were intervals of a year or longer with no priest in residence. Religious services did not cease. A deacon or psalm reader conducted simple prayer services faithfully and regularly. After 1924 three priests who followed each other were of pure Russian blood, for no longer were Aleuts of pure or mixed parentage receiving an opportunity for the necessary education.[8]

Local quarrels after 1867 between church and government agents were aggravated by the repercussions of the fierce religious war raging on the mainland of Alaska between the Russian Church, legally protected by the Treaty of Transfer wherever their parishes had been established previously to the Purchase, and the pioneering Protestant missionaries entering Alaska for the first time. Treaty clauses were weak defense against the charm of the new prophets who opened homes and schools for children and provided nourishing food and warm clothing. How the original inhabitants of Alaska ever survived the quarrels between their spiritual teachers is difficult to understand. Protestants charged the Russian priests with treason, with encouraging sloth, filth, and drunkenness. The Russian priests replied with equally fierce epithets, calling the ministers false prophets, infidels, and much worse. Christian ideals were hidden by the fetid smoke of verbal battles. The gentler voices of peace-loving idealists on each side were drowned out by the battle cries of the zealots.

The wild, exaggerated rumors reaching St. Paul aroused both priest and congregation to a fanatical devotion to their faith, making them more hostile to English education, more determined to cling to the Slavic services in defiance of the Protestant infidels. Government agents, even those most anxious to elevate the lot of the sealers, were affected by the same rumors. More and more they blamed the church for retarding the peoples' progress.

The struggle subsided gradually through the years. The Russian Revolution, which took away the political power of the Orthodox Church, made the Russian parishes dependent upon their parishioners for support, with some financial aid from the Russian churches in the States. The Aleuts showed no disposition to desert their religion. The priests busied themselves more with local problems, quietly trying to teach each generation the Slavonic liturgy at least. The bluster and fire went out of their speeches when no ambassador in Washington heeded their accusations. They became content to hold those souls that were theirs. And the Protestant missions, settled in untouched fields, had their hands too full of supporting their schools, hospitals, and orphanages to continue fighting another church. Gradually the new American missionaries had discovered that the evil social conditions were not the fault of the Russian priests but something all religious leaders were trying to remedy.

Locally on St. Paul the church remains the convenient scapegoat. Unaware that the church services are conducted in Old Slavonic, a nonconversational language, the island authorities echo the stale slander, "The people would learn English if they did not listen to Russian in church. If the priest would only talk to them in English, if the priest would not try to teach them Russian, if the priest did not tell them to refuse to learn English . . ."

Dear Father Baranoff was protected from being one of the main topics of social gatherings only by being present. A cultured, brilliant gentleman, he little deserved such criticism. He had to learn English late in life and was still studying his adopted language. Instead of respecting an elderly man for undertaking such a difficult task, the official colony pettily ridiculed his pronunciation and grammatical errors. Some of them never realized that their own speech was studded with glaring mistakes.

Aleut children, prodded by their parents, drifted in and out of Father's classes where he attempted to teach the mysteries of the Old Slavonic alphabet, the same alphabet in which Veniaminov had recorded their native tongue and therefore doubly useful to the villagers. When the alphabet was mastered Father helped them memorize the responses of the liturgy.

Once he experimented with an English translation of the Creed. His students were young people who had finished school. Almost immediately they were stumbling over the phrase *visible and invisible.* He asked whether they understood the meaning of the phrase. Every head nodded yes. When he requested individuals to explain, no one could define either word.

I chuckled when he told me the story. The evening before I had struggled to convey the meaning of *invisible* to Alice, the school's most advanced pupil. Only the voice of the radio had enabled me to clarify the word. Father, still studiously attacking English lessons himself, could not, he lamented, set himself up as an English instructor even if he had the leisure. If the children or people were conversant in English, he had no objection to using the English translation of church services, even though some of the sonorous beauty of the chants would be lost. When he occasionally preached a sermon, he spoke in English to his flock.

Not even Father Baranoff remembered to defend his church by pointing out that millions of Roman Catholics, whose worship is expressed in ancient Latin, have not been shut off from the speech of their country. I was not too popular when I interjected the fact gently during local conversations.

The Russian Church in Alaska, in the Aleut parishes, is no menace to Americanism. The loss of false power when the Mother Church ceased to be the State Church of a powerful despotism and the loss of the financial backing of the Russian crown have left the Alaskan missions bereft of all save their ability to minister to the spiritual needs of its communicants. If it provides them with solace and comfort to enable them to withstand the sorrows and limitations of their lives, it will remain alive and flourishing in Alaska. If its teachings fail to help its followers, then only will it cease to exist, not crumbling under the onslaughts of religious rivals but withering away from its own inadequacies. Meanwhile the church on the Seal Islands continues to conceal the defects of governmental policy from those officials who erroneously think a couple of hours' recitation of ancient Slavonic prayers once a week counteracts an entire week of English schooling.

Many local priests have not, it is true, been a great help to their congregation who looked to them for guidance in accepting American customs or for an example in obeying American laws. Father [Paul] Shayashnikoff was a saintly man, moral, firm with his flock, fighting drunkenness and dishonesty, but his fears that the church would be destroyed by the newcomers led him to excessive resistance. When he resented brutality toward members of his congregation, when he railed against libertine propensities of American officials, his heart was a true guide but his attacks on the "heretics" were marred by his outspoken, aggressive bitterness.

In 1885 he and a treasury agent became embroiled over wills, which had generally been written by the priest and presented to the office with no other witnessing signature. The fact that the majority of the sealers left their entire savings or the larger portion of their worldly goods to the church had aroused the suspicion that the priest was using undue pressure upon the will maker. Widows and children were left dependent upon the Alaska Commercial Company, who disliked the extra burden very much. Father Shayashnikoff was confronted with a ruling that no will would be considered legal unless it had been signed by two disinterested parties and submitted to the government agent for copying in the official records before the bequest were distributed.[9] The priest felt that the new regulation was a direct insult to him and was wounded by the inference that he had influenced people unwisely. Later wills, written and witnessed by laypeople, continued to remember the church's needs ahead of the wants of the bereaved family.

By 1887 island officials were charging Father Shayashnikoff with un-Americanism and the organization of a church party to assume control of local affairs by securing the election or selection of its own candidates for Aleut foreman.[10] This "Church Party" became a great bugaboo to the officials and seems to have been extremely nebulous. At one time an individual would be classified and reviled as a member of the "Church Party." At another the same officials would praise him as a cooperative workman. Whoever displeased the local government, protested against low wages, working conditions, high prices in the company store, or other matters was immediately labeled a "Church Party" member.

The Aleuts learned that they could best express their antagonism against local despots and unkindly policies, regulations and restrictions, as well as outright injustices, by appearing indifferent to the adoption of the English language and showing an increased fervid devotion to the church. During the regime of humane officials, it is noteworthy that the "Church Party" was unmentioned. A harsh agent created a unity of resistance championed by the priest, which provided the slight basis for such a term.

Tingle, a treasury agent, appears to have been the first to use the term "Church Party." He was probably the most overtly cruel American overseer the Aleuts have had. When the Aleuts elected foremen whom the Alaska Commercial Company did not like, Tingle stopped elections on the ground that the company was more capable of selecting men whom they wished to be the leaders of the work gang.[11] Naturally the company would prefer to select its own henchmen. Tingle's open support of the company seems almost a bid for employment. When the company failed to renew its lease and was unable to reward him for his loyal cooperation, he was fortunate enough to secure employment with the incoming lessee, the North American Commercial Company, as their superintendent of island affairs. The right to elect their own foremen had to be restored to the sealers by a Washington order.[12]

During Tingle's regime as a servant of the government, he levied heavy fines on the sealers for slight offenses, tossed them in jail on meager diets, and put them in irons.

Then came the great wood strike. During the October storms Tingle ordered the men to go to beaches miles from the village to collect fuel and tote the heavy, soaked driftwood back to the village on their backs. The Aleuts refused. Tingle summoned the men to his office. One by one they were called before him.

"Will you go for wood? No? Fifteen dollars fine. Next." So the court proceedings ran.

January 14, 1942
Up full of aches and tiredness from our devilish mattress. The dreams it engendered during the night seemed to deal with Mr. Tingle, an agent whom I had chuckled over a great deal yesterday because his notes betokened rather a pompous egotistic personality. Not with him much, but with his mother who was insane and kept doing outlandish things while Mr. Tingle protested that she was just as sane as he or I when I wanted her removed from the island.

I have been loosely commenting sarcastically on the fact that first men came up here working for Uncle Sam and the next time you ran across them, they were working for the lessee. But I begin to judge them more leniently now that I notice signs of their nervousness as presidential election time rolls around. They could not know in the fall whether their political party was in or out and had to worry until the following April or May to know whether they still had a job or not.

cont.

Finally one man weakened at the prospect of such a large fine and promised to go for wood the next day. Tingle was jubilant. The next sealer refused. In a fury Tingle increased the fine to twenty dollars. The harsh verdicts continued until the sealers became too frightened to resist any longer. One by one they crept shamefacedly back to the office to surrender. The last stubborn striker gave in. For two days the sealers scoured the cold, windswept beaches and tramped home bent under the heavy loads. Tingle rejoiced at his victory over the "Church Party," which he accused as the instigator of the strike.[13]

It is well to compare Tingle's conduct with the later report of Joseph Murray in 1891. Within that report lies the real explanation of the Aleuts' revolt and a devastating revelation of the meanness of Tingle's arbitrary demands and acts.

> I am well aware that you will be informed of the existence of plenty of driftwood strewn in large quantities along the beach, and of the laziness of the men who neglect to gather it for firing; but when one knows that the driftwood is not so very plentiful, and that it has been watersoaked for months, and that it is next to an impossibility to dry it in this damp climate, it is easily understood what a nuisance it must be to cook by or live near a fire made from such wood, which must be smeared over with blubber before it will burn.
>
> If for no other reason than of forever doing away with the use of blubber, the present quantity of coal ought to be increased. This blubber is stripped from the seals during the killing season of June and July, and is stored in

tubs, barrels, boxes, etc., until wanted for use in cold weather, by which time it has become rancid or rotten to such a degree that it is unfit to be allowed under the roof of civilized men, much less to be used to cook his food and warm his cottage.

Again, in order to obtain the firewood spoken of, it is oftentimes necessary to go across the island, a distance of 8 miles, through deep snow, for as much wood as a man can carry home on his back. That men sometimes sit down in despair and let their families suffer with cold, or that they squander their money for coal at the enormous price of $33.60 per ton, rather than undergo such hardships for a back load of wet wood is not at all to be wondered at.

They must have more coal. Two hundred tons is not too much for the natives of St. Paul Island if they are to have a fire every day, and since coming into [the] Bering Sea I have not seen a day when a good fire was not a necessity to every family. Indeed, I find they have bought and paid for out of their scanty earnings 153,650 pounds of coal from June 1, 1890, to May 31, 1891, for which they paid 1 1/2 cents per pound, or $33.60 per ton. Now all this was in addition to the 50 tons furnished by the lessees, under the lease, and makes in round numbers, for one year, 110 tons of coal in addition to the wood and blubber.

It is understandable that men who expected their job to end on a certain date would be preparing for future employment and what more natural than that they try to get one lined up with the only people with whom they had contact—and for work that they were already gaining experience of. They needn't be dishonest but there would be a tendency to treat the lessee nicely and to keep the head gently turned from subjects that might cause friction, etc. A bad system, indeed, that political appointee one.

A hard night as usual. But fortified with a cold shower and tea I'm finishing this at nine, will type a few of my notes, and then get to the office.

Good health depends very largely upon comfort and cleanliness, and no people can be comfortable who have to be constantly struggling to keep a miserable fire burning, made up from wet wood and rancid fat, nor can they be healthy long and be without plenty of pure water; nor can their children grow up to be robust men and women where drainage is unknown, and where the very air they breathe is poisoned by the accumulated filth of twenty years.

"But," we are told, "the natives will not try to do anything for themselves, nor attempt to improve their surroundings."

Admitting the truth of all this, if we apply it to a small minority, I deny that it would be just or right to leave them to their fate because of their want of knowledge of the true status of the case, and I insist it is our duty to teach while we assist and encourage them.

Every agent who has tried the experiment will say that the natives are docile and obedient, and can be induced to do almost anything when approached in a kind and rational manner.

For years the natives have been denied the right to buy or use sugar as an article of diet, because, forsooth, some man, long since dead, got drunk from quass made from sugar.

That there have been cases of quass-making, and that, even now, a native will take a drink when he has a chance, is undoubtedly true, but there is neither sense nor reason in punishing the whole community, young and old, men and women alike, for the sin of one or two men who know no better, and who can, very easily, be persuaded from repeating the act. There had been altogether too much said about the weakness of the natives for strong drink, so much so that it is commonly believed in the United States that they are in a constant state of intoxication, when the facts are the very opposite.

I was on St. George Island fourteen months, and a little longer on St. Paul, and I have yet to find the second drunken man on the islands.
Once, on board a steamer, one of the men got too much whisky, enough to keep him off work for two hours, and that is the only case of drunkenness I ever saw on the islands.

Besides, were they the inveterate quass-makers they have been represented to be, the want of sugar would be no bar to their business, for they can make quass out of nearly everything they use as food or drink, sweet crackers, jelly, yeast, etc., entering largely into the composition. And, lest there be objections raised, sugar can be prepared very readily so that it will not ferment, and yet be all right for ordinary use as food. Two per cent of powdered borax mixed with sugar will not injure it more than to prevent fermentation. The same is true of sulphate of calcium. I respectfully submit that it is worth trying.

Whenever a person is taken sick on the islands he is allowed sugar, but what is the use of giving him, at the eleventh hour, the very thing for the want of which his sickness originated?

Especial attention is called to the subject of schools on the seal islands, for if we are to succeed in teaching the English language to the rising generation there must be a radical reform, amounting indeed to a complete change, in the present system and method of teaching.

That the Lessees comply with the requirements of the lease in regard to schools and teachers is true enough, but the defect is in the system itself, which, owing to many causes, is not the one adapted to the conditions existing here. . . . It is not that the average native child is unusually dull or stupid, for he is not, but it is because the child never hears English spoken except what he hears in the school. . . . I advocate the employment

> of teachers of long and varied experience, men and women of character, whose blameless lives shall be a guaranty of the success of the school, and who are, withal, devoted to the work for the sake of the good to be accomplished, and who are not above stooping down to lift up the poor and lowly ones in whose welfare so very few take an interest.[14]

I include the whole dreadful picture from the printed government report so that the revolt of refusing to gather wood can be understood as a revolt against many other miserable social injustices. Handcuffs and irons, these were Tingle's immediate orders when the slightest infringement of his rules occurred. Years later when he was the superintendent of the lessee he inspired another strike, again a communal expression against more than the single incident that caused the revolt.

A vessel had just brought back a number of St. Paul men who had been working for the company at Unalaska for a long period. The men were tired from a rough journey and hungry and anxious to see their families. Tingle refused to let them leave the dock and ordered them to commence unloading supplies at once. They complied but as their hunger and fatigue increased their resentment increased proportionately. They notified Tingle that they would not return in the morning, which was Sunday and a Holy Day, to continue unloading.

Tingle rushed angrily to Agent Williams demanding that the men be ordered to work. Since this occurred before the sealers were treated as wards of the government, Williams calmly pointed out that the Aleuts shared the rights of all American citizens to abstain from labor on Sunday and attend church. He refused to coerce them or attempt to deprive them of their civil rights. He did invite the sealers to meet with him to discuss their grievances. How the Aleuts needed friends like Williams and how few they had.

January 15, 1942
Logging yesterday with forty-five minutes off at noon, during which time I threw some lunch together, ate, played with Tobyanne, and heard some news. Then back until Sam came for me with a flashlight to light my steps homeward, which thrilled me very much. Got a great deal of interesting stuff.

Have fallen in love with Col. Marston who fought the company agent tooth and nail during the winter he was in charge when Bryant was out on leave. His lush raving about clouds, walks on the ice in winter, about the wind, about the sun, which he calls Old Saul—and his admixture of Biblical phrases in everything plus some gentle skepticism and his fierce regard for the poor and his hatred of petty politics. Both he and Frances Lessen, a predecessor, who spoke Russian, speak so nicely about the Natives. Then along comes Blood and Thunder Tingle with handcuffs with which to put offenders in irons, with beatings for truants from school, with declarations after some such victory "that I guess now I will be obeyed."

After he listened to the sealers, he composed a gentle letter to Tingle that must have been a reproof hard for that vitriolic gentleman to endure because of its restraint and reasonableness. The sealers, Williams promised, would report to work Sunday morning because they understood the necessity of wasting no time during sealing season as well as the officials. Furthermore they would never have considered refusing to unload cargo had they been permitted to go home to see their families and eat supper before starting work. Most of all, they objected to being abused, called monkeys, jackasses, and other less printable epithets.

Between arrogant bosses like Tingle and zealous, unwise churchmen, the Aleuts were mere dice to be shaken first by one and then by the other. In the midst of the puzzling contradictions of life, the church building, the church faith remained a refuge.

Bewildered, smarting at real and supposed injustices, the Aleuts flocked to the church door. Once inside they were neither apes nor jackasses but human souls precious to a loving Father who forgave them their repented sins and threatened them with no chains or handcuffs. Gradually the Aleuts hardened themselves against physical punishment, learned to scorn fines, and, worst of all, to be more cunning in their propositions to island officials. No matter what rules they broke, they realized, they would not starve or be sent from the Pribilofs as long as they were wanted as sealers. Open rebellions subsided more and more into alcoholic escape from the nagging sense of being possessed and enslaved. Two means of escape! One led to prayer. The other to the kvass barrel.

One of the ugliest fights between spiritual and temporal powers developed from Bishop Nicolai's demand that no more orphans be sent to the Jesse Lee Home in Unalaska. When Murray pointed out that the children were not cut off from their church and merely received home care and English schooling in a kindly atmosphere, the bishop would barely listen to the interpreter. To provide for their bodies at the risk of having them become Protestants and thereby lose their immortal souls could not be countenanced by the church, the bishop insisted. No other orphans were permitted to attend the school after the Russian ambassador protested to the State Department.[15]

The record is a sorry one to review. The prejudice and bigotry of Orthodox and Protestant churchmen alike is unpleasant. Christ's teachings were lost in the welter of battles. The Russian language continued to die out but English did not grow healthily in its stead. Protestants on the island, people from the States, insulted the church and saw nothing but evil in its influence. Few critics tried to cooperate tactfully with the priests or genuinely strove to implant different ideals of conduct and make the community self-governing and self-respecting. Even had the priests all been as upright and honorable, as compassionate and benevolent, as Father Baranoff, even had the church eased its stringent bans, religion would still have remained fairly impotent as an ethical force because local factors too formidable to be combated with holy words constantly contradicted religious instruction.

In the minority, but overly successful in teaching outward obedience, were the Simon Legrees with handcuffs and beatings, were the masters who fed the sealers liquor to obtain their servile loyalty and thereby taught them contempt for law. Worst of all were the men from the States who trifled with the women and left piteous "strays" to be cuffed and beaten by people who had no interest in them, save as a means of increasing the household income by charity donations.

Yet despite the church's failure to alleviate their physical distress or to make their lives more "respectable" in the eyes of others, after all the years the Aleuts were still crowding into the church, whether the service was the short colorless prayer meeting led by a layman or the bright pageantry of the priest-conducted service. Toward the end of my stay I ventured to ask a few their real feelings toward the church. Two men who had worked "outside" and spoke English relatively well tried hard to analyze their sentiments.

"Of course, I know," said one, "there's a lot of bunk in the services. The church ain't done much to help us. But the way I feel about it, 'tis ours."

He expressed the conclusion I had reached by my own observations. The sealers had so little of their very own. The roofs over their heads were not theirs. Most of their food and clothing came disguised as a favor from the paternalistic caretakers instead of payment for labor. Nothing belonged to them except the church. Out of their sealing divisions the church had been supported for years. At least the high prices they paid for articles in their own Canteen, supervised and managed by the agent until it seemed just another government function, provided money for the upkeep of the church and the support of the priest. No government agent, no "white" crossed the threshold of the church save on a sightseeing trip on Christmas Eve and Easter.

It was more than their possession.

The church was a refuge when officials were stern or indifferent. It was a kindly mother who forgave them their sins. It gave them each week a few hours when they stood side by side clothed with the dignity of human beings precious to the God they were addressing. It gave their drab lives color, the beauty of painted icons, the gleam of flickering candles, the sweet savor of incense, and the harmony of ancient chants. It gave their purposeless lives a direction. For most of all, it gave them a destiny toward which to strive, not just to be sealers forever but to walk at last in eternal happiness, hand in hand, with a loving God. For in the eyes of God there are no "Natives" and no "whites." Before his throne there would be no more race prejudice, no more discrimination. In heaven Aleut and non-Aleut would be equal. The church alone gave the Aleuts a future.

Chapter 32

Autumn storms attacked the island frequently in October and November with frenzied winds and flashing bayonets of rain. We walked the beaches near home almost daily. The wind tired us quickly on longer journeys. Days inside the house glided by swiftly, the hours filled with studies of Aleut language and history. There were quiet days between gales when the clouds hung gracefully in low billowing curves and the hours were purple shadowed as at twilight. We rambled tranquilly in the subdued atmosphere. The island had become mystical in mood. Around it a roiling green sea reflected violet land shadows.

On such a morning in early November we visited Big and Little Polovina rookeries. Tobyanne slept in a nest of blankets in the car. A paragraph of Elliott's report had determined our destination. Too long the magnetic charm of Polovina Hill had drawn us to her summit and made us neglect her seafront. From the road we had looked across a plain that seemed to meet the sea at eye level, a vista tame and unexciting. Tricked by my eyes I had been startled by Elliott's lyric praise: "a very beautiful geological section of the simple structure of St. Paul. The ringing, iron-like basaltic foundations of the island are here setting boldly up from the sea to a height of forty or fifty feet—black and purplish-red, polished like ebony by the friction of the surf, and worn by its agency into grotesque arches, tiny caverns and deep fissures."[1]

Our immediate approach to the water's edge after we parked our car was checked abruptly. We walked engrossed in finding secure footing among scattered rocks and avoiding falling on the slippery surface where bruised decaying grasses broken by resting seals in the early fall had mixed with the hair they shed into a slimy treacherous greenish yellow paste. Then we realized that the apparent rough excrescences of rock at the limit of the plain were animate. Seal heads bobbed up and down like marionette figures. We walked over a mile parallel to the shore before we came to the end of the sentry line. Then we looked down upon a small half-moon shingle. A few seals were loafing on the jet boulders, fanning indolently despite the coolness of the air. Around them rose steep, vertical walls of black and plum-colored glossy stone, wrinkled in fine imbrications like imperfect glass. Even seals' sticky flippers could not ascend the glazed shear sides. We went from one arcuate indentation to another. Many were broken glassy bowls accessible only from the sea. Others were connected with the plain above by narrow slides of soil packed hard and smooth by flippers. Cautiously I essayed to go down one. Immediately my feet slid out from under me, and I arrived breathless at the bottom, narrowly averting fracturing a few bones on the waiting rocks.

Beyond the cliffs, a wide shingled slope led for half a mile along the waterfront to the broad sands of Webster Beach. At the entrance of the sands we turned back to the car and Tobyanne, who might be bleating like a seal pup for her bottle. We found her still sleeping and stole off to prowl in the neighborhood of the camp house. We sought traces of the old barabara community, one of the earliest villages. The years have obliterated the surface ruins of the old settlement and its adjoining cemetery. There are barabara ruins that belong to the early years of the century. I thought of Elliott's dismal picture of that ancient graveyard: "It was, when I saw it in 1876, in a melancholy state of ruin—a thousand young seals at least moved off from its surface as I came up, and they had actually trampled out many sandy graves, rolling the bones and skulls of Aleutian ancestry in every direction."[2]

When I had asked one of the oldest inhabitants of St. Paul about that cemetery site, he had looked at me in speechless amazement. A cemetery at Polovina! What crazy ideas some people from the States got hold of. John Hanson remembered old people pointing out the village site, not far from Polovina Lake, but he had only the haziest recollection of its exact location.

At last we really had to start homeward.

All summer the reindeer had kept to the south and west areas where few people intruded. The thinning vegetation was forcing them to spread out all over the fields where the crisp grey reindeer mosses had not been cropped too short. Loitering bands were visible wherever we looked. A large herd grazed close to

> November 23, 1941
> Walking in the famous Pribilof wind is exactly like wrestling with a slightly stronger opponent. Every step forward in the face of the wind is the result of great effort. Every step with the wind at your back requires great resistance to prevent being pushed on your face. It is great sport for a while as long as you wear clothing impervious to wind penetration. But it makes conversation on a walk completely hopeless. Also, it is more difficult than ever to walk and look at the scenery.
>
> We stayed at the Hellbaums for a couple of hours. Mr. Hellbaum was out and came in just as we were leaving. Sam told Mrs. she should stay in bed for some time yet with her injured leg. We chatted about the village affairs as usual and some about the world situation.
>
> We had planned to stay there only a few minutes and then go on to see Harrington but we left too late and had to hurry home to see her majesty. I suspect she had been summoning us for some time but her wails stopped the minute I slammed the front door and she waited patiently for me to come in and get her.

the lake. We stopped to watch them. A sentinel must have caught a whiff of gasoline and given an alarm. The animals began to move leisurely away from the lake southward toward the stone barrier of Kamenisti. As the herd gathered momentum the animals blended into a motley colored wave, a broad ribbon fringed raggedly with tips of tossing antlers. A cream and brown streamer fluttered across the bleached rocks of Kamenisti and was gone.

The reindeer live placidly on the Pribilofs where no predatory animals track them and man disturbs them only once a year. In turn the reindeer seldom infringe upon the privacy of the seals, probably because they obtain the salt they love from lakes contaminated by the sea. The reindeer are a domesticated species of the caribou, unique among deer because both males and females develop antlers. In the spring the soft tender knobs on their foreheads begin to grow and branch out into antlers, retaining a clothlike protective sheath until the horn is fully developed and hardened. Before the rutting season in the early autumn, the velvet peels off. Then the males fight terrific duels with their deadly sharp, many-pronged horns to secure the mates of their choice. The fawns are born about the middle of April and the females shed their horns. Almost immediately the new ones begin to sprout. The greatest hardship the island deer can suffer is to have the snow remain capped for weeks with a crust too hard to be broken by the deer's hoof so they can reach the reindeer moss. Their layers of fat from summer grazing help them to endure a leaner diet in winter.

Sam was feeling very tender toward the reindeer, for the scene of the autumn roundup of the animals was still vivid in his mind. I thanked my postnatal convalescence that made me miss the butchery of a hundred and fifty of them for food. Johnston had told Ruth Gruber and me that the Department wanted to decrease the herd, grown too large to be supported by island vegetation. Yet the Aleuts were given reindeer flesh only twice during the winter while official families had it often.[3]

The reindeer were imported in 1910.[4] In a press release issued appropriately on the twenty-fourth of December of that year the Bureau of Fisheries explained that the animals had been introduced to provide fresh meat for all residents, but particularly to supply the sealers with winter meat to replace seal flesh. The animals were to be domesticated to furnish dairy products and be broken in as beasts of burden. From their hides the islanders would obtain material for clothing and leather to make useful objects. The sealers were also expected to augment their income by the sale of trinkets made from the antlers.

Oliver Angelook, the Eskimo herder of the twenty-five reindeer that survived the sea voyage north to St. Paul, wintered on the island, supposedly to instruct the sealers in herding duties. Then the custom lapsed. The reindeer wandered at will through the island, until, just before the rutting season in the fall, they were rounded up, driven into the corral between Kamenisti and Telegraph Hill and counted. Always a few were slain, shot through the head as they passed down a narrow fenced alley.

Hospital patients were fed much reindeer meat during the winter. Otherwise, villagers had only the two issues on holidays. I coaxed Peter into making several horn souvenirs for me. He surprised me with the gift of a fan-shaped decorative comb. The creamy background was shot through with greenish smears giving it the appearance of a very primitive artifact corroded by age. Otherwise there was no local manufacture of horn trinkets.

In the fall we made the intimate acquaintance of another summer visitant, a young hair seal Ford Wilke brought into the village. Every time he was released from his box and felt the familiar earth beneath his body, he began to scramble instinctively toward the water, digging his front flippers into the loose scoria and dragging his fat little body along speedily. His flippers were divided into five quite wide flaps. The hind ones were useless for land locomotion. His tail was the most absurd little tip, seven centimeters long. He seemed proud of it for he had the habit of curling his two hind flippers into a circular position with the tail resting on top. He weighed twenty-six pounds and was seventy centimeters long (27 1/2 inches). Bored with attempts to measure his squirming body, he grabbed the tape in his mouth and held on grimly. No dull-witted fur seal would ever tussle so good naturedly with human beings. His monkey face was gaminish and appealing. His body was covered with a wrinkled dark grey rubbery skin oddly ornamented with tufts of his fine yellowish fur and guard hairs. No one knew whether his hair had been shed naturally because of some disease or had been rubbed off in some accidental fashion. The loss of both guard hairs and fine hairs puzzled visiting scientists. I picked him up to have our picture taken. His skin was corrugated slightly, like coarse leather, but the sensation of the roughened surface was pleasantly counteracted by the luscious rolling of the soft thick blubber under my fingers. It was like toying with a worn old silky balloon. Mrs. Stacy nervously picked him up to pose and dropped him. He bounced like a ball and seemed undamaged but a trifle annoyed.

Wilke and Banner opened up a rival hospital in the Government House basement and called in Sam to give pediatric advice to sick seal pups. Eventually every patient died, not, I think, because of the physician. Any sentient thing would die rather than be fed canned milk through an enormous rubber tube running into its stomach.

The scientific activities going on in the laboratory in the sacred dwelling consecrated to officials almost gave Mac apoplexy. He could be heard a block away complaining of the stench and dirt, not of the pups alone but the bird skins and other specimens being prepared for shipment. No odor was discernible on the first floor and even in the lab the air was mainly contaminated by chemicals and disinfectants. But Mac's dislike for those he dubbed "bug hunters" or "scientists" found an outlet.

Interbreeding among island cats had produced a species conspicuous for its ugliness. Kuska, our first cat, was one of the homeliest and seemed very aware of his unfortunate color scheme. He was too pathetically grateful for the slightest attention. We almost broke his heart when we agreed to shelter a pretty tiger-striped kitten until Wilke's wife arrived. We called him Kitty and waited for Helen to name her own pet. The war ruined the scheme for the Wilkes to winter on the island and Helen remained only long enough for us to know that we were going to miss some very congenial companionship in the winter months. We could not cast out the feline boarder that Heretina was already calling Wilke. Though the pranks of two young cats often upset the household, there was no question of evicting Kuska who had priority rights. Wilke had no inhibitions and where he led, Kuska followed timidly and clumsily as soon as he realized his pretty rival was no threat to his security. Except for their habit of inviting half the island cats to gay parties in the cellar, they added a pleasant zestful flavor to life.

Their sociability may have been copied from Heretina who entertained many of her friends after school. Sometimes they were asked in formally for pleasure, for her birthday, and other special occasions. Generally they were a tribute to Heretina's organizational talents as she shepherded them in at appropriate hours to help her with household tasks. Help is too strong an expression. Heretina commanded and the others obeyed and toiled. They were indirectly paid by supper or little lunches of cocoa and cake at odd hours.

As autumn progressed toward winter, our friendship with Father and Matushka Baranoff deepened. Father began to teach Sam Russian three mornings a week. They enthusiastically cooperated in taking and developing photographs. Father and I pursued our investigations of local history and wrangled affectionately over Russian place names. It was a social error to chose as our most intimate friends some Natives and the prelate who was a symbol of the island scapegoat, the foreign-language church. Not that we were reserved with other associates, for we grew fond of most members of the Service families particularly the Hellbaums and the Hoversons, Mrs. Mac, and the Elliotts, although we knew they considered us slightly daft. Mac's coarse language repelled both of us. Earl Oberg was a nice, good-natured fellow. His wife's fairly constant fretting, because of her isolation from a busier world, dissipated some of her potential charm. Roy Herd, the radioman during the winter, was a splendid person whose social life was nonexistent as he had to nap night and day in the short periods between sending out weather reports. The Stacys were young, immature, and very much wrapped up in their personal affairs.

The Baranoffs were our natural friends. Warm, generous, tolerant of their parishioners instead of being superior and carping, they had predilections and tastes that harmonized with our own. If the island had given us nothing more than the enduring friendship of the Baranoffs, Harrington, and R.H.G., we would have been sufficiently enriched by our experiences.

Chapter 33

It is ironical that the least known Americans, the Aleuts of the Pribilof Islands, should be associated with the most publicized animals in all history. In my innocent ignorance I had regarded the fur seal as a mere marine mammal, an uncomplicated creature of simple life habits, useful to man because of its furry covering against the chill of northern seas. It was not so. That warm coat had led to universal fame and tragedy for beast and mankind. Because of that soft sleek fur, the seal had acquired a past that began in the court circles of St. Petersburg. This rather feeble-minded amphibian had agitated the palace intrigues of Imperial Russia, motivated the backstage forces that supported the American purchase of Alaska, and upset amicable relations between four of the great nations of the world. It had occasioned serious international tribunals, aroused the most virulent savage fights on the floor of Congress and still more rancorous battlings behind the scenes in congressional committee rooms. Brilliant reputations, political and scientific, had been toppled by the fur seal and its human friends. Venomous feuds between persons in public life, the fragments of broken friendships, were but minor disasters it had caused. The stale stench of anti-Semitism spread out from its soft fur. Because of that fur, men had died in actual fighting, and wars between nations had been but narrowly averted.

In another book I hope to present the complete history of the fur seal.[1] For this story of the islands and its peoples I must strive to condense past events, to expose only the skeleton of the tangle in order to present the background of political warfare from which the present-day Aleut emerged. The public career of the fur seal began in the royal chambers of St. Petersburg. So many aristocratic families had shares in the Russian-American Company that Nicolai Rezanov's 1805 report aroused the court circles as much as humbler merchant stockholders with its account of reckless slaughter, ruined skins, and the decrease in the size of the seal herd. In 1803, for instance, eight hundred thousand seals had been killed but only one-eighth of them had been marketed. Some were deliberately withheld to maintain the sale price. But thousands of skins had been imperfectly cured and had rotted. Bales of skins, well cured or ruined, had been burned or thrown

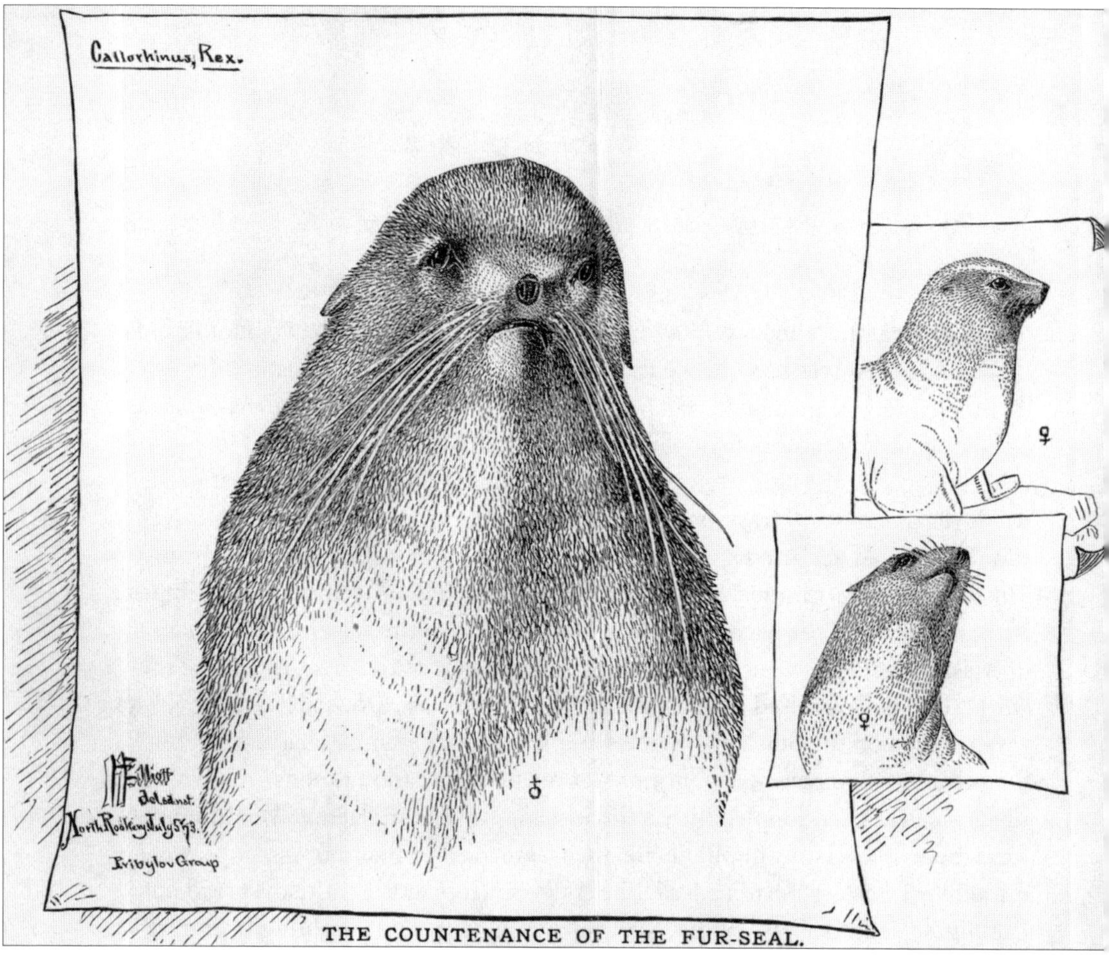

Elliott's drawing "The Countenance of the Fur-Seal" dated July 5, 1873 (*Fur-Seal Fisheries of Alaska, 1889,* Plate 5).

into the sea. The first *zapusk* or rest period to permit the seal herd to recuperate was instituted. In 1806, at Rezanov's order, the inhabitants of the Seal Islands were removed to Unalaska. The seals were left to multiply in solitude on the lava beaches.

The Russian-American Company agents experimented with many restrictions, forbidding the killing of old bulls, then ordering a number of young males reserved for breeding purposes each year, and finally forbidding the killing of young pups, the "spring chicken of the Aleuts." Just before 1847 they chose the seemingly natural conservation measure: they put a stop to the slaughter of females. By 1864 the annual take of skins had reached seventy thousand. The herd was flourishing and increasing in numbers annually. The Russians had solved the problem of reaping a yearly abundance of furs without damaging the fur bearers fatally.

Then in 1867 the United States bought Russian America for $7,200,000. The American flag flew over the Seal Islands, the seals, and the sealers. While the reports of the guns saluting the Stars and Stripes, just raised at Sitka, were still echoing, a far-sighted businessman, H. M. Hutchinson, was purchasing from the departing Russian-American Company manager, Prince Maksutov, all their properties, buildings, and equipment, even those on the Seal Islands. In the spring of 1868 sailing vessels from several companies began to converge on the Pribilofs, loaded with stores and ready to dicker with the Aleuts for seal furs. Trouble among the competing companies was resolved by judicious compromise. Hutchinson, Kohl, and Company had the advantage in bargaining because they were the owners of all buildings, tools, and stores of the Russian-American Company. The smaller traders who attempted to muscle in met with ill fortune.[2]

Rumors that the seal herd would be exterminated had forced a congressional injunction against further killings.[3] News of the law did not reach the Pribilofs until autumn. Fortunately for the male seals, one factor operated in their favor. Daniel Webster, stationed at Northeast Point on St. Paul, admitted that sealing stopped there only because the sealers were physically exhausted and the supply of salt had been used up.[4] Judging by the seal skins passed through San Francisco customs the total take from both islands by all companies was over three hundred fifty thousand, a total representing five years' sealing under Russian management. William Healy Dall, the American scientist, says, and other sources agree, that thousands more were sent to the Sandwich Islands to escape American custom inspection.[5]

May 22, 1869, the revenue cutter *Lincoln* landed a force of soldiers on St. Paul and a lieutenant of the Revenue Service to govern the island. The military and treasury forces together were to prevent sealing, except the killing of animals for food. Captain John Henriques commented on the cheerful compliance of the Aleuts with the orders he gave them. Through an interpreter he addressed them and ordered, among other things, that all guns be given to Lieutenant Barnes until the seals had left the island and they were needed to shoot birds for food. Ten minutes after he informed them dogs were not to be kept on the islands, every poor dog had been killed by his owner.[6] No one even complained at the destruction of his pet. The swift compliance indicates a subservience not complimentary to the Aleuts, but no one can surmise what pangs of sorrow were felt by the people who had learned for generations that open resistance to authority was futile.

The sealing of 1869 is shrouded in a cloud of statements and counterstatements. Captain Charles Bryant had arrived at the island to take charge as an official of the treasury with Dr. H. H. McIntyre as an assistant. Lieutenant Barnes gave permission for thirty thousand seals to be killed for food. But Special Agent Frank Wicker reported he had discovered four salt houses filled with skins.[7] The island officials had informed him there were but three salt houses holding only the designated number of skins. The sealers told Wicker many skins had been removed from the islands before his arrival. His explorations of the island of St. Paul were hampered by all government officials. He charged that skins were being shipped out on whaling vessels to the world fur markets via Hawaii.

In July 1870 Congress at last declared itself in favor of leasing to a single firm for twenty years and ironically entitled the measure as an act to preserve the fur seals. Secretary Boutwell asked for bids at once. He gave the lease to Hutchinson's new company, the Alaska Commercial Company. The act authorizing the lease did not require that the lease go to the highest bidder. Because of this peculiar circumstance, the Alaska Commercial Company won the sealing lease and permission to take a hundred thousand seal skins each year for a yearly rent of fifty-five thousand dollars and a tax of $2.62 per skin and the assumption of certain responsibilities for the sealers. H. H. McIntyre soon left government service and became managing agent for the Alaska Commercial Company for the duration of its lease.[8] The public protests of disgruntled bidders and other envious businessmen, mainly from the West Coast, increased to such proportions that six years later the officials of the company had to defend their rights to the lease and their conduct before a congressional committee.[9]

Among those testifying to the satisfactory state of affairs was Professor Henry Wood Elliott. Both orally and in print Elliott had defended the leasing system of sealing, praised the Alaska Commercial Company for its humane policies, and singled out Mr. Hutchinson for unusual adulation. Gossip among the Aleuts, Elliott had argued, would serve as the best natural check upon the lessee should the latter be tempted to take more seals than permitted or break the contract in any fashion.[10] How naive to believe that chatter among the Unalaskan friends and relatives of Pribilof sealers would ever reach or be listened to in the national capital or any circles that could act to protect the seals and sealers. Elliott honorably made up for his youthful misjudgments by an astounding devotion to the interests of seals and the taxpayers of the United States.

Henry Wood Elliott was an extremely young artist and naturalist when he secured the post of assistant treasury agent assigned to the Pribilofs.[11] He claimed that the great Spencer Baird, head of the Smithsonian Institution, had suggested his appointment in order that he should collect information about the fur seal, an animal of which scientific circles knew little. No one suspected, least of all Elliott himself, bubbling over with youthful enthusiasm for his intended studies, that another volcano had emerged on St. Paul when he arrived in 1872, a human volcano whose brimstone and sulfur would scorch many a reputation, whose explosions would shake the very foundations of government bureaus and topple bureaucrats.

I like to remember the description of his arrival when I contemplate the national furor he was to arouse years later. The steamer *Alexander* waited offshore two days because of storms. At last a baidar braved the high seas and brought Agent Bryant, his wife, and Elliott safely to land on Lukanin Beach. The Aleuts were waiting with a sled for the baggage. The storm-wearied Bryants and Elliott availed themselves of the transport. Perched on the luggage they were drawn slowly to the waiting fireside at Company House. Poor Elliott was appalled at the stench of the dead seals leaking out of cracks in the snow. He wrote in his notes, "I remember well the unmitigated sensations of disgust that possessed me when I first landed."

Four months after his arrival, Elliott married the daughter of Alexander Melovidov, a former agent of the Russian-American Company.[12] Eighteen-year-old Alexandra had been born in Sitka and had lived on St. Paul only a few years. She was beautiful and well educated. The swiftness of his courtship seems characteristic. They remained on the

December 5, 1941
Elliott in Aleut is known as *Iliyitax*, with the accent on the penult and a full *ch* sound for the *x*. He married Alexandra Melovidova. She is still alive as she was just a young girl when she married Elliott. She must be over ninety. She resides in San Francisco and can be located through the Russian priest. Her brother was Simeon Melovidov, who went out to the States after serving as teacher here in the company days for a long time. Rumor has it that he left in 1912. Or the year after. His handwriting is exquisite clear script. I saw a couple of school reports that he made out. Anna Stepetin says that he writes to her via Gabriel since he married her sister who is dead. She reports that he has five children. Actually, she does not remember the exact number. Two boys, she states, are not married. Simeon became a chicken farmer near San Francisco and apparently flourished. One of his sons conducts orchestras.

Another brother-in-law of Elliott was Anton or Antoine Melovidov, who was "chief" of this island in the early 1900s.[13] "Chief" refers to foreman responsibilities only and is not inheritable. Chiefs were appointed at some times, elected at others. Usually became company or government stooges.

May 27, 1942
Tomorrow we hope to resume hiking. While we were idling, I decided to exchange books from Government House and finally found Elliott's monograph. That made me forget all

cont.

possible doubts for the future and I have been busy with it since yesterday afternoon and finished looking it over before I had my shower. New Aleut place names, confirmation and contradiction of some Russian place names. A few yarns, some new and some old, a slightly clearer picture of early settlements here and some other crumbs of information for which I had been seeking.

In addition to the reading material we shall derive great help from little sketches of sections of the island in which he has hills and elevated spots marked. I shall have to get busy tracing some to take on our hikes with us so that we shall finally get some of the vistas regulated in our minds. Between maps to copy and several dozens of pages of text to type for myself, Baranoff, and Harrington, Elliott has provided me with much work to do for the next couple of months. His pictures in the book are the most amusing things I have ever seen. His faces are so ludicrous and unreal . . . I wonder just how seriously he took his art. He could do line drawing, practical stuff, but as a portrayer of persons he belonged to the office of an advertiser for freak shows.

Was he in earnest? Did people really look like that to him? How could he maintain the attitude that he has toward the Aleuts and still marry a girl who had at least some Aleut blood in her veins? Will I ever find out any details of that wedding? Why did not he and Bryant get along? I have a hundred questions buzzing in

cont.

island, except for a sojourn on St. George where Elliott surveyed the rookeries until the end of the next year's sealing. Of all his work Elliott was most proud of his system of estimating the number of seals.

In 1874, Elliott, lauded to the skies for his first report on the fur seal, returned to the islands with Naval Lieutenant Washburn Maynard to recheck his earlier findings and ascertain how the lessees were carrying out their contract. Elliott was pleased with everything, with the flourishing state of the seal kingdom, with the wooden houses that the company was erecting to replace the dank barabaras. Optimistically he declared that the large annual killing could in no way damage the seal herd. Elliott had lost his heart to the fur seal. Until the end of his life in 1930 he was their loyal, fervid spokesman and champion. His monograph on the seals sparkles in every sentence with his affectionate ardor. It gave him fame and prestige even though it was later reviled and jeered at by his political opponents.

In 1889, although the Alaska Commercial Company knew the seal herd had decreased, they entered their bid for a renewal of their lease, again offering to meet and surpass the highest bidder. They had new arguments to bolster their claim. They could point to the wooden houses they had built for the Aleut families, to the business buildings, boats, and stores on the island that they owned. Their lobbyists must have been overconfident, lulled by the ease of their first success. The treasury awarded the lease to a firm with more powerful political friends, the North American Commercial Company. Among its stockholders there were actually senators and other public officers. The rent was raised to sixty thousand dollars a year; the tax on each skin increased to $9.62. Obligations to the islanders were almost identical except to supply them with a little more fuel and food than the previous firm. The quota of one hundred thousand skins was lowered to a promise of sixty thousand the first year. The Secretary of the Treasury was empowered to decide the number for succeeding years, for something terrible had happened to the seal herd. Treasury agents had sent Washington few hints of it until 1889. Then Special Agent Goff and two of his assistants had submitted a report that caused Secretary Windom to open his eyes in surprise and call the Smithsonian to ask for the oracle of the fur seal, Henry W. Elliott, to assist him in solving the puzzle. Northward Elliott sped, appointed special investigator under a hurriedly passed congressional measure, to solve the mystery of the vanishing fur sea.

> my mind about him. I hope I get back to the States someday before he has been forgotten and I can answer some of them.
>
> I had hoped to send a letter out to Simeon Melovidov about getting in touch with Elliott's children on this boat-if there were a boat-and if he had children.[14]

In June 1890 Elliott stood on the rocks overhanging the seal beaches of St. Paul scarcely able to believe his eyes' testimony. Where had the vast seal herd vanished? His heart ached with grief as he saw only a few hundred thousand animals scattered thinly over the harem grounds. His anger against the agents of destruction was terrible. He and Agent Goff ordered the lessees to suspend operations. Elliott went back to Washington, unhappy but confident of restoring the herd by getting treasury confirmation for a *zapusk*. At a meeting with the assembled sealers, he promised that Washington would act at once to protect both the animals and the human residents.

Scarcely had he reached Washington before the political friends of the North American Commercial Company, many of them shareholders, were in full cry against his findings. Elliott blamed the herd's depletion on two causes, pelagic sealing and improper methods of land killing. He emphasized that the latter was the principal cause of destruction, thereby indicting the very company, the very individuals, he had so lavishly praised in his earlier writings.

Since the Alaska Commercial Company was still interested in regaining the sealing rights, Elliott was caught in a crossfire of violent nasty criticism. By one group he was smeared as the tool of the former lessee. Publicists of the former lessee raved hysterically that he was in the pay of pelagic sealers, a British agent, and a traitor to American interests. Both sides agreed that he knew nothing about seals, that his method of counting seals was ridiculous, and that he was a scientific faker. Men who had respectfully called him "professor" in accordance with conventional courtesy for the learned, whether they possessed framed academic degrees or not, attacked the title as self-bestowed and the mark of the pretender.[15] No mud was too filthy to be flung by his enemies. His report and his recommendations were kept buried in the official files. To counteract his conclusions, strings were pulled to send other more objective investigators who would have no previous reputation to protect. Every year men went north to spend a few weeks of the sealing season, principally scientists from various government departments. One and all reported the herd had suffered only from pelagic sealing.

Pelagic sealing is as old as the first man who speared a seal from his canoe. Hundreds, possibly thousands, of years passed during which the stone-tipped spear or harpoon wreaked no damage to seal life. Then almost in a season it became an industry of civilized man. Firearms replaced the primitive weapons. Immediately the seal millions began to decrease. About 1879, when whaling was declining, the captains of whalers were attracted by the rich profits of the increasingly fashionable fur seal. By 1880 pelagic sealing was an established and very profitable industry. From fifteen thousand skins obtained by the piratical sealers in 1882, the toll rose through the years until in 1896 over sixty thousand were taken in the ocean. Nearly a hundred small schooners, owned by Americans, Canadians, and Japanese, were operating in the Pacific, sailing in the spring in time to meet the seals coming north along the American coast. Killing as they sailed northward, the sealers entered the Bering Sea and hunted the animals off their breeding islands, sometimes coming within the three-mile territorial limit.

Pelagic sealers themselves testified that for every dead seal hauled on deck nine others had been shot and had sunk before the body could be seized. An unborn pup died with every female slaughtered in the spring on her way to the islands to give birth. If the sealers shot a female in the Bering, on one of her trips back and forth to her feeding grounds, not only did another unborn seal perish with her but her recently delivered pup died slowly and horribly of starvation on the Pribilof beaches. A triple murder was committed. Efforts to control pelagic sealing, prompted by discussions between Great Britain and the United States, resulted in a conference called the Paris Tribunal of 1891.

The tribunal stipulated that a zone of sixty miles around the island be closed to pelagic schooners during the summer. It was a futile measure since the females went more than twice that distance in summer. The schooners had merely to lie in wait outside that zone, safe from U.S. revenue cutters, and stock their salt bins quickly with female skins. The dates of the closed season from May 1 until August were the jaws of a trap that captured the females easily. By August 1, the date when the restriction was lifted, all the females had been delivered of their young. The whole female contingent was occupied in getting food and returning to nurse their young. With numerous females taken, thousands of wasted bodies of motherless seal pups lay dead of starvation on the rookeries.

The British cleverly utilized Elliott's description of improper land killings and gave his enemy fresh ammunition for further attacks.[16] Stubbornly Elliott stuck to his thesis. Clean up our own house from within, first stop all seal killing on land and when the herd is partially restored, begin again to negotiate with the British. He argued that the United States could not ask the British to refrain from killing seals in the free waters of the earth unless it were willing to nourish and protect the animals when they landed on American soil. Unless we respect our own property we cannot ask others to, he repeated patiently over and over again. The supporters of the North American Commercial Company reviled him because they were losing money on their contract. They bolstered their arguments for permission to take more seals by pleading the rights of the Aleuts to make a living. Congress was forced to vote $19,500 a year to supplement the meager earnings of the Aleuts. This expenditure, in addition to the upkeep of revenue vessels to ward off poachers, the cost of outfitting investigators and sending representatives to international conferences, and the damages paid to protesting seal pirates changed the Seal Islands from a public asset bringing in a rich revenue in rent and taxes into an immense drain on the taxpayers of the country.

British diplomats asserted that pelagic sealing would end as soon as the herd had decreased so much that sealing voyages were profitless. Some Americans became wearily willing to agree to that callous opinion and let the fur seal follow the sea cow into oblivion. The men who wanted to garner wealth from the seal on the islands and Elliott who wanted to keep the seals alive and flourishing kept the fight going. Elliott was grimly determined that the fur seal should not perish from the face of the earth, at the hands of either greedy lessees or piratical poachers, as long as he had a voice with which to challenge the forces of greed.

In 1896 the investigation to end all investigations was launched with David Starr Jordan, the great ichthyologist, at its head. After two seasons' study four monumental tomes were published.[17] The former lessee was officially cleared of guilt. The decrease of the seal herd was attributed to pelagic sealing alone. The study asserted that because Elliott's manner of seal computation had been false and infantile there had been no such enormous assembly of seals as he claimed in 1872 and therefore no such catastrophic decline as he asserted.

In certain political and commercial circles there was satisfaction. The great seal authority was silenced. Their gratification was short lived. Before the final volumes were off the press Elliott was on the warpath, a road he never deserted until his death. During the first years of his crusade the seal herd continued to disappear until by 1903 there were about two hundred thousand seals left. In that year a senatorial committee visited Alaska and returned to fight for legislation for a vacation from land killing as a prelude to inviting further negotiations with Japan and Great Britain. Their proposed legislation died quietly in committee.

In 1905 Secretary Hay, on the eve of consummating a treaty with Great Britain to protect the fur seals, died. His successor, Elihu Root, failed to continue the negotiations. Even Elliott was discouraged. From the descriptions of furs put on sale in London he believed the lessee was breaking many regulations in choosing the killable seals in order to scrape together an annual take of a few thousand pelts. Chiefly he believed that females and very young seals were deliberately being slaughtered.

At this moment of discouragement, attacked on all sides by politicians and men whom he always alluded to in quotation marks as "scientists," strong forces came to his aid. The redoubtable champion of the wild animals, Dr. William T. Hornaday, decided to battle for the seals. He was backed by the powerful Campfire Society. Hornaday believed he could achieve the conservation of the fur seal more easily if Elliott remained in the background and made bullets of the facts he had amassed in his long, vitriolic campaign. A familiar figure disappeared from the halls of Congress, from the offices of the senators and representatives. Now Hornaday sat in the witness chair in Elliott's stead at congressional hearings trying to negotiate what he and his supporters had rashly predicted would be a love feast.

Despite Hornaday's efforts there began what he described in his own words as "the bitterest and most brutal fight ever waged around the fur seal." In 1910 the first victory of the fur seal was won. The system of leasing the island to a private concern was abolished by congressional actions over the protests of officials of the Department of Commerce and Labor, which had replaced the Treasury Department as caretaker of the Pribilofs. The measure would not have passed had not Senator Dillingham cannily waited until certain of his colleagues were absent from the Senate. When they returned it was too late to protect their own interests. The Secretary of Commerce and Labor immediately began proceedings to pass a bill giving his office the right to determine the time and number of future seal killings.

In 1910 the long years of international negotiations ended with the agreement of Russia, the United States, England, and Japan to end pelagic sealing. As owners of land where fur seals came ashore the United States and Russia were to divide thirty percent of their annual sealing proceeds equally between England and Japan, either in furs or cash. In return England and Japan were to prevent their nationals from poaching. Japan was to exchange fifteen percent of her small Kurile Islands annual harvest of pelts to the two principal seal-owning nations. The waters of the ocean became safe for the fur seal after thirty years of piracy. With a gentleman's agreement the fur seal hearings were ended. Secretary Nagel gave verbal assurance that his department's policy was to enforce a rest period on land to enable the herd to multiply. A congressional committee had promised a fifty-thousand-dollar appropriation to support the sealers during the forthcoming *zapusk*. The fur seal bowed its thanks and departed from congressional chambers.

The armistice lasted a few months. In May the Commissioner of Fisheries announced that commercial killing was to be resumed. To the protests of Hornaday and the Campfire committee, the officials replied defiantly that they knew best. The gentleman's agreement was forgotten. In the late summer, reports from the island showed that over twelve thousand seals had been killed. Elliott studied the table of weights of the furs. He declared that many of them were illegally slaughtered yearlings and females. Hornaday released Elliott from his promise to remain behind the scenes and summoned him forth to the "fight to the absolute defeat of one side or the other."

With Henry Wood Elliott back in the arena, the battle flared more intensely. Relentlessly he battered down the weaker arguments of his foes with patient repetitions that began "the facts are." When the hearings from 1911 to 1914, collected in two heavy volumes, were ended, many reputations were lost, officials were dropped from offices, and the frenzied vituperation that curdled the air of hearing chamber had set new patterns in picturesque epithets. The outcome of the fight was a congressional act to halt seal killings for five years.

In 1913, during the hearings, Elliott and a secretary paid a brief visit to the Pribilofs.[18] He was an unwelcome guest and a churlish visitor. He and Agent Lembkey had crossed verbal swords too often in Washington to abide by the rules of conventional politeness. A telegram had already informed Lembkey that the investigating committee had reached a partisan decision. The Democrats, in the majority, had decided in favor of the holiday from sealing. The Republican minority was opposed to it. The fur seals, the fewer than a hundred thousand that still had their pelts, had become a political football. The unfortunate seal, neither Republican nor Democrat, not even possessing a vote, would have been fated to pass out of existence if the Republicans had the major representation on the committee.

Many incidents of that last visit were never recorded by either island official or Elliott himself. I heard them on St. Paul. Elliott had insisted for years that hundreds of seal skins sent to market were deliberately poorly blubbered in order to have their weight approximate the true weight of well-flensed pelts of older animals in the legally killable classification. Fierce denials met this accusation, which he never withdrew. One day on St. Paul while Lembkey sat eating his lunch, Elliott entered the dining room and flung down a fresh bloody skin in front of the agent. Overcome by the actual proof of inadequate blubbering of a small skin, the stench of the unpalatable bloody pelt, Lembkey put one hand over his mouth and dashed out of the room. "He could not eat for a week," said my informant, laughing uproariously at the remembered scene. "I was working as a mess boy then. I remember good. Gee, it was fun."

"But what about the blubber?" I inquired. "Were the men really told to leave lots of blubber on the skins?"

He looked amazed at the silliness of my question. "Sure thing. Not many seals then. Had to kill little ones. The company say they send the men off St. Paul if they tell. They afraid to talk."

That seemed to me the final disproof of Elliott's optimistic assertion that gossiping Natives could prevent the lessees from breaking the clauses of their contracts. My informant went on talking of Elliott. "The man with the pencil," he called him. So did other Aleuts who remembered him.

"Once Elliott come in where I wash dishes and say to me, 'Why don't you Aleut boys stop being cheated? You know I married a girl from this island and I don't like to see the way you get cheated and knocked around.'"

This was incendiary language for a scientific investigator, but Elliott had long since ceased being objective. His words could not stir up the sealers who were bound to silence by years of lessons in obedience to authority, made helpless vassals by the fears of generations.

The fur seals were safe on land and sea by 1914. Elliott might return to his "vineyard in Cleveland," happy and content though his victory brought him no public acclaim and the smears of his opponents still clung to his public reputation.[19]

It would be so nice if that were really the end of the story and "they lived happily ever after." Only the peace again was not completely won as far as the benefits to the taxpayers from their island livestock was concerned. The seal herd grew apace during the *zapusk*. And in 1919 killing recommenced, carried on by the government alone.[20] The first skins were turned over to a firm, Funsten Brothers of St. Louis, to be processed and auctioned as finished pelts. The firm collected a major share of the returns from the sales. Then the president of Funsten Brothers, Philip Fouke, became the president of the newly created Fouke Fur Company. He secured a contract guaranteeing payments for additional work in handling the skins.

There would be little left for the public treasury. Elliott was aroused from his rightfully earned peace and returned again in the 1920s to the congressional hearing chambers. This time he was a spokesman for the taxpayers. He strove to prove that the government would make more money from selling raw salted skins directly to the market than financing the dyeing and processing procedures and paying high fees to an auctioneer. In 1930 Elliott was living with his son and daughter in Seattle, busily engaged in sketching Mount Rainier. At eighty-four he was alert, keenly interested in every public event, in touch with men of affairs all over the nation through a superhuman correspondence. After

January 12, 1942
I managed to finish Elliott's notes Friday. Or rather Saturday. And Paul left Gov. House unlocked so we could lug up the tons of books we had borrowed and get some new ones in return. I had to discipline myself very much to avoid copying most of E. whose charm is great and whose nonsense is most charming.

January 21, 1942
I am going through the recent logs rapidly. There is a gap between 1919 and 1925 and Carl thinks the books are at Gov. House. I never saw them there and am worrying about them. But the logs beginning 1925 are dull work lists with the barest notices of other sorts. Some death and birth notices, an occasional accident, etc. but all the drama and color of life has been squeezed out even of the few disorderly cases mentioned. It would be difficult for a historian to put the pieces together. He would know how many days two men managed to spend painting radiators in the hospital but that is about all. And could conclude that the men had made

cont.

a brief illness of a week he died, unmourned by the beasts he had given the best part of his life to save or by his fellow citizens whose interests he had protected so vigilantly.

A few months before he died he wrote to his brother-in-law Simeon Melovidov, a resident of California, "I only did what any right minded citizen would have done." Hornaday paid him great tribute in a book published soon after his death: "By the year 2000 Mr. Elliott's great-great-grandchildren may receive for him 'the thanks of Congress.' But I doubt it." His opponents were men in high places. Where their influence reached in recording posthumous credit, there is no mention of the man who loved the fur seals. And few people will ever accidentally come upon his barbed wit, his persistent practical arguments, his searing, caustic epithets within the covers of stodgy-looking congressional hearings.

ca' canny a fine art-which is true. He would not have acquired the liking for McMillin that he and I can have for Judge or the dislike for Tingle, etc.

An hour's work tomorrow will finish the books in the office and I will ask Paul to leave the door unlocked in Gov. House for me to look for the missing ones. And-what annoys me is that Tobyanne's birth is not entered in the log. Must speak to Carl about that for in these warring times it may never be possible to get her birth certificate from Juneau, and according to the log itself she was never born.

Eventually the seals did win their deserved holiday and today the herd is again a mighty host of two million seals. And of the ninety-five thousand seals taken in 1941, sixty-two thousand have already been sold for over two million dollars, by auctioneers, the Fouke Fur Company.[21] Had there never been an Elliott, the fur seal would have been an amphibian wraith like Steller's sea cow.

Chapter 34

One dark bloody tale remains to be exhumed from the seal's tragic history, a chapter from the blackest years of pelagic butchery. Contrary to gloomy predictions that pelagic sealing would ebb as the extermination of the seals grew nearer, the poachers faced the decrease with boldness, resorting to shore raids. Again and again raiders landed on St. George beaches far from the village. Protected by overhanging cliffs they slew their helpless prey with ease. A broken club, skinned carcasses, or blood-splashed rocks were the only traces the visitors left.

Harassed government agents posted guards at the rookeries and begged for boats with which to reach poaching vessels not far from shore and weapons with which to frighten off the pirates. Watch houses were built at the rookeries to house parties of guards. There were hardly enough adult males to guard all rookery shores effectively, particularly since the men were all needed for routine work. It became commonplace for a sealing schooner to drift at ease close to the island, launching small boats to kill swimming seals. When the mists were densest, the islanders could hear the sharp crack of rifles, the deep-throated roar of fog-signal guns. One revenue cutter could not watch the waters around the two islands. Furthermore, the cutter had to go back to Unalaska at frequent intervals for refueling. The poachers had a nose for keeping track of the cutter. No sooner was the cutter out of sight than the pirates came into view.

Toward the end of pelagic sealing more and more schooners were registered from Japanese ports and carried Japanese crews. Some were legitimate property of Japanese merchants. Others actually belonged to citizens of other countries.

John Fratis is still alive. He can relate the story of those July days when the sounds of cannon and rifle fire rolled ominously landward through the fogs that walled off the sea from the watchers on St. Paul. He can tell how his heart beat and his knees trembled as he lifted his hunting gun to shoot at the retreating marauders. He could not believe his eyes when he saw men topple into their boat and realized that he had killed a fellow human being. But John's and Metrofan's memories became blurred during the years. The number of dead Japanese became ten, twenty, thirty, forty.

"The water," said Metrofan, "was full of dead bodies. We couldn't count them all." Fratis repeats, "There was a lot of dead Japs didn't get ashore."

Old men's embroidered tales brought back the atmosphere of the minor war waged from July 16 to 18, 1906, which even extrudes from the dry factual reports of government agents.[1] Both John Fratis and Metrofan had taken part in the battle.

The cutter was absent at Unalaska although the breeding season was just reaching its climax. At least sixteen Japanese vessels were within the proscribed zone, insolently anchoring within the three-mile limit. Helplessly the guards on St. Paul rookeries listened to the poachers' gunfire. Occasionally through a rift in the heavy mists the alien boats were visible but too far away to be alarmed by rifle shots. There were only thirty-eight able-bodied males armed with twelve rifles to protect the forty miles of coastline. Had the combined crews, averaging thirty men apiece, of the four Japanese vessels sighted on July 16 and 17 landed simultaneously the guards could have protected neither themselves nor the animals.

Early on the morning of the sixteenth, three guards posted at Northeast Point spied a large schooner drawing close to shore. A guard went back to summon Agent Lembkey who soon arrived from the watch house with reinforcements. The islanders hid behind natural rock ramparts and watched a small boat, outfitted with mainsail and jib, put out from the vessel and pull directly toward the base of Hutchinson Hill. Six unsuspecting Japanese sailors climbed out of the boat and were immediately surrounded. One sailor pleaded in broken English that they had come ashore for freshwater. Sealing clubs, skinning knives, and other sealing gear in their boat gave the lie of his excuse. The boat contained a five-gallon cask full of freshwater. The six oars, bound with greased cloth, rested in padded oarlocks, that no sound of clashing metal could betray the boat's unwelcome presence. The prisoners were immediately marched off, under guard, along the twelve-mile road to St. Paul Village. Through their clumsy interpreter, the prisoners revealed that they were sailors on the *Toyai Maru No 2*, part of a crew of thirty-two men, sailing from the port of Hakodato, Japan.

During the day guards at every rookery waited alertly while guns barked eerily behind the curtain of fog. By means of cannon the marauding schooners communicated with each other and with their small butcher boats at intervals. Guards at Reef Point glimpsed a vessel close to shore. At Polovina Point, other watchers saw, for a few minutes, still another sealer at work.

At eight o'clock the next morning, a second band of Japanese land pirates, in three small boats, approached the western side of Northeast Point, taking advantage of the thick morning fog. Suddenly the wind dispersed the fog and the Aleut guards, Michael Kozloff and John Fratis, saw the lead boat at the shoreline. Two sailors were busy with the sail. A third sat facing landward with a rifle in his hands. Kozloff and Fratis leaped to their feet and shouted, "Hands up." Hastily the Japanese abandoned the sail and grabbed their oars. Kozloff fired three warning shots in the water close to the boat. The frantic sailors bent to their oars. The guards fired six more shots, aiming directly at the boat and its occupants. The Japanese slumped in their seats. The strong wind swept the boat back to the beach. Kozloff and Fratis ran to haul it up on the shingle. Inside lay two dead Japanese. The third man crouched in fright, nursing a wounded shoulder. The other boats had escaped back to the schooner when the alarm was given. The wounded sailor disclosed, through the English-speaking captive, that his ship was the *Mei Maru,* sailing from Hakodato, also, and had, before the morning's misadventure, a crew of thirty-two men.

Offshore rifle fire rent the fog at Zapadni Rookery in the afternoon. Suddenly the clouds of mist rolled away and the two astonished shore guards gaped at three boats, holding eighteen or twenty sailors, a few yards from them. Excitedly the two guards, frightened at the sudden appearance of such a large force, shot wildly toward the boats. All three swerved immediately and pulled vigorously for the open sea. The guards could not discern what damage, if any, their hastily aimed fusillade had effected.

The captains of the ships off Northeast Point were determined to carry out their thievery. All day long, the staccato of rifle fire beat against the ears of the shore guards. Again and again the deep voice of the signal cannons spoke through the murky atmosphere, the threatening sound echoing and reechoing among the rocks. Until eight in the evening the fog protected the marine marauders. Then the guards could see a schooner anchored in the dangerously shallow water, three hundred yards from the shore, on the western side of the Point. A messenger ran hastily for the agent who was waiting under shelter, not far away. He soon arrived with a squad of Aleuts.

Just then the fog bank was pushed farther west, disclosing a number of Japanese on the beach, hastily preparing to embark. Lembkey called out to them to halt. But the Japanese rowed frantically to get their boats to safety. Lembkey signaled his men to fire. As the bullets pattered over, around, and into the boats, all three turned shoreward to surrender. Then Lembkey realized his own forces were too few to ensure the capture of so many armed poachers. He permitted the first returning boat to land, then waved the others back to their ship. This was not cowardice. The fifteen Aleuts of his party had but six rifles.

Gunfire from the schooner had answered the attack of the Aleuts on the landing party but the bullets fell harmlessly into the surf. The casualties among the Japanese were serious. One dead sailor lay in the boat that was captured. A sailor in one of the fleeing boats was seen to topple overboard. His body floated from sight. A third body was tossed overboard from the schooner, with callous disregard for the Japanese rites for the dead.

The five living prisoners, one wounded, huddled together while the guards inspected the rookery. The ravages of the vandals had been frightful. One hundred and eighty-three seals had been killed. The skins of one hundred and twenty were in the surrendered boat. Sixty-three seals, either dead or wounded, lay scattered among the stones. Some seals had been merely stunned by a blow on the head and skinned while still alive. These denuded animals staggered piteously to their feet, dragged themselves on mutilated flippers first in one direction, then another. Their cries rose above the breakers in bewildered wails of pain before the horrified Aleut guards could end their misery. No danger can frighten the big bull seal of a harem from his homesite during the breeding season. Only in death does he forsake his watch over his cows and their young. Ruthlessly the Japanese had beaten the threatening bulls across their slightly protruding eyeballs until the eyes were destroyed. In the midst of the carnage these intrepid blinded males roared and plunged to meet imaginary dangers and drive off possible intruders. These, too, were mercifully killed by the Aleuts.

Only two of the slain seals were male. The wanton slaughter of nursing mother seals caused the death of 180 seal pups from slow starvation.

The five prisoners were escorted to the village by guards whose hearts were full of hatred toward them. On the afternoon of July 18, the unwounded prisoners returned to Northeast Point to dig the grave for the three dead sailors. There, near the scene of their crime, where lupine and pedicularis wave gaily in summer among the lichen-splattered lava rocks, their bodies were hidden from the eyes of accusing man, from the sight of heaven.

The prisoners, taken by cutter to Valdez, Alaska, for trial, received sentences of three months apiece for their depredations. The sentence was light because these men were only hired sailors obliged to carry out the orders of their officers.

The flotilla of Japanese sealing schooners that surrounded the island, until the last skirmish at Northeast Point frightened them away, represented a potential threat, not only to the seals but to the human inhabitants, too. Had the schooners sent their men ashore simultaneously at various points along the coast, the Aleuts and government agents would have been vastly outnumbered. The poachers could have repeated the invasion of the Commander Islands where Japanese attackers had held off a large armed defense for two weeks while despoiling the herd of seals. The Japanese had killed and wounded many of the Russian defenders. Had Agent Lembkey and his Aleut guards failed to drive away the raiders, there would have been no end to the thieving, murdering activities of the Japanese sealers. Neither would the Japanese government have been forced at last to sign the fur seal treaty of 1911, which she finally abrogated in 1941.

It was not only Metrofan and John, the only living survivors of the battle of Northeast Point, who kept the incident alive. Others remembered the butchery because of the incredible mutilation of the seals. If the Japanese could so torture helpless and harmless animals, their vengeance for their sailor dead would be unpredictable.[2] John Hanson told me some island doctor had dug up at least the skulls of the poachers and that they had been rolling around in odd corners of the attic of our house for years. When we had cleaned out the last dark corner under the eaves we still had not found them. They may have been taken off the island as souvenirs. They more likely were tossed into the rubbish heap by some good housekeeper.

I never wonder about their ultimate fate without recalling the anecdote of the mysterious skull. Workmen were repairing the road just above the hospital and dug up a head. Elary Gromoff ran down to the dentist's office with it because he thought the dentist would be interested in the skull's fine set of teeth. Apolon Bourdokofsky heard of it and was shocked. He warned Elary, "You done wrong. Take that head back and put it in bone yard, else you will dream of it nights." Elary rushed back, reclaimed the head, and buried it in the cemetery. Legend makes the single skull into the entire skeleton of a female and there has been much speculation as to just what the lady was doing in such a nude condition on the public highway.

There could hardly be much reverence for old bones on an island where huge fields are nothing but thin soil over thick layers of undecayed seal bones on old killing grounds and where human graveyards had been dug up and ruined by living seals.

Chapter 35

Because of the earlier invasion of Japanese pirates, it is easy to understand why, of all people living under the American flag beyond the borders of the southern Pacific area being attacked, the Aleuts of St. Paul were the most frightened when their radios spoke on Sunday, December 7, 1941. The old people said, "I told you so." The young shivered for they had been nourished on the tale of the July attack. How the villagers were certain the Japanese would come for the fur seals they coveted. Now they would avenge their sailor dead. The fur seal had given warning of Pearl Harbor. There were statesmen in America who knew what Japan's abrogation of the fur seal protection treaty in October 1941 meant.[1] Just as Metrofan on St. Paul, tensely listening to the clipped English speech of a Japanese announcer, knew and trembled when the voice declared that from now on war would be waged against the fur seals of the Pacific. Metrofan said slowly aloud, "Against us, too."

War! War in the Pacific! Tobyanne! The words were clinging in my heart. The *Penguin* was off St. George waiting for high seas to subside to finish unloading cargo. In a few days she would return southward. Should Tobyanne go with her? I thought of the bereaved mothers of that first day's brutal

December 7, 1941
These random notes were broken off by the entrance of Vivian who had come to cut Sam's hair. Now it's Sunday 2:00 p.m. and like living in a new world-for the war shadow we felt closing about has at last reached out to engulf the Americas. So I will jot down the items briefly that I intended to do yesterday and return to the advent of war later and more.

Vivian stayed so long that I asked whether she would like supper here. We sent for Earl and ate about six. A very dull evening. I wanted to come type, feeling the hours slip by so slowly doing nothing. After ten they left and we walked down to West Landing. The moon and clouds were wonderful. Back to bed where we lay long talking. Consequently it was hellish for Sam to rise to feed the baby. At 8:45 he came back to bed and we napped until quarter to eleven when I rose to feed Tobyanne. We had a struggle as she preferred play.

Tobyanne had at last finished her eleven o'clock bottle. She sat playing on the sofa beside me, trying to catch hold of my moving

cont.

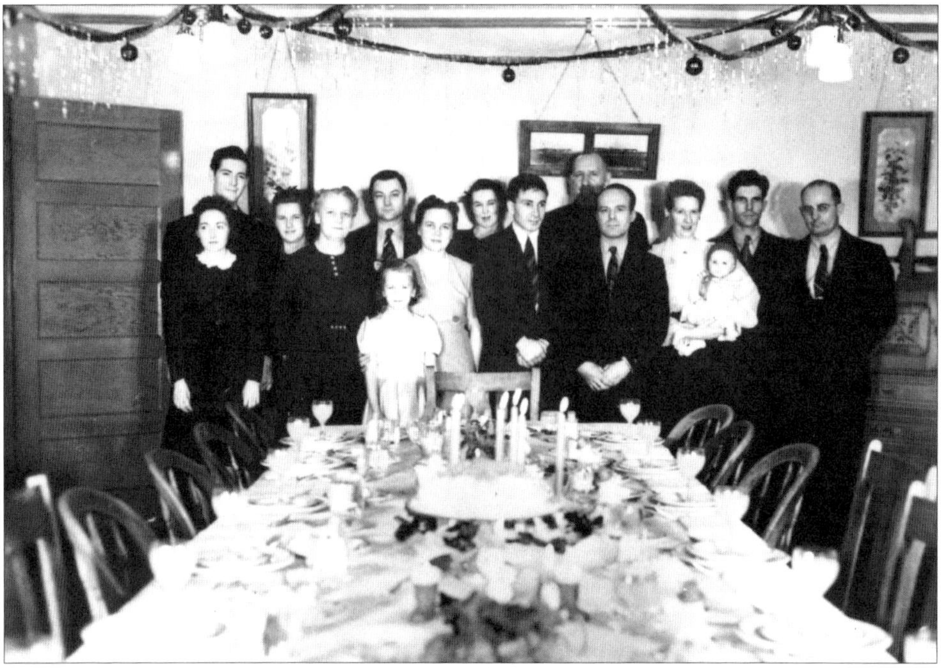

Christmas dinner with the government employees, 1941 (from the Martin Collection, USUAF210, Archives, Alaska and Polar Regions, Rasmuson Library, University of Alaska Fairbanks).

fingers and gurgling ecstatically when she managed to clutch and hold on to one of them. No serener scene in the whole world than the two of us, mother and daughter, playing together, laughing together, while a tired father napped in the other room, enjoying the luxury of no office hours for patients on Sunday.

Suddenly Hank Banner burst into the house and demanded, "Have you heard the news?"

"What news?"

"The Japanese bombed Pearl Harbor this morning."

"What!" I tore to my feet and rushed to waken Sam. We turned on the radio and sat tense, trying to sort some coherent sounds from the cacophony of static.

cont.

warfare and of other mothers on Pacific outposts who were also crying out, "How can I save my child?" I had seen Spanish mothers weeping over the pitiful remnants of their children's bodies. Was it my turn now?

There was no question of our leaving, but the day and night until the *Penguin* pulled away the debate went on. Should I entrust her to others on the ship or were the radio rumors of enemy submarines off Kodiak true? Would she be safer with us? And in the end the *Penguin* went without her.

Nightly blackouts were ordered. Planes were heard at night. Whose planes no one knew. In the dusk, a ship's lights signaled near Otter Island. At daybreak the seas were empty.

There is a quality about an island that breeds a sense of security. Accustomed to being isolated from the world, it is difficult to imagine the world arriving at one's doorstep with a machine gun. For awhile the Aleuts were agitated, remembering the desecrated graves on Hutchinson Hill. Then the routine of normal life calmed fears and restored emotional stability. Until spring we all agreed we were safe from attack.

Briefly we discussed the irony of our situation. Seeking a respite from the clamorous world for a year, we had settled too close to the dragon's tail. Firmly we resolved to waste no time in futile anxieties but to continue our studies and activities with renewed zeal and enjoy our island sojourn to the full.

So we welcomed midwinter holidays, a double round of them. First we celebrated Christmas on December 25. Festivities commenced conventionally with a play at the Community Hall presented by the schoolchildren. It might have been any school entertainment in the States except that some of the costumes were shabby and dull. Down in the audience the smallest children squirmed, torn between the action of the play and the pyramid of gifts piled about the artificial Christmas tree.

Just as the play ended something happened to Santa Claus' trousers. He disappeared. Necks grew weary supporting the anxious heads straining backward to watch the door. Welcome were the harsh clangings of a cowbell that announced his entrance. Capering carefully, because some rather conspicuous slits in his trousers threatened to expel his padding of cushions, Santa reached the tree. Peering through the extremely narrow slits in his mask he slowly read a typewritten greeting to the village children. He was a real Pribilof Santa, wearing the high rubber boots of the sealing profession.

The most attractively wrapped packages came from the Fouke Fur Company. Sears Roebuck had sent a mass of damaged toys

The whole day passed without much activity. Huddling near the radio, turning the dials from station to station, listening to the screeching tumult of static until darkness cleared the airways. Then the voices of the outer world came clearly into our rooms, narrating disaster after disaster or reading the defiant editorial opinions of the country's papers.

December 11, 1941
We stayed at Lukanin until a little after eleven and then came back to feed Tobyanne. We sent Heretina out to see the sights. We had waited in vain for Harrington. Hoverson arrived there, in search of Harrington whom they could not find in the village. I have not yet had a chance to find out just where he was located. On our way into town we passed a truck loaded with Natives. I pictured Harrington sitting in the front seat and mentally waved him good-bye. Mrs. Hellbaum told me he arrived standing in the back jammed in with the crowd of Natives, but positively not taking notes. It must have been nearly one when the *Penguin* upped anchor and set out for St. George, off whose cliffs she has been sitting, but, oh, so bumpily, ever since.

That evening, when we were relaxing after supper, we both confessed to a nostalgic emotion, compounded of regret because we knew neither Hank nor Harrington might drop in anymore and a longing to be in safer territory just now and where we might feel a bit more inside things than here.[2] The *cont.*

isolation would please me very much for a long time to come if we were not helpless militarily and if we were not so sure that Dutch Harbor cannot offer us much help if the Japs come over. However, there is not much sense in expecting them until spring or summer when the weather is more mild and whatever sudden storms sweep up will be of rain instead of snow and hail and sleet . . .

December 15, Bill of Rights Day
The hospital [patients] listened to the *Penguin* over the radio this evening but we were confused by the words they heard. Peter reported that he heard Elliott who is working during the day on the *Penguin* say, "Merry Christmas and A Happy New Year" and took this to be a farewell. But who knows? The person who had been on the *Penguin* from Seattle to here and was remaining to return would have material for quite an amusing yarn. It can't be very amusing for the poor passengers who went out of here last Thursday morning and have been tossing up and down on the rough waves ever since-getting seasick for nothing and making no progress toward their goal. I can picture Dr. Harrington at work, with his papers all spread out about him, putting the poor half-seasick Aleuts through his third degree, himself too enthused to pay attention to his own innards. We never said good-bye to him. He was back and forth in the house all morning and we promised to see him on the beach. The loading was being done at Lukanin. Earl drove us over

cont.

that had been reconditioned on the island. There was one of these gifts for each child. Each one, even Tobyanne, received a small brown paper sack of nuts and candy from Uncle Sam.

Stacy had wrapped up a Sears machine gun for Sam, which evoked much nervous laughter. Even a toy gun seemed ominous and reminded people of our unprotected shores. It proved very useful at home. Its spluttering racket was one noise that overawed the cats. We kept it propped near our tree and foiled all feline attempts to nest in the branches or toy with swaying ornaments.

We staggered home under a load of gifts from our patients, the kind of gifts that bring lumps to one's throat. Hand-crocheted doilies, over two dozen baby dresses for Tobyanne, toiletries from the Canteen, cigarettes; each carried a significance beyond the gift itself. The remainder of the evening we spent at home, trimming a real tree that the Hoversons had secured from Seattle by the last *Penguin*. Its nostalgic scent made us homesick for wooded hills for a moment.

Visitors came early on Christmas morning, both Aleut and government people. We had to inspect the hospital. Peter and Mary were beamingly proud in an atmosphere that sparkled.

The visit of the village children in the afternoon is a tradition dating back to the pleasanter social atmosphere when the Americans first arrived. The natural instinct to give gifts to small callers invited to Government House in those days to see the decorations had become a rigid custom of preparing edible tidbits for every child from the toddlers to the sixteen-year-old youngsters. The children gathered in crowds and waited for the magic hour of 1:00 p.m. before rushing swiftly from house to house to collect their swag. I watched them gathering on the road above our house as I hastily stuffed small bags with nuts, fruit, and candy and small trinkets like marbles and balloons. Two advance scouts ventured down to our door. We rashly gave them our contribution. They rushed back and shouted to the crowd above. Like an avalanche the others poured down the slope, some falling and rolling in the mad descent. I hadn't enough ammunition so Sam got the camera and coaxed them out on the porch to pose. A second wave flowed in a few minutes later. Only when the stragglers came later did anyone have time to sit down, admire the tree, play with the baby's toys and the cats, and talk to us. The person who prepared no gifts would be unpopular forever after. Though housewives of officials fuss and fume, they make the cakes and cookies every year for a ritual that long ago lost personal meaning and warmth.

In the evening, again in concordance with tradition, the Service families dined on turkey in the Company House. Christmas, New Year's, and Washington's birthday, we had the same formal gathering. All of them were dull, conversationless affairs, lacking the usual chatter and animation of social hours at the employees' houses. Perhaps the enormous task of tackling the big turkey dinner was reason for the unnatural solemnity. The party was gay enough when we moved on to the Hellbaums to walk back home at midnight in mellow moonlight, in moist spring air that made our Christmas tree seem out of place when we opened the door. On New Year's Eve we Service people welcomed 1942 together at the Hoversons' home and met again at the Company House for dinner the next evening.

A few days later church bells were ringing in the Orthodox nativity celebration.

with Vivian before ten. Just as we were leaving we heard that Wilke had a telegram telling him to leave at the first opportunity. Alas, if the wire had only been delayed a few hours, but it came just in time to rob us of some really pleasant winter companions. They packed in a mad whirl. Of course, that leaves us with their cat. But I would have preferred them.

Hank Banner was anything but gay, worried about the war, worried about the trip down, anxious to see his wife, and worried about his future since there will be a cut in appropriations and most surely the present seal investigation is off, for now and for a long time after. As Hank said, the projected trip of the *Black Douglas* and the related work, preliminary work that Hank and Ford Wilke were engaged in here, were but a part of an appeasement measure toward Japan.

December 12, 1941

I know my tummy felt very chilly Friday evening when Sam came home from a professional call on the Obergs about ten o'clock and reported that he had met one of the Melovidovs who was on watch and was searching for Hoverson to report the movements of a light at sea that was being watched carefully. Sam called Hoverson later, found him at the radio station, and went down. Hoverson was making no effort to report the presence of lights. He is the official man responsible for reporting planes. But he said Dutch Harbor was not answering any messages. That is sensible but surely they have a listening

cont.

post as well as the Army at Anchorage and should be notified of any unusual sights and sounds at sea. Elinor Hellbaum saw the light first about seven, looking from her attic window. At that time it was near Otter Island. The general conclusion was that there were two vessels of sorts out there and the lights, which did not burn steadily but flashed occasionally, were signals. Probably our own ships in this instance. But it still seems as if Dutch Harbor should be notified and if a time comes when they know where all their boats are they can send out planes to investigate such events. The lights seemed to be going off, nearer and nearer to St. George, and were last seen at 12:40. St. George saw nothing but they seem to be asleep in so many ways that that means nothing. Nothing has been seen since.

We keep our shades down and the village is not a pleasant place to walk at night now. Our flashlight is growing weak and we are hoarding it carefully. It will not last the winter.

December 22, 1941
We stopped at the office and no one was there. Next stop the Company House. Hoverson, whom we were seeking, was not there, but Stacy was busy repairing and wrapping the toys sent by Sears Roebuck. Such cheap free advertising I never saw. When I heard that Sears sent Xmas presents for the children, I believed they were being amusingly generous in thus keeping in good favor with the island inhabitants who give them twenty-five

cont.

Sam and I fought through blinding rain and wind and blackest darkness to attend the services. We stood in the back of the church, listening to the fresh voices of the youthful choir, the cadenced chant of Father Baranoff. We watched the bright pageant of the service, stealing glances from time to time to watch our laundryman trying to cling to the wall to stand upright. The odor of kvass he emitted overcame the strong scent of incense.

The next day the "stars" went around the village. Small groups of children and adults went from house to house. The parties came thronging into our living room without a greeting. Grouped in a corner of the room, they solemnly sang a short Russian song while the leader kept a large colored pinwheel spinning at the top of a stick. The song ended with a chorus of Merry Christmas greetings. Once the "stars" collected money donations for the church. Once, too, the parties visited the barn and sang to the animals and marched to the cemetery to pay their respects to the dead. The habit died out as the adopted Russian customs began to lose popularity.[3]

Next came the "beggars." Night after night they flocked to our door, mysterious bulky figures wrapped in blankets padded out with pillows, wearing masks of salt sacks. The rubber boots that peeped out from under the blankets gave no clue to the suppliants' identities. Each rattled a tin pail or a kettle until a contribution was dropped in. We used up several pounds of lump sugar, which were satisfactory donations. Anything was acceptable from a lump of coal or an onion to a slice of bread or a cake, though the last was most welcome. We were told that begging was a custom imported from our own western states.

Russian New Year opened up a week of dancing and masquerades. Sometimes the maskers simply dressed fancifully, held a grand parade, and then mingled with the dancers. The more dramatic maskings revealed a depth of imagination, a sense of humor, and a wonderful gift of mimicry that the Aleuts rarely displayed in public on ordinary occasions.

At one masquerading performance, in between interviewing applicants in a recruiting skit, the officers lounged in their chairs, with their feet on their desks. When an applicant wandered in, the feet came down with a thump. The officers became military rectitude personified. How did the isolated Aleuts think up that amusing and natural touch? When the Army doctors examined the recruits, slapstick entered the hall. One chap had a toothache. The dentist, after much exertion, extracted a huge sea lion tooth. A man with a vast protruding abdomen was operated upon. The doctor hauled out an amazing quantity of tools, tin cans, bottles, and other rubbish. A third man was too tall. The surgeon lopped off his legs and passed him off as fit for duty.

Another masking was a complete take-off of the village at work. No mannerism of the officials was overlooked. Every habitual gesture of Stacy or Hoverson was perfectly imitated. The man who played John Hanson twitched his fingers nervously and paced up and down with jerky impatient steps. I thought Nikita Hapoff, the carpenter, must be impersonating himself. It seemed as if no one could ape his way of holding a cigarette constantly in the corner of his mouth or mimic his peculiar hopping gait. Mechanic Oberg and Teacher Hellbaum were personified almost too perfectly.

thousand dollars a year of business or more. It seemed like one of the usual hypocritical gestures of a good business firm. But today I discovered it is even worse. A large proportion of the goods are marked defective goods. So poor Tracy was trying to repair some toys and the job looked very difficult. At first view the room seemed a veritable Santa's workshop with animals, building sets, dishes for dolls, tiny ironing boards, toy automobiles and airplanes, and a half hundred other objects scattered around. But when I saw the little signs "Defective Merchandise" scattered everywhere, I began to feel slightly nauseated. I brought one along for a souvenir. Cheap. Cheap. Cheap.

On the other hand Fouke Fur does a neat job, sending a nicely wrapped present ready for presentation.

The radio informs us that Churchill has landed in the U. S. A. today to help plan for an interallied military strategy council. They better hurry up. Only the Russians continue to advance and report over a million dead Germans on the Moscow front. Hitler has taken over the German army. There are hints that he will turn his back on Russia and advance toward Africa, via Spain. I hope the Nazi leaders start fighting among themselves and the German people get some inkling of what is really going on. We listened to Mrs. Winston Churchill speaking over a shortwave this afternoon, appealing for more money for the million-pound drive to

cont.

give comfort to the suffering Russians. Apparently the drive is going along very well. It must be distasteful to her to use all her charm and appeal to ask for funds for this purpose, but politics are politics . . .

December 31, 1941
Last week the Navy wired for information from us: if it were necessary for them to send a boat up here, where could she anchor? That took away my last remaining kernel of faith in the Navy. With supply boats coming every year, with the head of this part of the fleet looking us over this very summer, and Dutch Harbor—which should be our guardian—does not know how to come here. They must have read the *Coastal Pilot* and decided we were safe from the Japs, as safe as we are from help from our own side.

My opinion is that in the spring the Japanese may move on this area, if not before, in order to protect the fishing fleet. Fish is too basic a staple of the Japanese diet for them to permit their fleet to be bottled up and they probably know how inadequate are our preparations in the Alaska waters. I wish I could shake off this feeling that the Japanese will take over the islands and we will have no chance to get off ahead of them.

The last war I was in hurt me enough. Yet psychologically I was very safe in that war. Voluntarily I had chosen to be part of it . . . Now we are trapped here, above the unarmed Aleutians with Japanese craft between us and home. Since this war has become partially

cont.

The costuming was good. The props, created from junk in the afternoon, before the performance, were extremely clever, including trucks built from orange crates and old wheels and an airplane let down on ropes from the balcony. The performances were the more remarkable because the sequence had been improvised and pieced together a few hours before by the actors and rehearsed only in the creation.

Coming home from the Community Hall we were full of regretful thoughts. What a wonderful people the Aleuts really were. Creative, imaginative, and fun loving, they possessed the opportunity to display their true characters for only one week of the year.

One day in late January a dark unfamiliar craft steamed into Village Cove. Radio had bespoken the *Penguin*'s arrival but the camouflage made her somber and alien.[4] Temporarily in the service of the Navy she was doing errands among the islands. She brought us the last mail we ever received on St. Paul. We learned from a coded cable that the Elliotts and McMillins, who had gone out on leave, that Dr. Harrington, Banner, and the Wilkes were safe in Seattle.[5]

anti-Fascist, I no longer want to sit on the sidelines. Still less do I want to sit on this rock where we cannot strike back a single blow in self-defense against an invader. . . . I have no psychological armor now that I have a daughter.

January 2, 1942
I spent most of the evening typing notes from Jordan's report and we did not join the clan at Hoversons' until ten thirty. We played or watched games and enjoyed a nice lunch. We were just tackling Mrs. Hoverson's excellent apple pie, with superlative ice cream atop it, when we discovered that the fatal hour had struck. I suggested we sing Auld Lang Syne but the chorus was rather weak. We hung on there until two or after. Some piano banging and then Carl and Elinor provided some music.

Home through gorgeous moonlight. And so gladly to bed. Sam crawled out heroically to feed Tobyanne at seven but was back as soon as possible. I managed to wake up at eleven and fed her. Sam finally got up at noon. By one we were dressed. We had a lunch of fruitcake that Mrs. Hoverson had given me. And lazed around a bit. I went back to my typing eventually and banged away most of the afternoon, until nearly six when we had to get dressed for dinner at the Company House . . .

Manila a little closer to capture added nothing to evening's joy. The war was a constant topic during dinner. The two hostesses, Mrs. Hellbaum and Mrs. Stacy, had worked very hard. They made crepe paper hats, lovely ones for the ladies, silly ones for the men.

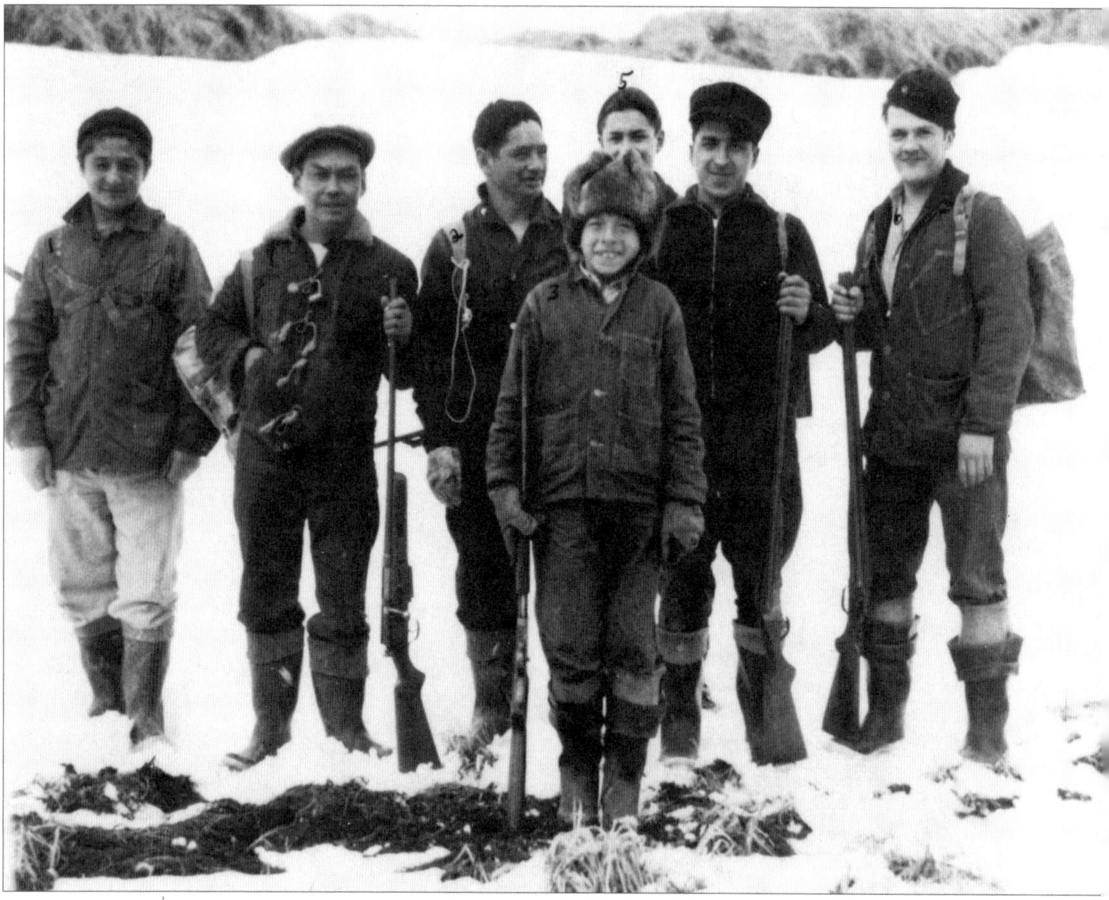

Men ready for a day of winter hunting (from the Martin Collection, USUAF210, Archives, Alaska and Polar Regions, Rasmuson Library, University of Alaska Fairbanks).

Chapter 36

As part payment for sealing, the first lessee had contracted to supplement the Aleut seal meat diet with smoked and salt salmon and salt beef. Its successor in 1890 was to supply the same foods in amounts decided annually by the Secretary of the Treasury. By that time the decrease in seals had led to strict restrictions against killing pups for food. In trying to plan how much Congress should contribute to the support of the sealers after the small fur killings reduced their cash income almost to the vanishing point, Agent [Charles J.] Goff prepared a list of daily supplies needed for one sealer: two pounds of seal or canned meat; eighteen ounces of soft bread or flour and biscuits; two ounces of tea and one of salt; two each of sugar, rice, and butter; three ounces of condensed milk, four of tobacco, and two of soap. That access to a company store had accustomed the Aleuts to other foods, to fruit and vegetables, was not even considered. Congress appropriated $19,500 for annual relief for both islands.[1] When a sealer exhausted his meager earnings, the agents authorized the company to extend him credit to be charged off against government funds, the amount depending upon his [sealing] class and the size of his family. In 1910 the government began to provide food and clothing in addition to continuing the feudal arrangement of dividing up sealing shares of cash.

July 19, 1941
I rested until two with two tiny catnaps. Then we went out just as the sky was clearing and the sun was pouring down. We talked awhile with McMillin about using a car and he promised to try to get us one as soon as the Easts were gone. I hope he lives up to his word. He kept talking about the Natives. He said that people made mistakes treating them as their equals but that the safe way was to treat them just like thoroughbred dogs or cattle. That is often quite a regal fashion, if I mistake not. He said that as wards of the government, no one could beat them. Fortunately.

The provision of food as part payment for work was an insidious factor that bred the idea that the sealers were wards of the government and not citizens. So firmly did the notion become entrenched that even officials were puzzled when we asked whether the sealers were actual wards, completely dependent upon the government and unable to arrange their own destinies, or were they like all Alaskan Natives.[2] The fiction was not exposed until the fortunes of war took the Aleuts away from the Pribilofs.

The food allotments were inadequate for normal appetites as well as very limited in variety for constant diet year after year. When an opportunity offered, the Aleuts ordered food from Seattle. In 1927 the sealers, guided by the agent, financed a store entitled "Native Canteen" to avoid the nuisance and expense of buying individual stocks in the States. Individuals lent part of their sealing division to buy the initial stock of goods. The Canteen is proudly referred to as a community project under official supervision. The supervision seems to have been of doubtful assistance in keeping food costs down. And in other ways. A few years ago the Canteen was bankrupt. No one knew what had happened to several hundred dollars. The officials we met made sly wisecracks about their predecessors. The Aleuts raised their eyebrows suggestively. Clearly no Aleut had the opportunity for theft or such gross carelessness.

More insidious than a single loss or misappropriation are the everyday prices. No agent has ever helped the Aleuts purchase goods at wholesale prices despite the large size of orders. The sealers had agreed that it would be easier to support the church and rent movies and provide funds for other communal benefits by paying higher rates on merchandise than by direct levy. So food and supplies purchased at retail prices in Seattle are sold for still higher prices to the Aleuts. Though the Aleuts are well aware of their right to purchase from wholesalers, they are powerless to alter the arrangements. They continue to pay much higher prices than they would by ordering directly from the States, although many try to get as many clothes as possible from Sears Roebuck. Odd methods of deciding prices come into play. I bought in November a couple of gay, rather sleazy sweaters. Mrs. Hellbaum decided after Christmas to buy a similar one for her daughter. I paid $2.25. The prices had increased over two dollars. Elary explained that the jump was occasioned by the necessity of making money to meet expenses, and clothing had been arbitrarily made more expensive so that more vital food products should not be increased. For officials it was unimportant. For the people whom the Canteen had been supposed to benefit such juggling was a hardship.

Contents of the crowded shelves included canned fruit and vegetables and soups, tinned meat and fish, delicacies like canned mushrooms, and such modern preparations as canned baby foods. Every known brand of candy bar was on display. Coca-Cola led as favorite among the hundreds of cases of soft drinks. Slipshod economy made the bottle unreturnable. Consequently a modest sum of money was scattered all over the island. Abandoned bottles often shattered the mood of isolation of beautiful spots far distant from the village. Testimonials to the powers of advertising wizards were the shelves of Alka-Seltzer, Castoria, and various vitamin pills. Incidentally, I could never understand how Dr. Migliori arrived at his exaggerated conception of the local desire to guzzle cod liver oil. We had great trouble with patients' reluctance to take the vile stuff. We did discover that almost every family was either buying vitamin capsules at the Canteen or ordering them from Sears.

It was disturbing to see the sealers paying such high prices for food out of their limited earnings. We were puzzled by the quantities of food purchased by people supposedly issued an adequate weekly ration each Friday from the government stores. Various inexplicable dietary problems in treating patients led Sam to inspect the official diet code. As an outline for a lifelong diet, the foods were appallingly monotonous and questionably adequate to support life. It allowed no additional food for a child under two and nothing but cereal from that age until four years old. Obviously canned baby foods on the Canteen shelves were vitally necessary.

> February 20, 1942
> During the winter the Natives get no fresh meat except birds they can shoot, which means ducks mainly, and sea lion. Yesterday about ten men went to Northeast Point to camp out and go sea lion hunting. Two weeks ago someone got a big one. And Mamet Emanoff got one last Thursday. I had always thought that the Natives got fresh reindeer meat from the carcasses hung in the cooler after the fall killing. But it seems they got only two issues of that during the winter, because the cooler is too small.
>
> It can hardly be cheaper to buy and find space for salt beef, salt pork, and fish like herring and cod than to build and maintain a sufficiently large cooler. Such messing, always.

The recorded diet schedule provided the following weekly amounts for a family of four with no child under the age of four: 2 1/2 pounds of butter, one bottle of catsup or hot sauce, 20 pounds of flour, two cans of fruit, one can jelly, 2 pounds of onions, 12 pounds of potatoes, 1 1/2 pounds of rice, 3 1/2 pounds of sugar, two cans of vegetables, 5 pounds of fresh root vegetables such as beets, carrots, and turnips; 10 pounds of salt fish, two cans of meat, either corned beef or roast beef; and 1/2 pound of tea. The monthly items were: 1 pound of coffee, one can of fish, 1/2 gallon of syrup, 10 pounds of salt beef, 4 pounds of lard, and 1 pound of cornstarch. Six times a year the family was entitled to a gallon of vegetable oil.

The schedule was definite about the bottle of catsup or hot sauce weekly. A former agent had arbitrarily limited the issue to twice a year lest the people drink the stuff straight from the bottle. Condiments such as pepper were lacking. In summer, seal meat replaced the canned meat issue. Then in winter there were the two holiday rations of reindeer. At Easter, eggs for baking traditional Russian cakes were distributed, just the one time a year.

Our patients informed us that canned fruit and vegetables were not actually issued weekly. Inspecting articles brought from the government store as the carts or bundles were dragged by our house, we satisfied ourselves that the people were telling the truth. After Andy went south and no one at Company House could

August 19, 1941
After our late breakfast the sun that had been tempting us all morning decided to withdraw itself but we went out anyway. We hung around the Canteen for awhile, chatting with Elary. Elary now says that he likes the sound of *Ellery* when Sam talks to him. I suspect because he has grown to like Sam who has been chatting with him quite often recently. Yesterday Sam was sympathizing with him over the tendency to let the Canteen buy so much canned food that, if it continues, the Natives will be buying most of their food there. Elary admitted the Natives asked for the various types of canned goods that are stocked, that often delegations came and asked for certain articles. He explained that Gabriel [Stepetin] was one of a committee that made the actual orders. The only food I could see that might be classed as a luxury was canned mushrooms. Canned meat, fruit, dry cereals, and jellies, fresh fruit such as oranges and the special treat of grapes. The latter may be luxuries. The oranges are something very vital to the diet. Coffee and tea are carried because so few people like the grade handed out to them. Since I think our brands pretty foul and they are a much better grade than the Natives are rationed, I can sympathize with their desire to buy better kinds. The pity of it is that only the first two classes of workmen can afford to augment their diet. The injustice is that for their labors, which are certainly strenuous, the men are
cont.

wangle leftover foods for hospital patients, their daily meals showed similar dietary deficiency. Week after week, despite pleas to the acting agent, the four tubercular patients, who needed not only nourishing food but also food to tempt invalid appetites, ate alternating desertless meals of canned meats and reindeer accompanied by potatoes, turnips, macaroni, and rice. I know I shall never see anything more dismal in my life than one of those plates of greasy reindeer chops and soggy, mushy lumps of potatoes, rice, and macaroni. They did enjoy the luxury of an egg for breakfast and sometimes a sliver of ham. Even cabbage and carrots for salad were denied them.

Tradition, Hoverson informed us, had sanctioned the decisions of previous agents to withhold canned vegetables until all root vegetables were gone or to give them canned fruit only on holidays and to dispense various other foods at less frequent intervals than designated in the official diet code. The pretension that the people were issued an adequate diet was shattered. The criticism that the sealers wasted their money in buying extravagant and unnecessary foods at their Canteen was convicted of being unfair and unjust. If the islanders were to get enough to eat, a canteen or similar device was necessary. Once a canteen was established other tastes developed to be satisfied. A normal selection of foods, confections, and soft drinks was put in and testified to the modernity of the Aleut appetite. Probably Dinty Moore's canned Irish stew, a prime local favorite, was a toothsome delicacy to alternate with salt beef. A can of good red salmon or tasty sardines broke the monotony of the eternal salt herring and cod.

As for clothing. The allowance was skimpy. Even clothes for workmen were not sufficient so the sealers bought overalls, slickers, shirts, and canvas gloves from the Canteen. Issue clothing was so ugly that even men pored over the pages of the Sears catalog, wistfully studying the attractive suits, overcoats, and shoes. The natural instincts of the Aleuts responded to smart clothing. Their liking for pretty clothes and good things to eat differed no whit from any American's. The clothing supply in the government stores had not been replenished for a long time. Even if people hesitated to spend money on Sears' or Canteen garments, they frequently found no government clothes to fit them. They were told to try the Canteen.

When the sealing money came in on the *Spica,* the village throbbed with excitement. First, the Canteen debts were paid off. The orders for Sears were reluctantly completed. The last painful decision was made. So familiar were the contents of the Sears catalogue (their most beloved book) that most villagers could quote page number and article as if they were repeating Scripture verses. All orders were handed in at the office. The staff pruned and regulated them in an effort to keep sufficient cash for each family to carry them through the winter without making too great inroads on the next summer's income.

The crowd at the Canteen jammed the hall and clustered around the door. Every few moments a violent motion indicated someone laden with bundles was trying to break through the mass. Customers emerged, flustered but beaming. The children squeezed under elbows and between legs more easily. They ambled round the village, cheeks and pockets bulging with candy bars, arms filled with Coca-Cola bottles.

Soon the shopping splurge was over. The cash had melted away. By Christmas most people had to return to credit charged

supposed to receive adequate food and clothing for their families, plus the cash bonus. It is not fair that the bonus should be used almost completely to supplement their diet. The Canteen can become—and what official will guide it in another direction?—little more than a sort of inverted company store. While the government will receive no direct benefit as companies do, indirectly expenses will be cut down at the expense of the Native workmen and their families.

The Canteen should provide an outlet for the sort of goods now obtained through Sears Roebuck: clothing, furnishings, etc. That part of the stock at present, clothes, is skimpy and of the worst grades. Out of the proceeds of the Canteen have come the movie equipment and the maintenance of the church. The priest, when here, receives his food from the Canteen and six hundred dollars a year in cash.

Yesterday Sam had discussed the same trend with Elary. Last night Mr. Elliott had mentioned that when he commented on the amount of goods the Canteen had purchased, Elary had said to him, "I wish the other store down the hill had as much and as good food."

"Someone must have been agitating among the Natives," said Mr. Elliott.

I looked at my "agitator" husband's tranquil face. He didn't mind the name calling. He does want to see the Natives get proper diets. Either from above or through their own efforts.

against the next summer's sealing proceeds. Regulations permitted a first-class sealer $2.50 credit per week. Fifty cents was deducted from each succeeding class in order until the fourth-class man had only a dollar's credit.

During the months of February and March Sam gathered his facts for his annual report. A large proportion of the families who filled out his questionnaire about household furnishings added a postscript plea for more food rations because of hunger in winter. Their articulate requests contradicted the pleasant official fiction that they were indifferent to creature comforts, protected by some mysterious inherited primitive stoicism.

> January 12, 1942
> A grey rawish day but not wintry. Our open weather continues. . . . How pleasant life would be here if this sort of weather continued, if only the houses were modernly heated and air conditioned. Or, to begin at the beginning, if they had been intelligently constructed by someone who knew how to combat northern weather and winds, and if the material had been of a better sort, seasoned wood, for instance, instead of green wood that shrank, leaving wide gaps for the wind's easy entrance. And windows might be constructed that would let in some air when wanted and not too much air around all the joints, when a gale is in progress.

Gradually we learned the Aleuts had no love for their own store, that they had no sense of communal ownership. Rather they felt that its existence jeopardized their remuneration for labor, which was supposed to be paid for in food and clothing, as well as in cash. More and more, officials were expecting them to buy their necessities from the store instead of depending upon government stock.

For instance, the government had once furnished shells to the men in winter to enable them to hunt birds to make up for dietary insufficiency. It was a subtle admission that the regulation diet was not ample. There came a day when the Aleuts were told to buy their own ammunition at the Canteen. An extra credit was extended to them. Two dollars a week could be spent for shells during hunting season.

House furnishings are hardly ever issued anymore. All householders strive to stretch their cash to include at least one furniture order each season. If there were stoves in stock the agent could assign one to a newly married couple who were fortunate enough to get a house to themselves.

Had the government issues been designed as charitable relief only there would be no reason to cavil at the tendency to decrease the kind and amount of goods. The food issues, however, were specifically intended as payment in goods instead of complete payment in cash.

During the period of lessee control, the companies had paid a certain amount of cash per skin divided as at present, had provided housing, medical care, and schooling, some fuel and food, for the killing and skinning of seals *only.* Seal killing took up a very small portion of the villager's time. Any other labor performed was paid for in cash. Such labor included making baidars, loading and unloading boats, cleaning up the village, carpentering, painting, and all other maintenance jobs. Sealers who killed sea lions were paid for the skins. Their wives were paid for treating or sewing them, for cleaning the throat and intestinal membranes. All work except sealing was voluntary. If a man worked, he received money. If he preferred to loaf, he got along on his sealing division. He had, in those days, a partial independence. Usually no man refused an opportunity to work. Supplies were expensive. For a long time the company sold coal to the sealers for thirty dollars a ton although government employees purchased the same coal at exactly half the price. It was years before a government agent noticed the discrepancy and reported it to Washington.

As soon as the government appropriated money to assist the sealers in 1890, it was decided that the sum was not a dole. The men must give their services for road work and village maintenance for the credit at the store. The custom developed through the years into the present work arrangement. Every male from the age of sixteen, until disabled by illness or old age, was to work an eight-hour day, with Saturday afternoon and Sunday off. At first there were many religious holidays. Not every worshipper went to church services. Gradually the number of *prasniki* were lopped off. During sealing the men worked on Sunday morning just as on weekdays. During the sealing season even younger boys were given jobs. Except for a few specialized men, the majority of sealers worked the hours that each day's take demanded, reporting back for other work later in the day. Throughout the rest of the year they followed the regular schedule, beginning work at nine in winter, earlier when the days were longer.

Their labors were compensated by the single cash payment of the sealing division plus the minor sum from fox trapping, housing, electricity, medical care, schooling, and supposedly sufficient food and clothing for their needs. The one cash payment a year, the retention of that feudal hunting share at the heart of a complicated million-dollar business, is ironical and psychologically unhealthy. Inevitably the sealer feels that the nebulous total of cash, supplies, and utilities is not sufficient recompense for his labors. And because so many services are rendered as partial support and supplies are issued, the stigma of ward of the government taints the actual payment for labor.

Since the sealer dare not protest openly, he has found a simple means of self-defense. He adopted the motto, "Don't work too hard. Take it easy." Why should he care if his "white" supervisors curse him as lazy, inefficient, inept, and stupid? Behind his poker face he chuckles with delight at outwitting his overlords, at protecting himself from being underpaid by giving the least possible amount of his services.

Yet his self-defense pleases himself least of all. He wants regular wages. He wants wages more truly representative of the value of the labor he could perform. Over and over we heard people say they wished the government would "stop

[From a letter dated July 24, 1941, and incorporated into the typed journal]

We have a lot of social problems here we would like to tackle but are wondering just how to go about some of them. I think we can do no better at present than collect facts and pictures and perhaps not use them until we are away, firstly by presenting them to some of the top boys in Washington and secondly by publication. We have a patient in the hospital who just came across a copy of the Constitution in the World Almanac and is very excited over the clause of right of assembly, which he says cannot be done here. There is some question over the exact legal status of these people. They are called and treated as wards of the government and yet a number of years ago an act of Congress gave citizenship to *all* Natives in Alaska. So I would like to have some legal light thrown on the problem. Once, the Natives voted. Alaska had a candidate whom the bureau running the island at the time did not like so that Natives were primed and permitted to vote. They voted for the wrong man and never got another chance, but I doubt whether voting would have been permitted did they not actually have the right to. But meanwhile it is profitable to keep permanent seal catchers here so civil rights are not mentioned above a whisper. But the Natives themselves are not unaware of the trap they are in, but awfully afraid to speak to a "white."

fooling them with things instead of cash" and let them manage their own lives and enjoy their work. They want more frequent paydays as well as the right to work out their own budgets. They are starved for an opportunity to release their potential workmanship capabilities and to savor the pride of independence. As long as hunters crouch in the cold wind popping away at ducks in the bay watching their supper carried farther from instead of upon the shore by teasing currents, or seeing it sink out of sight, partial payment in food rations will remain an indignity and an insult. As long as hunters prowl day after day for a laggard sea lion wintering in the Bering and are unable to bring their prize inshore and instead go home to a meager meal of crackers and tea, so long will that one summer payday be meaningless and a constant irritant.

Maybe no Aleut would starve if he lived on the rations and saved his money instead of buying Canteen foods. I am sure he would not be very healthy, although human bodies are wonderfully tough. The general health of the villagers is poor today. Most of them have few of their own teeth after adolescence. When one gets "outside" by a miracle, his ill-nourished body succumbs to contact with the virulent bacteria lurking in city air. Before his body can develop an immunity, the Aleut is in bed. His body is not strong enough to resist the disease. And official wisecracks nod sagaciously and pull out their favorite platitude, "These people just can't stand the climate."

I wanted to test out the diet, to see whether I could eat just what a sealer did and have energy to help Sam in the office, run back and forth to the hospital several times a day, spend two or three hours typing, and enjoy a moderate walk. I planned to limit us to the experiment for a week. One day was enough. Or rather too much. We had to calm our surprised protesting neglected stomachs before we could go to sleep. It was not only the kind of food but the small quantity that ended our test.

I no longer wondered why kids sneaked around the garbage cans and ate some of the filthy refuse. I started trying to fill some of the smaller two-legged bottomless pits that I had seen gathering for raids on the garbage cans behind the Company House. I had to limit my generosity. Each youngster brought his friends to be fed. Though I decreased my gifts they still hovered around the house for crumbs or waited for handouts from Heretina. For months, one or two and sometimes more of Heretina's friends arrived just in time for the evening meal. She made them pay for their punctuality and food by helping her with dishes. It was a very satisfactory system . . . for them.

Chapter 37

Next to the Canteen on the lower floor of the Community Hall were the recreation room and the Aleut library. The pool and ping-pong tables were always popular and in use. The magazines and newspaper comic sheets were well used in the library but few books were withdrawn. The few hundred volumes were principally the light fiction of forty or fifty years ago that no one could enjoy reading. The community piano stood in the library except when moved upstairs for dances. Both Mrs. Hoverson and Mrs. McMillin had a few piano pupils, some of whom practiced on the library piano. A few practiced in their teacher's home. During Lent the village women met in the library to sew and talk, after playing basketball and doing exercises. I went to their weekly meetings to give health talks. Some topics I picked out myself. Most subjects were chosen as a result of their questions, very sensible, natural, and intelligent questions, too. How to reduce was a problem that interested many. Their comments about overweight sounded like the chatter of any woman's gathering in the rest of America. It was another indication I was constantly bumping into that the Aleut women were no different from me and my old neighbors in the States, not even in their most superficial reactions.

The second floor was the large hall for games, movies, and dances. I can almost see some of my arty friends leaning back in satisfaction, saying, "Ah, at last the Native dance." Only it was not the Dance but dancing. I had hoped there might be someone who remembered an ancient tribal dance, a symbolic ritual of movement. I was just as silly as the average newcomer to Alaska who hopes to trade a handful of beads or a box of matches for some fine carved ivory or a fur. He is usually met at the boat by Eskimos taking Kodachrome movies of him disembarking for their own souvenirs or to sell him copies to take home if he can pay their high prices. His disillusionment is harsh and immediate. Since my hope had been slight, my disappointment was a mere shadow of regret.

I came to my first dance while the floor was crowded with moving couples. In the far corner, an Aleut orchestra of piano and stringed instruments beat out a familiar tune, "Deep in the Heart of Texas." Most of the players had picked up their repertoire by ear from the radio or records or talkies. They had a fine sense, a good beat but not much melody. As soon as the music ceased the males escorted their partners to the benches along one wall and returned to the masculine side of the room for the interval. During the few minutes between pieces the couples marched slowly in a circle around the room, a style imported from the West Coast and, although new to me, by no means a tribal hangover. The girls looked so fresh and pretty in bright frocks, their hair curled like the beauties of the latest magazine pictures they had seen. Some of them had homemade permanents set with equipment from Sears. One girl that first evening wore a green evening gown that went well with her pale skin and light brown hair. She as well as several others wore gold dancing sandals. She looked brilliant on the dance floor.

Every holiday was a dance night and usually Sunday evenings, for their religious day began on Saturday at sundown and ended early Sunday evening. Only during the forty days of Lent were there no dances. But I did wish profoundly that there were more grandmothers in the village so that fewer babies had to endure the movies and dances.

The dances brought an illusion of democracy, for the male officials danced with many Aleut girls and women and a few of the more confident Aleut men asked the officials' wives to be their partners.

Curiously enough, such social mingling was once natural. For a number of years after 1870 island records constantly spoke of the officials having dined and remained all evening for dancing in some Aleut home.[1] No trace of superiority or contempt for a racial minority tinged the entries, which elaborated on the charms of the hostess, the warmth

January 13, 1942
How news gets around this town. Last night we learned that about five days ago the office received a wire stating that Mr. McMillin says there are so many tires. This was the signal agreed on that McMillin would include his name in a message, whether it made sense or not, to signify that they had arrived in Seattle. But whether by *Penguin* or other boat still remains a mystery. They probably transferred mail sacks if they transferred passengers so by now our friends in the East should be reading the stale autumn news and remain just as worried as ever about our safety. But when will we hear from them?

It is a gorgeous fresh bright morning, with a gilded eastern sky. I did not notice the thermometer when I stuck my head out the front door but it must be up in the forties.

Yesterday was a fairly satisfying day. After I finished typing, I read some more history of this place until lunch. After lunch I went to the office and began to delve into the logs, the records of the past. I have not yet run across a book that has information before 1877 and have gleaned but few notes for my own information although some medical stuff for Sam. The logs are haphazardly written—a funeral will be mentioned but no death recorded. I think there is a separate book for such stuff. So many threads of untold tales. So many hints of dissension between company agents and treasury agents—but only hints.

January 14, 1942
At ten Sam and I left the house and took a little stroll to West Landing and watched the ducks bobbing up and down on the tranquil waters. Sun bright and air brisk. Back to the office where Sam dropped me and I went in to work on the log. At twelve home for lunch and a few hugs with Tobyanne. Then back to the log. I was overjoyed to find the log that began in the late spring of 1872 where Elliott comes to the island. When I finish here I will be typing up those notes so shall include nothing here. I am about half through that log. Came home at five, whipped up a gingerbread after Heretina burned the soup-a nice big pot of soup that I hoped would sustain us today while she was off celebrating New Year.

July 17, 1941
The next night when we went up to listen to the news, I was informed that there was a clump of heather outside the door for me. It was exquisite. J[ohnston] said it grew only on the one spot in the island. Carrying it in my hand, dirty and disheveled, I went to the dance. We must have stayed about an hour despite our decision to just peek in and run away. The women sit on one side and the men on the other. Except the married white regulars who sit down at one end of the hall if they intend to dance and up in the balcony if they intend to observe. I broke all custom by sliding on to a vacant male bench near the door as soon as it was empty. The orchestra had good time but not much music. The airs they learn

cont.

of the host. Perhaps the fact that many of the earliest officials bore military titles because of their services during the Civil War accounted for their democratic behavior. They had come so recently from battles to make a small racial group free that they had no imperialistic instincts or thought patterns. In turn they invited Aleuts to dine with them at the official table. In 1941 there might have been more afternoons devoted to me by officials' wives except for the almost certain danger of finding me entertaining old Anna or some other Native.

To hark back to the past of the Aleuts once more, there is one tribal dance that was dimly remembered and recorded.[2] It was a midwinter religious ceremony of which the significance had been lost. Only heroic people could have participated. Men and women, clothed only in masks, danced in a long double line, back to back. It was sacrilegious to lift the mask and peek over the shoulder at the nudity of the opposite sex in the other line. Their poor bodies must have suffered from the wind oftentimes and cruel biting snow. Religious fervor alone protected them from the elements. Their masks were highly unwieldy, greatly decorated wooden creations, too heavy for the bodies to keep warm by the liveliest motions.

Basketball was a Lenten sport for women when Russian tradition confined them indoors. Walking for pleasure only, even up and down the village roads, was irreligious. To meet to sew and play and hear instructive talks kept the letter of the religious custom intact.

Baseball was the masculine sport. The baseball club was THE CLUB on the island. The men practiced hard to be able to win the summer series against Fouke Fur workers. They fought so bitterly to win and grew so surly when defeat seemed imminent that it seemed as if the sport symbolized an effort to prove themselves the equals or superiors of the "whites."

At some place in this book I have to discuss drinking. I would like to omit it completely. Suppose I express myself so badly that defenders of certain prejudices sniff and say, "I knew the Natives were a bunch of drunkards"? Or some of my late Pribilof associates would accuse me of trying to create a false impression of my pet Natives?

The Christmas before we arrived over forty barrels of kvass—a fermented concoction made from anything and everything edible, from jam and condensed milk and canned vegetables and old bread, were taken from the houses and dumped.[4] Forty-one barrels from forty-nine houses. Slavic people knew the potency of real kvass. But the effects of fermented garbage are something illustrated only by an explosion.

The first Americans brought new liquors. Then Congress made the Pribilofs a special reservation and prohibited liquor. The law was offset by the smuggled spirits of officials after 1870 and by liquor bribes handed out by company agents. The years the naval radio station was in operation provided the villagers with examples, gargantuan in magnitude, beyond their own simple capacities. The villagers enjoyed earning or begging supplies from the naval men. Priests drank without concealing their vice. Doctors drank and were unable to take care of patients. Agents drank and fined the Aleuts caught indulging in the same recreation.

Blasts from Washington about suppressing drinking among the sealers were only momentarily effective if at all. Denying them sugar and jams and imposing fines and jail sentences were temporarily beneficial.

by ear from the radio or the movie. After hearing "Alexander's Rag Time Band" at the movie one night, they were playing it the next day fairly accurately from the one hearing.

January 31, 1942

We have the painters still with us in the kitchen to start the week off. We expect to rip off the top linoleum in the center that is wrecked beyond decency and see whether whatever lies beneath it cannot be painted grey as the closet floor has been. The table that belongs in the nook has been painted a rather uninteresting orange but it was the best shade available.

This is being continued after supper. Roy said that last night he heard someone trying to speak to Bristol Bay Army post, which is supposed to have listeners on several frequencies constantly. But this voice was pleading for someone to answer him because he had information about landing conditions that might prevent a plane accident. When Roy spoke to Bristol Bay at midnight, he asked whether the fellow finally made a connection and [this] was the first Bristol Bay had heard of it.

Tonight at midnight, Roy starts sending our weather reports to Bristol Bay. He has already been relaying Sand Point's for several nights. Stacy is having lots of trouble figuring out the codes that were sent him. But is supposed to be ready to start tonight.

It seems that we have only three friends to count on to protect us for a few months: fog, wind, and ice. For tonight our huge moon is

cont.

rolling up the sky beyond Black Bluffs in radiant glory but the wind is blowing a gale of over fifty miles an hour. No planes would like to buck such winds. It might be a good title, but "Wind, Sand and Stars" is too new in the public mind.[3]

February 1, 1942
Gabe [Stepetin] admitted most of our charges against the Aleuts. We asked him to explain it and he had some theories about causes but none about improvement. He says all of them fear a white man even if they are digging a ditch with him. He says a few years ago he would have been frightened to talk to any white person the way he talks to us. He says another reason people have no ambition is that the weak get punished and the strong get away with murder. Finally, he explained that statement as meaning that the office had favorites; also he said the people had no responsibility. But he admitted that he told people that they were working for their rent and light, etc. and were better off economically than many people in the States. Drinking is their curse. It was ironical to listen to that and remember his record in the log. I shall ask him about that some other time. . . .

Earlier Sam had been asking Peter and Heretina some Aleut words from Geoghegan's list and many they did not know.[7] It is more and more obvious that they do not know their language well. And then to hear Gabe saying that they did not know Aleut well or English well or Russian well was most amusing-but certainly a tragic *cont.*

Dire consequences of drunkenness made but slight impressions. When the second chief Bakoff and his family were suffocated because they had gone to an alcoholic sleep without extinguishing the lamp, the community met to discuss fire hazards. Without one dissent, overlooking the real cause of the tragedy, the villagers decided that kerosene lamps were dangerous and should be cast out of their houses.

When Russian-speaking Agent Lessen translated an order to stop manufacturing and drinking kvass in 1874, the villagers were indignant that exaggerated reports of their drinking had been sent to Washington. Lessen confessed that he had a delicate duty to perform in comforting them.[5]

Kind agents like Judge and Murray tried to institute reforms. Murray bewailed his inability to influence them because so weary were the majority with their isolation that they mocked handcuffs and hoped to be exiled. He also lamented the tendency for a drunken sealer to start beating his wife, rarely stopping until the poor female was seriously injured.

Various robberies were due to the desire to get liquor. The dispensary was broken into at one time, at another the camp house for the officials at Northeast Point. Old Metrofan was mixed up with one raid on that building. Apparently the officials kept plentiful stocks on hand. A larger boy bullied Metrofan, then a child, into allowing himself to be pushed through a broken window and opening the door. Liquor bottles were not only in cupboards but even stuck conveniently under the bed. Cigars were abundant, too. The older boy drank himself to sleep while Metrofan experimented with a cigar. He became ill and frightened. He ran home in the morning before the other was awake and reported to the office. He went unpunished, save for the beating the bully gave him for telling tales. On another occasion, the foremen broke into the building where scientist Townsend had alcohol for pickling specimens. They started imbibing immediately. Reeling, they tried to find their way out carrying the remainder. They could not find the open window in the dark and lit a match that flamed far enough to touch alcohol. The culprits were discovered by their burned hands.[6]

In 1896 the islanders formed a council of nine and resolved to end kvass making and drinking forever. That was February. In September Peter Oustigoff and his mother were tried by the council. Peter was sent to jail to a bread-and-water diet. His mother was ordered to walk up and down the village wearing a sign on her back that read, "I made kvass."

For long periods there were no drunken disturbances and apparently complete abstinence. Then some individual would get bored or too unhappy with his lot and try to drown his sorrows in the kvass kettle. First one individual would have his fling and then another. A man went to Mac's house one night while intoxicated and told him what he thought of him in very brutal profane English. He was probably speaking from his heart what he lacked courage to say when sober. He had seemed one of the quietest well-behaved workmen. I sympathized with him.

Sobered up the rebels took their punishment without protest and went on living in the same horizonless rut.

Considering the influence of the civilized respectable "whites" and the knowledge that, as wards, they have no future and a present controlled by others, it is remarkable that the people are not drunk more frequently.

fact to have confirmed. He spoke of the superstitions that are still rampant, belief in ghosts, of the many who see Devil's Fires.

I gave him the story of the "Forgotten Village" to read.[8] That ought to do more than anything we can say. Of course, Gabe is afraid to take any action. People are afraid to follow him because he has a record. Once he went off the island and was made to stay there and had a hard time to get back. Allowed back for summer work, he led a demand for better food and more wages—a minor strike that was quickly smashed and he was sent off the island with several others for being a ringleader—and it was years before they let him come back. We suggested his getting a few people together and starting a current events class, which would be interesting but would also be a means of improving the English they already know.

He pointed out that the Natives resented most cultural efforts made in their behalf as being forced on them by the whites. How to raise the demand and the desire in his people is the problem. He speaks to many but gets little response. Peter says the same. And even if Gabe could get a few to follow him, he would be singled out again as ringleader and exiled at once, unless the whole population was behind him. We gave him various subversive suggestions. Even that the Village Committee should wire out a petition for military protection or evacuation. That he would certainly like to do.

February 11, 1942
Have just taken Tobyanne up to the roost, running through the icy spaces of the large attic. Sam is shut up in the office with the Rev. and the Russian grammar. Heretina splashes about in the kitchen. And the painters are actually busy in the bedroom. There is a faint hope in my breast that we may be able to move in there tomorrow.

Sam came dashing to find out whether I could spare some paper for the Rev. who dare not ask the office for much. The Rev. is pouring out his heart to Sam: "They ask me why I don't change the services to English from Russian. But the Jews use Hebrew, the Catholics use Latin, the Arabs use old Arabic, the Greeks use old Greek and we use Slavonic, which is a thousand years old and not Russian. Why should we not? Does the Constitution not say there shall be religious freedom in this country? Even the English Bible is written in old English, in Elizabethan English. Why should I change the language of the church? It is the Church. I am speaking to God, not to the people."

And while he mourns his sorrows, the greater part of the world must be, not merely mourning, but must be angry that the Japanese are so close to Singapore. The corrosion of empire has worn through to the vital heart of the imperial organization. The empty excuses are not even worth laughing at for the sad state of affairs.

But back to our island, which will never know siege, because the Japs can come ashore when they wish.

cont.

Orders from Washington will not stop kvass making. Punishment will not. Real citizenship, opportunities for advancement, and the right to possess and strive to accomplish ambitions will.

As one man wrote on the bottom of a questionnaire returned to Sam, "I admit I like to drink. I also make my own drink. But my Doctor tells me it's very bad for me. Still I make my own homemade, after all I'm human, like to celebrate once in awhile on holidays. For this reason why can't I have a real beer up here? As I know and we know they are drinking all over the world and telling me and us not to drink. Again there is nothing going on on this lonely island anyway."

If the Service colony constantly topped off grumbling remarks about conditions with the half-serious witticism that there were three federal prisons on the Pacific coast, Alcatraz, St. George, and St. Paul, and Alcatraz was the best because it had regular mail service, it is not difficult to realize how confined and hopeless the Aleut felt at times and sympathize with their alcoholic rebellions.

Yesterday afternoon I went to the women's club, which was holding its organizational meeting. The women in a group are far more at ease and act like a normal group of females anywhere. Twenty-four of the thirty-four women who had signed up for it came. Mrs. Hoverson marshaled them up to sit on three benches and Vivian began to play for them to sing. There were only three songbooks. The women seemed to like singing. And most of them seemed to know several verses of songs like "America," "Juanita, My Bonnie." Asked to suggest numbers, Mrs. Paul Merculieff suggested "Columbia, Gem of the Ocean." Someone else asked for "Long Long Ago."

I gave a brief talk about exercises being useful to make women look pretty . . . Mrs. Mandregan with her excess weight wanted to know whether she could do exercises. I told her to try. She is not eating bread or potatoes since Sam told her not to a couple of weeks ago. She asked me hesitantly whether I would eat some of her cooking. I said I surely would. Her rich smile blossomed and she promised to send me something when her birthday came, maybe some chicken. She is a very sweet, happy-go-lucky person, with a pretty face, wild hair, but a wonderful smile. I recognize her children easily now by their mother's smile. . . .

Last evening I read a little, and then helped Sam with his Russian for a couple of hours. We were just ready to get off to bed a little after ten when we struck a news broadcast with the bad news from Singapore. That made us victims to the Bob Hope hour that followed and kept us awake until eleven.

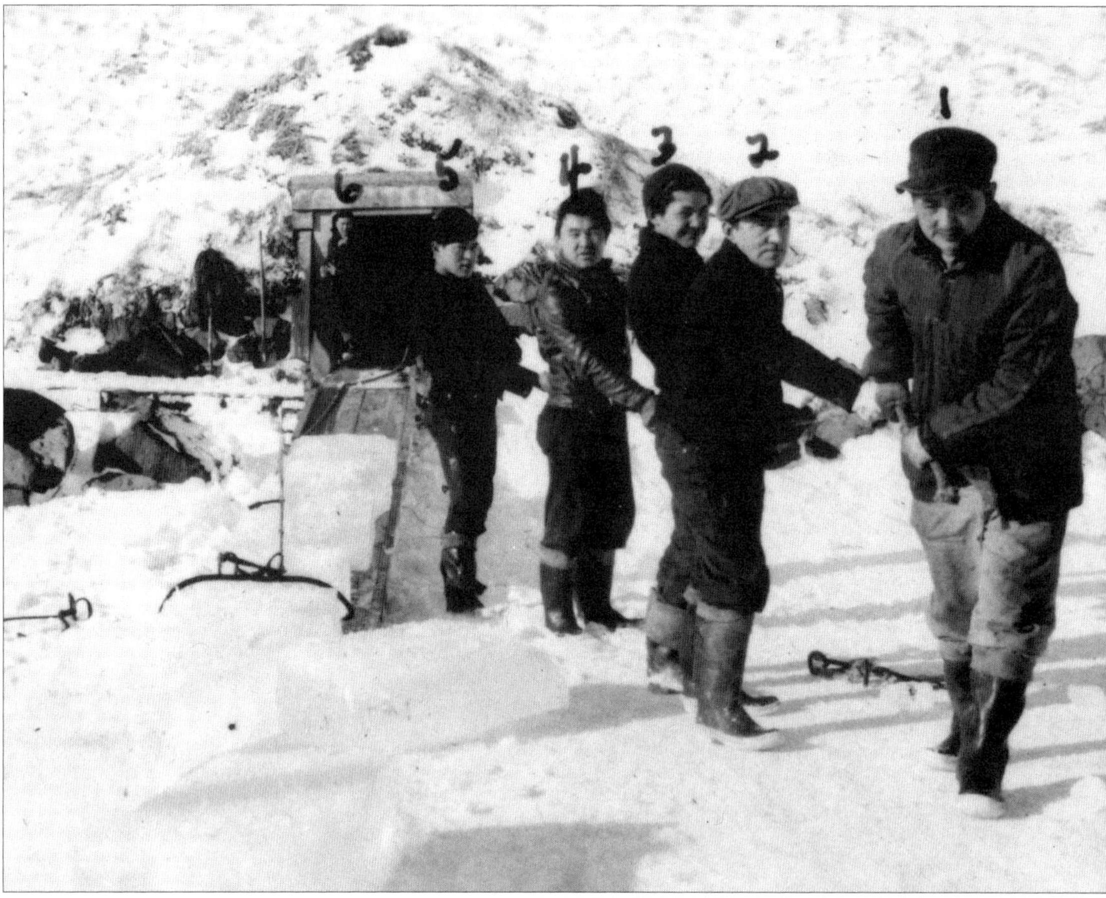

Men preparing to store ice in the sod house (from the Martin Collection, USUAF210, Archives, Alaska and Polar Regions, Rasmuson Library, University of Alaska Fairbanks).

Chapter 38

So profound was the ancient reverence for the wind's government that from infancy early Aleuts were taught not even to whisper a complaint against the weather. The sun's rare warmth must not be heralded in speech. The tempests must not be reviled. When the hunter waited in his unheated lair, held captive by the churning, wind-whipped waves, he would comfort his hunger pangs with the consoling phrase "the wind is no river."

The winds of the Bering Sea, so often called the cradle of the winds, are the wildest, craziest winds of the universe, invisible whirling dervishes that brush against your left cheek gently and turn back fiercely to smite you rudely from the right a little later. Surely Aeolius and his sons dwelt in some niche among the volcanic rocks of St. Paul, running in and out to torment the air and water like restless mischievous children.

When for a few hours the winds rested, the island was so quiet, so motionless, that the landscape seemed painted and unreal.

In winter the wind blows most steadily from the north and northeast driving before it the great white islands of the arctic ice floe, packing the whining jagged fragments against and upon the island's shore. Sometimes the ice has been driven south as far as St. George. Rarely has it failed to encircle St. Paul.

All summer I was undismayed by the local tales of the harshness of winter winds because I expected them to bring me the glittering ice formations I had seen shimmer before the crimson ramblers of our Maryland garden, the vision that had lured us north. On the doorsteps of the Arctic, how ridiculous to complain of hostile winds, of frozen seas.

Winter began lazily. November, December passed with only a few breaths of snow drifting earthward. The snowless Christmases were over. In February I comforted myself, the ice would come.

Presently there were snowstorms. There were quiet days when the snow came as gently as the proverbial goose feathers. Flakes winged gracefully earthward, a migration of ghostly butterflies dancing over the planes of air, across the brown earth to the smoky sea. On fiercer days the archers of the sky leaped from the ambush of purplish swollen clouds, firing a shower of twinkling quartz darts. The sharp points stunned and pierced our faces while we stumbled unseeing, our eyelids closed against the attack.

How various and picturesque were the pranks of the winds with so little snow. Thin slips of white lay sheltered by rocks for days until a teasing wind sought out their hiding place, gathered the crystals, and flung them upward in fresh storms. Many days, watching from the windows, we puzzled whether it was snowing or just the wind romping with last week's snowfall. So madly danced the wind with its fragile partner that day after day it was dangerous to sit close to the window to study lest the book lie forgotten while my eyes followed the fascinating drama in the air. Schottische, polka, foxtrot, and saraband, stately minuet or acrobatic exercise, the figures of dances new and old mingled in the air. Madcap pirouette and winsome glissade of foaming air gave the dullest day a holiday mood.

Truly the wind was no river. It chose its mood, its channel, at will all winter. It blew from the south bearing rain, from the east or west and only occasionally from the north. And presently winter was over without even the distant ghost of icy turret on the northern horizon of the seas. No gleaming bracelet encircled the island.

A half dozen days the village pond was frozen hard enough for skating. The ice cut from Ice House Lake and stored in the scoria pit in the hillside for next summer's ice cream was only nine inches thick. The mild winter affected the Aleut cash income, for fox trapping yields were small. There was too much food in the open for the foxes to be enticed into the box traps for seal meat mush. The men went in small parties to camp out at various cottages, those near the rookeries and others at Marunich, Southwest Point, and Tsammana. They idled their days away, hunting birds and playing cards because so few foxes were found in the traps each morning.

February 1, 1942
The wind is blowing over seventy miles an hour tonight. When we left the house to go to supper, we faced the wind. I have never been knocked about so. It is difficult enough to keep footing on the glaring ice in the road but with the wind blowing so furiously, it is more than a miracle to stay on one's feet. As if that were not enough, the wind just shovels sand into eyes and nostrils and mouth. Somehow we reached the Company House without damage. As I turned about to go up the steps, with the wind at my back, zip, I found myself being lifted up the steps and flung into the hall.

Roy had been out to Northeast Point with Carl who had to pick up one villager who had been out there to hunt. Of course, shooting is impossible in the weather. The roads were free of snow but the sand was blowing so profusely that it was impossible to see more than a couple feet ahead of the car. Above Big Lake the sand was drifted so that it was necessary to get out and shovel the road free. "One to drive and one to shovel," said Roy, because the sand blew back so swiftly.

I have retained more pity for the Pribilof fox at execution time than for the bachelor seals. Not that I ever was in at the death. Nothing could persuade me to watch the process after hearing the vivid description of the method. Lifting the victim from the trap while controlling his dangerous snapping jaws and agile head with a forked bar about his neck, if the pelt was saleable, the trapper set his heel firmly upon the poor beast's abdomen, crushing heart and lungs and suffocating him. Then the hunter snapped the neck and broke it to make sure the animal was dead.

The ancestors of *Alopex lagopus pribilofensis* first reached the Pribilofs on the drifting winter ice. From time to time fresh immigrants arrive. Interbreeding for countless generations had differentiated the present animals from their arctic cousins and they are classified as a distinct subspecies. For many years the pelt of the Pribilof blue fox was popular in the fashion marts. Then the style taste swerved to white fox, which still reigns as the favorite.

Blue and white are merely color phases in the animal's life. Since summer pelts are commercially useless, no one mentioned the color of the summer fur within our hearing. I was amazed and disappointed when I saw a small brown and cream-colored animal regarding us from a heap of rocks a few days after we arrived. He was beautiful. He looked almost friendly, like a curious dog watching us. He was the only island animal who returned man's interest. During trapping season he was elusive but too curious to run far away. When he caught sight of us, he would race off, turning at intervals to observe our actions, and usually settling upon a distant ledge to play Paul Pry. His running was perpetually delightful to watch. He bounced like a rubber ball on all four feet at once. The impetus of each bounce swerved his body from side to side. Had an intoxicated hunter pursued him, he would have proved as elusive as pink elephants. How I envied those skillful bounding paces that carried him over the steepest hillsides of tumbled rocks with the swiftness and directness of bird flight. Where he skimmed the earth, we stepped clumsily and cautiously like snails.

The white fox is more common on St. George. I saw but one or two on our island. One winter day when there was scarcely any snow on the roadside near Zapadni, I heard some tall grass crackling. Then I saw the muzzle and gleaming amber eyes of a white fox protruding through the sedge. When I stood still he whisked away in snowy dignity but stopped on the crest of deep black lava blocks, a perfect alabaster statue on an ebony base. Although no fox ever invaded my house to steal his dinner, we had many amusing encounters on our walks. One afternoon we crept very close to a litter of young pups beneath Hutchinson Hill. The dozen or more whelps were as busy as bees, romping with one another, popping in and out of numerous burrow entrances, and gnawing chunks of seal carcass that loving mothers had dragged home. Despite their youth and activities, they kept careful watch of us as we crept closer. When we were very near, a female, curled so close to a rock that her bluish grey fur had blended with the stone tint, displayed herself to us provokingly. She trotted audaciously close to us, right up the slope we had come down, tempting us to follow her. When we refused to be duped, she took her station on a rock above us. Through the hour we loitered she kept a steady watch. Though we knew her exact position as she sat motionless upon her perch, we would have failed to see her when we looked back save for the two poised pointed ears cocked alertly to catch our movements.

Callously we disregarded her fears because it was so delightful to watch the young ones at play and occasional rifts of sunlight promised us a chance to get clear photographs. Motionless we stood. Sam gripped his camera tightly. I stood at his right because brief gusts of fine cold rain spit from that direction every few minutes. Protecting the camera, my right ear filled with rain, I dared not move to shake out the water that seeped slowly down my neck. My martyrdom was worthless because the sun withdrew and our films were "shot" in murky atmosphere between gusts of rain. Nor were our lively subjects cooperative sitters. They darted too fast for the camera to catch them. As soon as the last of the film had been used, the sun poured out of the clouds in blinding brilliance and the rain ceased for the afternoon.

Off to our left from the hilltop a sharp barking commenced. A second mother coming home from a hunting trip discovered us near her young. She charged furiously downhill toward us as if to wipe us from the earth's surface. Almost upon us, she swerved and mounted a rock pile a couple of hundred yards away. From this vantage she continued to assail our ears with sharp vindictive remarks and to warn the pups to go underground. The pups were interested in her clamor but completely disobedient. They felt quite able to protect themselves. Some bold ones came almost to our feet, sniffed, squealed, and raced back to their brothers. The ground under our feet was vocal with the voices of many more furry babies squealing and yelping as they played and tussled with each other in their dark warrens.

Jordan narrated the travail of an overcurious fox who accepted the offer of a bit of chewing tobacco. Immediately the poor beast was shaken with convulsive tremors and became unconscious. In a little while he woke, staggered to his feet, and retreated drunkenly and hastily from such a dangerous neighborhood.

Fox bites were commonplace during the trapping season. Sam learned to his sorrow not to trust even a dead fox too far. Wandering through the sand dunes above Marunich he found a fine clean fox skull. Most of the tiny knife-sharp teeth were in place in the jaws. He thrust it into his pocket. Half an hour later as we tramped along the beach I heard a profane sound behind me. I turned to see Sam ruefully surveying some bleeding fingers he had just withdrawn from his pocket. I could just imagine a little fox ghost chuckling gleefully at his posthumous success in annoying his enemy.

The foxes have thrived on the Pribilofs because of the seal carcasses, birds, and bird eggs. On St. George they dine well on shrews and lemmings. Attempts to introduce the latter two rodents on St. Paul have failed. Always we encountered foxes skulking in the rocks above the cliffs where birds congregated. In the spring we leaned over the steep bluffs of Einahnuhto and watched breathlessly as the foxes ran swiftly and sure-footedly down the seemingly straight face of the seawall. Surely a rash beast would drop into the angry waves three hundred feet below. A few seconds later he came skimming up with a limp bird in his jaws, bounding contemptuously past us to find a less crowded spot to eat.

The impish leer of a fox face must be an indication of his character. On the road to Zapadni a large building with a big wire-enclosed yard was built as a modern trap designed to supplant the small box traps. There were several entrances in the wire fences through which the foxes were supposed to enter during trapping season. Not a single fox obliged the designer. One morning, when trapping had ended, Hoverson and John Hanson were driving past the pen. Inside were five foxes, frolicking merrily, so cocksure that both the men were able to enter the yard and stand close to them. John, fortunately, had his camera and was able to film this superb effrontery of *Alopex pribilofensis.*

If the Pribilofs sometimes took on the guise of fairyland, certainly the foxes deserved the role of leprechauns or impish good-natured Ariels.

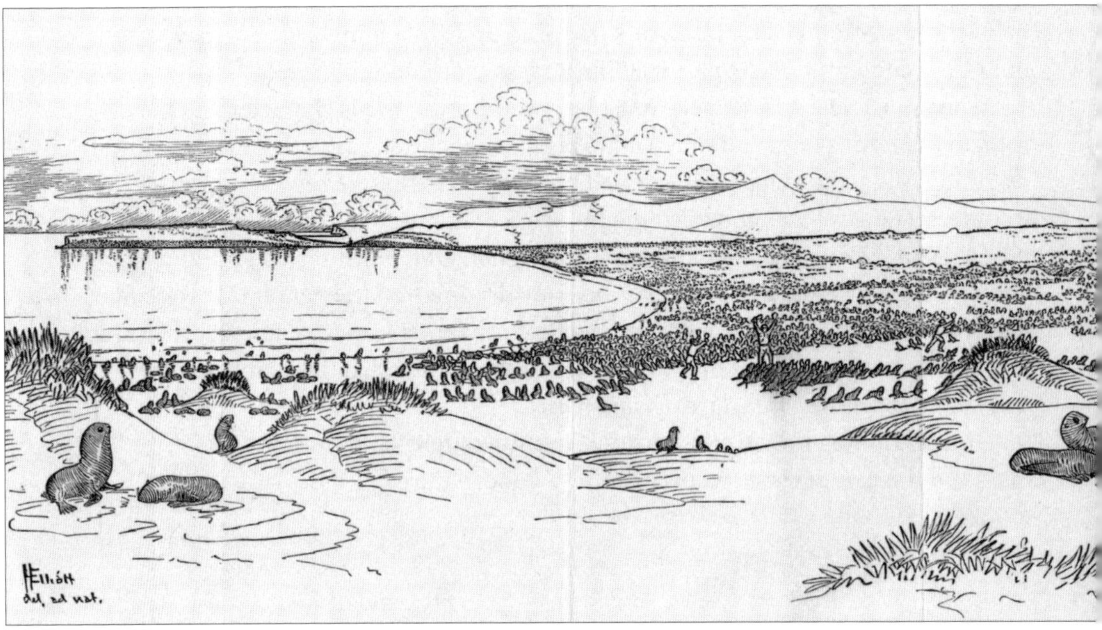

Elliott drew "Natives Selecting a Drive" showing the hauling grounds at English Bay. It shows the landscape to the west of the village (*Fur-Seal Fisheries of Alaska, 1889,* Plate 9).

Chapter 39

Spring came stealing from the smoke-green sea. No sudden fanfare of burgeoning green gave warning. The winds were less harsh. The sun shone more frequently. No seagulls loitered over the village yards in search of food. The snow buntings forsook us and started north. The ducks, which had thronged the lakes and bays during the winter months, were disappearing. Early in April we began to explore the island thoroughly. Before June came we had tramped every inch of the shore, climbed almost every hill, and crossed and recrossed the lowland stretches. Every physical feature of the island was engraved on our memories for our lifetime. We knew the most delicate details of the land. We had absorbed the beauty of a thousand landscape moods.

Often Tobyanne accompanied us, to remain asleep in the car or to be carried on our backs, stuffed in a knapsack. Heretina and Alice (Alexandra) Gromoff, who had come to live with us to study English, or other village youngsters shared many of our outings. As the days lengthened we rose earlier and earlier to enjoy the first gleam of dawn. We were able to use a car until 8:30 a.m., when the work gang needed it. Into the brief morning hours we crowded vibrant impressions of the island's awakening from winter torpor.

At Zapadni one afternoon with Alice and Heretina we started up a grassy slope to reach the Russian cross we thought marked the old cemetery. The ascent seemed direct and snow free. Abruptly we found ourselves on the brink of a deep gully choked with snow. We walked almost a mile until we found a narrow spot where the snow crust was firm. We crossed safely and came to the lichen-embellished cross. The bare ground revealed no trace of grave mounds. On our way back by a different route, we found several steep slopes where the snow was packed hard. It tempted us to sit down and slide to the bottom. Alice and Heretina rolled in the snow like puppies, delighted at our lack of adult dignity.

There were hunters in the watch house and we invited ourselves inside to warm up. Nikita Hapoff was a gracious host and offered to care for Tobyanne while we hiked toward Kursoolah, the "place where someone is angry," the Aleuts say. He also pointed out the battered, faded cross on one of the projecting fingers

April 11, 1942
The road to Zapadni has some badly gutted spots that do not show up in the red scoria until the car is plunging in and out again and the occupants are trying to get their breath, even driving very slowly. We missed the hard crusted snowbanks that we used to charge and glide across. The few large banks that remained were under the hills close to the watch house and were too soft to navigate. We parked the car and Tobyanne, packed in with pillows and blankets and very indignant at our desertion. It seemed as if we might easily ascend the steep slope that Elliott calls Cemetery Ridge on his maps. On the top of it is a Russian cross and, as his verbal description of the site of the first cemetery is not very clear, we had taken it for granted that the old graves must be up there on the rocky summit. . . .

For some time I pursued fragments of snow and ice as they slid down my back and legs but most of them managed to stay out of reach and melt at their own leisure. I couldn't let that disturb my search of the beach but found no treasures and finally sent the others strolling while I went back to the car to feed Tobyanne who had her hat awry and was complaining to nature of her cruel parents. As soon as she had eaten, I packed her in the knapsack and joined the hikers. We intended to take her with us but when we reached the house at Zapadni, we found old Nikita Hapoff and his youngsters installed for the weekend were glad to share

cont.

of Zapadni Headland that marked the old graveyard site. Prowl as we might on other excursions among the protruding rocks and grass-covered mounds, no mark distinguished an old grave. Few villagers knew what the cross on that low site stood for. I was pleased when the men sent to repaint the rookery markers stole time and paint enough to freshen the cross.

But that afternoon when we arrived at Kursoolah over behind Antone Lake, Sam found his first Japanese souvenir, a lovely pale green hollow glass sphere, a float from a Japanese fishing net. Those who know the currents claim that a float, broken loose from nets in the usual fishing grounds, must travel for at least seven years to reach the coasts of the archipelago. How much longer to reach the Pribilofs is unestimated. A capricious wave had flung Sam's first find across the mighty barrier of rocks into the soft grass near the lake.

I found my first float in the sands of Lukanin a few days later. We went often to the southern end of Lukanin. In mid-April we made the first of many hikes along its whole extent. The day was warm. A coat was a nuisance in walking. We were intoxicated by the sweep of the half-moon beach, by the tumbling snowy manes of the incoming waves. We drew pictures in the sand and wrote messages to each other. We rolled sea-soaked barrels down the sand slopes into the sea. Halfway along the beach we came upon a great field of amber kelp, coiled in fantastic patterns on the sand. Gleaming among the loops of the seaweed were a dozen Japanese floats. Could Sinbad have enjoyed his emeralds more than we as the sun burned the brilliant green globes with fiery gold flames?

Near the upper end of the beach the sand dunes became hillocks. Narrow passages between them led to cool, shadowy circular vales. Their floors were littered with sea debris. Brittle orange crates mingled with the great uprooted trees that powerful waves had jammed through the slender entrances. The mighty bleached ribs of stranded whales grounded by a careless sea were awesome fragments of the ocean's greatest monarchs. Ghostly bubbles gleamed wanly from tangled sprays of seaweed, the glass floats become as insubstantial as globules of seawater. As soon as we had found clear globes, we coveted one still braided in the rope of the net. Presently Sam whooped with delight as he came upon one half buried in the sand. Soon I had found another.

The slender promontory at the northern point of Lukanin possessed many names. The Russians called it *Tonki* or "thin." The Americans christened it Stony Point, a descriptive term suitable for many peninsulas. On a foggy night in July 1910, the revenue cutter *Perry* cruising offshore in the fog, ran aground.[1] No lives were lost. Most of the goods were recovered. The rather gaudy picture of Theodore Roosevelt that hung in the dining room of the Company House was a souvenir of the accident. Even at high tide, the rusting bulk of the *Perry*'s boiler, wedged between rocks a few hundred yards from shore, loomed out of the waves as a bizarre metallic sea monster. Since that fatal night the spot is frequently termed Perry Point.

From Tonki, Polovina Point appeared temptingly near. We continued strolling until we had to cut inland to the road, that we might hurry more quickly back for morning office hours.

At Tonki Sam had waded into the sea for a delicate pair of antlers still attached to the cranium. Unbroken and pale from soaking in the brine, they were a perfect memento

his fire. Nikita showed us how far up into the fields the rookery of 1890 had extended. I could hardly believe it since that was the year when the first notice was paid to the diminishing herd and Elliott had returned to have apoplectic fits over the small number of seals remaining. But Nikita stuck to his story despite my unbelief. He is one of the oldest men on the island today. He also showed me where the old cemetery is, a cleft in the hills opposite to the point shown as Cemetery Ridge on Elliott's maps. But the cleft was filled with snow and must be investigated later.

We abandoned Tobyanne to his care and started out to walk around Antone Lake on the flat side. At least the ground looks fairly level. In summer the walking from one clump of tall grass to another is practically impossible and even now the trip is not a pleasure stroll. . . .

When Sam and Alexandra reached the beach, Sam stumbled over a small Japanese float. How magical it seems to find one of these green glass spheres on the boulder strands. How did it skim to safety over the lava edges? It was the first one found by a member of our family and Sam was as elated as if he had found a bar of gold and I was nearly so. We sat on the rocks and watched the sea's antics and hoped that Japanese net floats would be the only Japanese invaders of St. Paul.

to bring back to the States. Most discarded antlers that littered the island were too broad and massive to display in a modern home. Sam, laden with a knapsack bulging with Japanese trophies and imperfect shells, bore them home on his shoulder. The horns projecting above his head imparted the dignity of a druidic priest or Teutonic knight. Peter polished them and we brought them safely home to hang over my desk while I write nostalgically of island days.

That evening Tobyanne sat on the living room floor playing with the lovely glass balls, the brightest toys she had known, and permitted us to take a photograph of her smiles for the first time. A few days later we went to Marunich. No one told us the road was impassable so we rode happily through pool and mud and crusty snowbanks. Once we skidded and stuck in a mud hole. We filled the ruts with scoria chunks and were soon on harder ground, safe and mud spattered.

The tall grasses of the past summer were sere and recumbent so that we could explore the old barabara sites. Four of them were half choked with fallen timbers. Remnants of driftwood planking still lined the lowest part of the pits. Other grass-grown hollows might have been dug by man but certain proof was lacking. Even as temporary habitations, two of the definite barabara depressions were extremely small. The relics of the wrecked *Alexander* were naked in the dead grass.

We spent the morning strolling the shore toward Tsammana and returning to the camp house where we ate lunch. The steep red and purple scoria of North or Marunich Hill lit up with gold and copper radiance in the sunlight. After lunch we tramped along North Point. Facing Northeast Point we had to battle a strong wind. It blew so vigorously and steadily that we seemed constantly pushing against a thick, tangible but invisible substance. Our feet slipped backward in the sand. The wide skirt of my parka gave me more wind resistance so that at times I became breathless as I trudged defiantly on. Sam snapped my picture, looking like a real arctic traveler in the garment. The faint fringe of the waves in the background gave a slight illusion of snow.

We loaded our pockets and knapsacks with Japanese floats and shells. Toward the Point the dunes began to rise up as hills higher than Lukanin's dunes. We penetrated the recesses that winter waves kept battered open between them. We pawed through piles of kelp and examined heaps of driftwood, finding our treasures. A pale ghost of a faraway woodland, a silvery birch whose bark was ecstasy to inhale, was a graceful castaway in one valley. There were long blanched ribs and massive vertebrae of whales and walrus skeletons stripped of their prized tusks. At the water's edge, crouching in the sand picking up pearly boat or slipper shells, I heard a blood-curdling shout of triumph from Sam, who was peering into sand hollows. I ran madly expecting to see him emerging with a walrus head still decorated with gleaming tusks. He was waiting for me empty handed. Ahead of him a huge float of rich green glass rested on the grey earth in a pool of sunlight.

Our arms could hold no more sea trove. We turned back from Vesolia Mista, the Happy Place, named by the first Aleut.

Behind the dunes lay Big Lake and Sheep Lake separated by a narrow strip of land known to the Aleuts by a foot-long term that simply meant "between the two lakes." On a sandy knoll a Russian cross leaned drunkenly. Not far from it Vasilii Sedulik had a barabara where he and his family camped to pick berries and hunt birds. John Hanson had a particular reverence for that cross.

When he was seven years old he lived with his grandmother. Like the other village children he was warned never to leave the village alone lest raiding poachers kidnap him. While his grandmother was berrying, John grew lonely and set out to find her. His spindly little legs followed the crude winding footpaths and occasional wagon impressions in the soil until he reached Polovina Point. He went inside the barabara but ran out frightened by the network of cobwebs. The peak of Polovina attracted him. Up its steep slope he plodded. From the height he hoped to catch a glimpse of the berry pickers. Instead he saw a large vessel not far from shore. Childishly he thought the pirates could see him as clearly as he viewed the ship. Panic stricken he ran blindly over the hill and lost all familiar landmarks. He wandered about the region between the lakes. At times he trembled thinking he heard the pirates approaching. Then he forgot his fears and played happily. He ate berries and drank water from Sheep Lake. When he accidentally wandered out on North Point Beach, he fashioned toys from the sticks and stones on the sand. Before it was dark he was back in the neighborhood of the lakes. He investigated the Sedulik barabara. The wooden sleeping bunk looked uninviting. He felt safer out on top of the earth. Close to the foot of the cross, he dug a hole in the sand. His cap made a pillow. He lay down and scooped the

April 23, 1942
If I were to write the story of today, I should be forced to entitle it "Two Ducks and Quack Americanism." . . . I ought to know how calloused human beings can be. I do know. But every fresh example of human cruelty whether petty or on a grand scale continues to shock me.

Four days ago Sam was talking of the traditions of Patriot's Day, which is a legal holiday in his home state, and just four days after I am wondering if that "shot fired round the world" should not have passed a little closer to the Pribilof Islands—but not to kill ducks for sick people. Oh, no, that might cause an inter-island crisis.

The hospital diet nauseates me to think of. We have lists of diets for weeks. Breakfasts are fair when they occasionally stick in some fruit. But month after month of corned beef and roast beef, canned, of course, for lunch and reindeer, either in steak form or in stews, for those tuberculous men on the top floor and the little girl with rheumatic fever and heart disease on the lower floor—with no desserts, a rare can of vegetables not even every two weeks, a well stomach revolts at the monotony as well as the mind recoiling from the obvious deficiencies for people who need nourishing food to fight disease. How can tuberculosis be cured on a diet of canned meats and potatoes? . . .

Early in the season of hunting, Sam asked the foreman to ask the men whether they would be willing to donate

cont.

a duck or two to the hospital whenever they were fortunate enough to shoot a large number. Nothing ever came of the suggestion. Sam has asked individuals. No luck. Today our janitor announced that he shot twenty ducks yesterday, and Sam asked him why he did not give one to the boys in the hospital. He said all right, with apparent cheerfulness. And we thought no more of the matter. At eleven o'clock Peter burst in breathlessly to announce that John Misikin, the cook in the Company House, who has two assistants to help him cook for one man who eats there and for the hospital patients, usually averaging ten people, refused to cook the ducks. . . .

The next disturbance, oddly enough, although it concerned us more personally and is aimed at someone I have come to love very dearly, seemed anticlimactic. After the awful smallness of the morning's example of "man's inhumanity to man," the wire stating that the Washington office did not approve our adoption of Alexandra Gromoff seemed a fairly natural happening. We immediate wrote out a wire and asked Carl to send it. It read, "Berenbergs request Washington Office please explain how Christian Americans can attempt to debar young, intelligent, lovable, crippled child from only opportunity for health, education and happiness." That should put their action in the correct light so that they realize that they are in the wrong and that I am going to fight this with every means possible. I shall start in easily, contacting public

cont.

sand over the lower portion of his body. He drew his jacket over his shoulders and face. Before he covered his face he looked up at the guardian cross, whispered a prayer, and made the sign of the cross. At once he fell peacefully asleep. The next day he played and dined on berries and lake water. And the next and still the next day. Each night, comforted by the cross, he slept well in his sandy nest. Sometimes at night he heard the voices of searching parties and saw distant lantern light. He kept silent because he feared they might be the horrible kidnappers.

After the fourth night he went down to the lake, stripped, and went wading with a couple of sticks for boats. While he was engrossed piloting his play craft, two searchers came across a trail of broken grass too wide for a fox path. They had trouble finding him even then because the grass was so high and John was so small. It had been above John's head as he wandered through the fields, a constant assurance of safe hiding. John heard them approaching and fled naked toward the other side of the lake. Breathless he lay on the ground, hoping the grass would hide him, that the men would leave. His heart pounded so loudly he could not hear footsteps. He felt someone leaning over him, picking him up. With relief he looked into the friendly eyes of a St. Paul man.

The successful searchers fired their revolvers and those who heard the welcome sound fired theirs. The sounds repeated all along the island and across it. The agent and doctor who were near Tonki Point hastened toward the agreed meeting place at Polovina. All the searchers bore provisions but nothing tempted John.

"They tried to give me apples and oranges," he told me. "But I couldn't eat. Not sardines either. Then the agent, he took somethin' out of his upper pocket which looked kinda' red and offered it to me. It was whiskey. I took a drink and said 'more,' and everybody laughed. He gimme three drinks and then I could eat sardines. Everybody thought it was so funny they talked about it for a long time. They carried me home in a mule cart and took me right to the dispensary for an examination but I was all right. I was lucky it was berry time so I didn't freeze and starve. After that my gramma wouldn't let me away from the house." Then he shook his head and added, "I often wish that I knowed more about writing in those days so I could wrote it all down while I remembered it all good for it would'a made a good story."

To the first inquiry in the village on our return from Marunich, we responded that we had been on the north shore. "You didn't drive to Marunich," the wife of an official asserted positively. "It hasn't been opened up yet. No one is allowed to drive there. You must have had a long walk across the island." We trespassers on an officially unopened road forbore to contradict her.

Polovina Hill drew us dawn after dawn to her summit. We never wearied of sitting in a windless pocket of the eastern slope, just under the guardian cross, as the sun came out of the sea and stained sky and water with passionate flaming radiance. Condrat Krukoff claimed the Aleuts had called the crater *Adagum Kayach* and the slightly lower peak behind her, known in English as Little Polovina, was *Adagumalak Kayach* or "son of *Adagum*." Polovina heads the procession of little red hills that straggle unevenly back across the tundra to the coast of Marunich. She is the grande dame of them all, sculptured in flowing lines from the bottom of her encircling green skirts to the queenly dignity of her scalloped red tiara.

people who are friends of mine to write or see Gabrielson and Ickes[2] and meanwhile have the legal right of the bureau to refuse investigated. Letters to newspapers, touching on other undeniable social evils here, will follow. Mrs. Roosevelt, of course, is one to rally to Alexandra's support. I shall not omit her. Then as soon as I get back, if nothing has been accomplished by mail, I shall get some congressmen and senators in action.

January 25, 1942

John Hanson . . . revealed that his father's name had been German, Garriman, or something similar. That his father had been adopted by Capt. Hanson. When John went out to school in Juneau, the old priest showed him the papers that proved that he had an aunt and uncle. The aunt was supposed to be in Seattle and the uncle, Zachar Herman, was and probably still is in Sitka. Until 1939 John heard from him and has since written to the priest at Sitka for information. In his search for his aunt he had less luck. She had not been at the Orthodox church for two years but the priest gave him an address of some trust company that held real estate and ten thousand dollars of hers. John lacked a few papers to prove his identity but back on the island he and McMillin filled out many papers and John sent the only picture he had of his father and his aunt and uncle and some other people. Apparently he had known none of the people in the picture except his father before that time.

cont.

After waiting over a year for a reply they wrote again. A receiver answered that the business was messed up and the oldest of three Mr. Phillips, the president of the company, was in jail for stealing funds. So not only did John and his uncle receive nothing from her estate but John lost his only picture.

January 26, 1942
I forgot to record yesterday that we learned from J. Hanson that it was Mr. Redpath, a company agent, who died and left about ten thousand dollars to some of the people here. He left four to Nekifer Mandregan's old blind mother, foster mother, or mother-in-law (I'm not sure which). And some to a Merculieff family on St. George who still have some according to the yearly publication.

Among the sparse short grasses, alpine plants decorate the queen hill's breast in the earliest days of spring. One dawn, heads literally in the clouds as we walked within the morning mist along the scoriaceous brow, a purplish haze underfoot attracted me. I knelt speechless to assure myself of the miracle. A tiny cluster of green leaves resembling embroidered French knots framed minute magenta flower cups. Tenuous hairlike rootlets grasped the rocks. The summit was festooned with the audacious *Saxifraga oppositifolia* or, more prosaically, red moss. The plant has both modesty and boldness to choose the windswept elevations for a home.

In the heart of the wide crater lay a pool, child of winter snow replenished by summer rains. The thirsty reindeer had worn paths around the waning circle. The beaten red walks alternated with circular bands of grass into a large colorful wheel of concentric circles.

Under an outcrop of rock inside the crater, Johnston showed us the hiding place of the only known patch of alpine or trailing azalea. At the tips of the recumbent leathery-leaved stems hung umbels of wee pink campanulate blossoms. We had regarded the site as a secret lest the single clump be uprooted by a greedy flower lover. One afternoon I raced breathlessly over the rim of North Hill and dropped down to rest. I found myself in a garden of azalea, trailing profusely along the upper slope. I wished I had an appropriate marker to set in the midst of my discovery. I might have been tempted to shift the cross but the winds had been ahead of me and its rotting parts had been blown far down the hillside.

Chapter 40

The last day of April was crisp and bright. We were wandering up and down Tolstoi headland and cliffs. We sat at rest on some boulders facing English Bay. In 1847 an English vessel was edging inshore toward Zapadni when it struck a hidden reef and sank. A number of the crew drowned. Their bodies were not recovered. According to the Aleut account to Elliott the men were "*mass-lucken*." The word is still a handy term to express a multitude of situations, principally a fatalistic "What of it? So what?" attitude. Elliott translated it as meaning in his day something beyond human ken or lost.[1] The whaler's nationality was memorialized in the bay's name. The sands of the bay usually offered us brilliant shells of several species of clams and sea slippers. Some lucky people gleaned a few fresh edible clams but our shells were always tenantless. Here and there a duck made a dark stain where it rested on the waves. Suddenly there was a dark blob of color that grew larger and larger. A seal was breaking the surface of the water. A bull had been reported offshore there two days before.

We were excited as if we had a special rendezvous with him. On the third of January we had encountered a young bull ensconced in a cave of piled rocks near the same spot. He had been annoyed at our approach, spitting and fuming at us. As the last seal of the 1941 season, he was a hermit who felt entitled to complete solitude.

Now the first herald of the incoming beasts was landing in front of us. Our joy turned to concern when we saw how the beast hauled his huge bulk with such effort. He seemed ill or wounded. Slowly he dragged himself over the rocks with a rolling drunken motion. As he passed us going high up on the beach, we realized he was no stricken creature. He was the monarch of harems, replete and bursting from his winter's gluttony, padded with thick layers of blubber on which he must subsist during his mating fast. The first bulls we had seen were already shrunken from their vigil. This enormous monster was in his spring prime.

He changed his mind about staying on shore. Repassing us he caught sight of our motionless figures. He stared with his rheumy eyes for a second and then

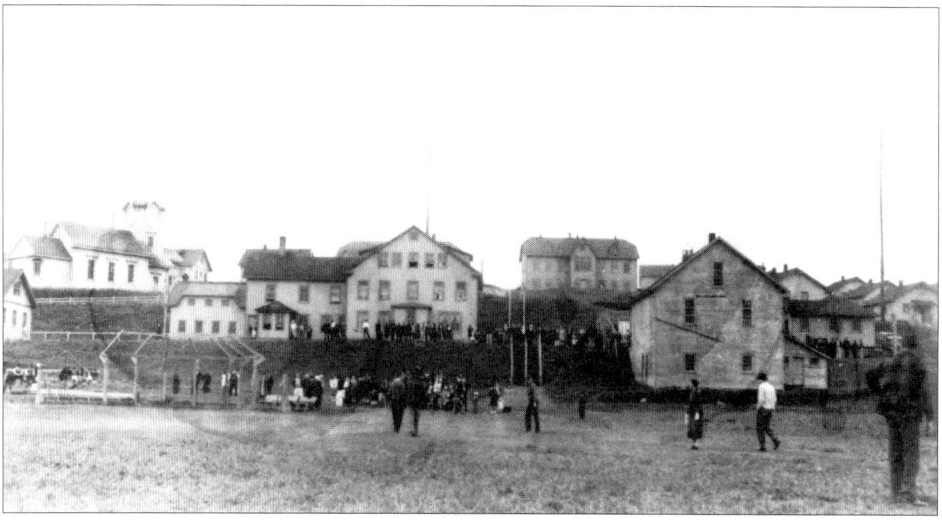

A baseball game between the St. Paul men and employees of the Fouke Fur Company, July 4, 1941 (from the Martin Collection, USUAF210, Archives, Alaska and Polar Regions, Rasmuson Library, University of Alaska Fairbanks).

lunged with the speed of a bullet over the remaining boulders and splashed into the sea. Despite his obesity he could, at will, travel swiftly.

That afternoon after many short inland sorties we cut homeward across the Zapadni road to the summit of Telegraph Hill, christened by a company official lonely for the steep streets of San Francisco. From the flats near the reindeer corral the slope rose gently into a level wedge-shaped plateau. On the village side, the hill fell more abruptly to the juncture of the Zapadni and Northeast Point roads and Ice House Lake. On this brow, the cross from the old church stood mounted on a large wooden sphere. Time had fractured the wooden globe but encircling bands of metal kept the pieces in place. Gaudy scraps of yellow paint still showed on the weathered wood rivaled by saffron shades of encroaching lichens. An evil American custom had pursued the cross to its solitary eminence. Cross and ball were studded with initials, even the conventional heart and arrows and a few dates. I wonder still who "Bride, 1936" might be and why the groom was not mentioned.

We had struggled uphill through the fury of a brief hailstorm. Abruptly the spasm was spent. The sun flashed from behind the clouds and brought every detail of the island into clear-cut lines. The village, reef, and even the humped spines of Gorbotch, on Reef Point, seemed within hand's reach. Behind us the landscape as far as Polovina seemed to have crept close to us.

At home Heretina and Alice confessed they had never climbed Telegraph Hill. We helped them into thick clothes and sent them off. Unintentionally we made them truant from church services that Saturday evening. They came home jubilant at dusk. Alice could just find strength to tumble into bed.

The next afternoon we took Alice to Lukanin, another place she had never been. We spent hours on the rookery grounds climbing up and down the basalt steps. One curved section was called the Amphitheater. Some terraces were simple steps built of fairly uniform blocks of glassy purple-black basalt. It seemed as if a mighty ebony temple had crashed there, its pillars cracking into small lengths that folded upright upon one another forming new oddly jointed posts and shafts. Coils of purplish reddish lava writhed liquidly from tier to tier in adjacent descents. A nosy hair seal caught sight of us and swam easily along the coast as our guide.

We met Merculieff youngsters out for a walk and left Alice with them while we ran home to feed Tobyanne. No Alice arrived for supper at seven in the evening. Finally I caught sight of Alice and Julia rounding the Lagoon. They had been lost among the dunes trying to find the road and had walked almost to Polovina. During their long ramble, Julia had been expounding her religious faith. Alice had escaped into daydreams uttering monosyllabic sounds from time to time. Then Julia began to discuss Father Baranoff. His soul was in danger. She had asked him whether God really made the earth in six days. Father had replied, "Perhaps six days or perhaps six hundred years. The time period might be a symbol." We relayed the story expecting Father to be amused by Julia's concern for his soul. Instead, it revived his apprehension.

One of our outings resembled a crime wave. Driving past Polovina a Pribilof sandpiper flew from the roadside and struck the car, dying immediately. Beyond Big Lake the winter winds had piled a thick layer of sand over the roadbed, as they refashioned the neighboring sand dunes. Every spring workmen had to clean up that road across the isthmus. One sandy waste had been named "Death Valley" by the road

May 1, 1942
What a different walk to the one I took on May 1, 1937. Five years ago—and so many of my companions that day, tramping the muddy road to Castillejo from Villa Paz, are dead or "missing" or lost in concentration camps. The same red handkerchief is in my pocket that I wore then in my uniform. I could not keep back tears thinking of them. The world was a sad enough place then, but how much more horrible today. How many more must die before this horror will be overcome? . . .

Father Baranoff was telling about Dr. Collins this morning, how he knew nothing of photography when he came here with a box camera and started but that he took over five thousand pictures of the island before he finished. He had no regular office hours and spent most of his time in his darkroom, which is now our bedroom, and ran down whenever anyone drifted in; furthermore, that he was frightened of the agent who cried economy constantly, never asked for anything, sent only the most vital cases to the hospital because of lack of cooperation of agent and economy slogan. No wonder his annual report was only a page long. . . .

I finished *Arctic Village* yesterday.[2] A swell study. Wish I could write that way about this place but it would be too disgraceful for Uncle Sam to have the complete truth told so I have to sugarcoat it with personal experience.

May 7, 1942
The island is crisp with a thick coating of snow and the air is filled with flurries every little while, some so dense that it is impossible to see far from the window. Yet yesterday the spring season was officially opened by the practice of the two baseball teams. For ten evenings the members of the baseball club have been working on their diamond. Really working. Shovels tossed heaps of dirt in a rhythm of very rapid tempo. Ashes and scoria were packed into the deep trenches dug beneath the baselines and then for several days the boys used the big roller to pack the soil. They did a swell job. Last night they appeared decked in their baseball costumes and after some warming up the blue socks played the red socks. They are getting in trim for the arrival of the Fouke Fur boys, who are expected around the twentieth. The baseball game, which I only surveyed for a few minutes while passing and from our windows for a short interval, was the conclusion of a very exciting day. We are not getting up as early as we used to for the change to War Time on Sunday has robbed us of an hour of daylight. [*St. Paul Island Log Book* noted on May 3, "Advanced local time one hour to conform with Bering War Time."] It is just greyly light at four.

workers and another was called the "Valley of Ten Thousand Smokes" in honor of a foreman who had spent most of his time loafing.

The fox feeding gang had slung loose planks across the shifting sand so they might more quickly transport food to the Point. The boards looked stable and we were tempted to drive across them. Just before we reached the corduroy section, a plank slipped from under a rear wheel. We were safely caught trespassing where we should never have ventured. The more Sam shoveled, the deeper the car sank. Machine and sand seemed diabolically determined to outwit our efforts to escape. He dug so deeply that the car almost sat back on its hind wheels, its nose pointed straight up to heaven. Finally we decided to hike two miles to Webster House, hoping workmen had completed repairing the winter damages to the telephone lines. Both cottages were locked. Having begun the morning with manslaughter, continued our career of crime by trespassing and getting trapped, we proceeded to do a good job of breaking and entering. Sam built up a precarious pile of lumber, pried open an unlocked window and climbed into the Aleut camp house.

While he cranked the phone handle I wandered off to the site of the old chapels used by sealing gangs who summered there before the era of roads. Legend reports a crude chapel there in the days of competitive Russian trading settlements. A level mound marked by a cross is supposed to be the site of all. Below the elevation were the depressions of two barabaras. All traces of others had been obliterated. We tramped back loaded with rotting burlap as soon as Sam gave up all hope of putting a call through. Before we had tunneled much more of the earth Hoverson and Nekifer arrived to rescue us. Not even the chunk of walrus ivory I had found on the beach while Sam dug with the one shovel recompensed me for the death of the sandpiper.

The excitement of the day was not over. As we ate lunch I heard a low thrumming sound. A plane seemed to rise right over the brim of Black Bluffs like a nasty black beetle crawling out of its shelter. It came directly over the village. Hoverson thought he identified it as an American plane. Its sudden approach and low flight almost over the houses were a fresh reminder of our situation. From the States a wire had come ordering bunkhouses prepared for summer workers for the twentieth of May. The news had been a tonic to the whole village.

Doubts and fears we thrust determinedly from our minds. The early flowers were beginning to bud. There were signs of green in the landscape. At first the reef turned vernal. The tiny algae and the mosses made the distant slope of Gorbotch and Ardiguen a soft velvety meadow. Standing in the fields looking down at the earth the tiny spears of hearty new blades were solitary and insignificant, piercing the mat of last year's sere recumbent grass. But when my eyes traveled across the landscape there was the soft shimmer of secretive green running beneath the brown crust. Every day the shadow deepened, grew more intense as the shoots pushed up past their predecessors.

The plateau and inland slope of Tolstoi Headland formed a lovely rock garden near our home. To walk by road around the curving Lagoon meant a tramp of three miles. At low tide there were fords across the narrows of the Lagoon that Sam could traverse dryly in his hip boots. My knee boots were too short so Sam would hoist me over his shoulder like a sack and wade across. In this position I arrived quickly at a flower lover's paradise. Early in the spring the sun shone on the mossy ledges and coaxed the rock jasmine, the scentless violets, the arctic coltsfoot, and

May 6, 1942
Out on the road when we were trying to lift our lagging spirits with jokes, I said all that we needed to round out the day was an air raid.

I remembered those words with a cold chill a little later. I left the lunch table while the others were still eating and came into the study for paper. I heard the unmistakable sound of a plane and, telling the others to get wraps, dashed to the door, saw that it was a pursuit plane and not a bomber and was already passing over the row of houses in which we live. I also thought I could descry the red and white and something else of a star. But just to make sure I grabbed Tobyanne and wrapped her up and got outside. Hoverson had strong glasses and he said he could see the star plainly. But I almost wish that our own planes would not come over if they are going to give us that tense moment of fear before we descry the star. The street was crowded in a moment and the joyful cry "Ours, Ours" went echoing along the street. It reminded me of that joyous relief I used to listen to five years ago, "Nuestras, Nuestras." Ours, too. The plane flew very low but made no dipping greeting as last summer's visitors did, flew out across the Black Bluffs, and by observers on the hilltop was seen to recross the island at Polovina toward Southwest Point. The afternoon seethed with conversation about planes, air raids, Japanese attacks, and the destination of the plane, whether it was Army or Navy.

other flowers to bloom. The blossoms of *Sibbaldia* and buttercups were pools of molten gold between jet rocks. The first pussy willows ran in a velvet network over the level headland. On Tolstoi alone the dark lily, the *Fritillaria camschatcensis,* which throve so lustily in crowded masses on St. George, grew in a few secluded nooks. The spring before, Dimitri Tetoff's wife had scoured the hill to get a mess of roots to eat. We poked into every corner of the hillside in our spring outings and found not one remaining plant. The first silvery furry spikes of lousewort stood up aloof from the soft moss cushions on the shelves of rock.

A touch of poignancy brooded in the air over the lovely flowered upland. The familiar Russian cross bore a metal plate on which had been crudely cut the epitaph:

Venedict Tetoff
Born March 27, 1907
Lost his life by drow[n]ing
In Village Cove
St. Paul Island
Dec. 29, 1932

The other men had clung to a capsized boat until rescued. But Venedict, Peter Kochergin's brother, was unable to swim and holding futilely to an oar had been swept away. Searching parties combed the island beaches constantly until late in January, but his body was never brought back by the waves. Graveless, the marker to his memory stands in the midst of beauty.

One evening we went in search of sea biscuits, fresh ones, for we were anxious to taste the yellow roe of the *echini* shellfish that had been a staple of the prehistoric Aleut spring diet. Peter and Heretina accompanied us to the Lagoon. It was an old tale to Peter, but Heretina had never searched for them before.

When we planned the outing, Peter had mentioned how rarely villagers gathered urchins or looked for clams, reputed to live in a curve of the Lagoon, in contrast to their habits when he was a lad. Idly, I asked why. The answer shocked me. "Because," said Peter in a matter-of-fact voice, "we Americanized now. Not work too hard." I preached for a quarter of an hour on the qualities of real Americanism, stressing industriousness and damning laziness and shiftlessness. How could my speech overcome the example paraded for seventy years until Americanization became synonymous with laziness?

Sam borrowed a rake. The rest of us were prepared to be Spartans and pick our shells from the icy water with bare hands. Sam seemed very superior, standing at ease raking while the rest of us waded back and forth bending ungracefully as we groped among the rocks. Heretina secured the only biscuit. In her excitement she stepped unwarily into a deep hole and was soaked exactly like the famous Doctor Foster. We rushed her home to dry clothes and realized she was already late for the Girl Scout meeting. So stern had Mrs. Hoverson been to her group that Heretina's teeth chattered more at the prospect of a scolding for being late than from her cold bath.

Peter had disappeared very quietly from the Lagoon. He came in about nine to explain why we found no urchins. Several villagers had been at the same spot just when the tide went out and had gathered several bushels. Peter's sure instinct had taken him from the cold water to George Kozloff's house where he had regaled himself on dozens of roes. With much ceremony he showed us how to slit our one lone urchin. Both Sam and I enjoyed the sweetish, rather clamlike flavor. It was still early in the season so it contained only a tiny cluster of eggs, hardly enough for a taste apiece. Later we found many of them on our walks, their brittle, spiny shells almost strained to the breaking point by the mass of eggs ready to be spawned.

We tried, too, on Peter's recommendation, to eat some dark curling seaweed that grew attached to the rocks. He called it sea lettuce or sea spinach in English. It could be eaten raw or cooked. The latter method I never tried. Fresh it tasted like nothing but the seawater it grew in.

The village men had little leisure that spring. They hunted more than other years because of food shortages caused by the *Penguin*'s failure to arrive. I liked best the red-legged kittiwake. It was much tenderer than either the puffin, the murre, or other gulls. Toward the end of May fresh eggs from owners of chickens were no longer available for Tobyanne. All eggs were being hatched so that the villagers might have chicken to eat if no boat reached us. We fed Tobyanne both murre and kittiwake eggs.

May 7, 1942
Alexandra came in from her name's-day party laden with tapioca pudding, coffee, Jell-O, pie—made of crowberries and very good—cookies and two kinds of cake. For two days people have been telling her and rejoicing that Washington had forbidden her to go with us. She had finally asked Elary who told her not to worry. Us she told last of all. She admitted this morning that some of the girls taunt her with being old fashioned because she does not go to the movies. There are other things but she seems reluctant to tell us. Sam thinks her reticence abnormal, a sign of indifference but I am not so sure. We told her to pay no attention to gossip and keep reiterating that if she learns to pronounce the alphabet by July 17 her going is assured.

Tuesday we did not go out in the morning because the weather was abominable early. I sterilized goods and kept Heretina busy—no, that was Monday that I kept her at work all day. And Tuesday morning we did go out. We drove up to Big Lake, stopped halfway along it and went down to Webster Beach and hiked toward Tolstoi, did not go quite to the rocky beach. Glorious morning after we got started. Stopped in at Vivian's and had coffee with her. Spent rest of morning at Gov. House exchanging books. Reading in afternoon and trying to find out more about shells. . . .

Monday a wire came from Mac with messages for most families and ours was "Tell Berenberg not to melt his collar about Alice," whatever

cont.

that means; we shall have to wait until the boat arrives, I guess.

May 11, 1942
I went to the greenhouse and plucked Swiss chard for supper. It was marvelous. I could have eaten tons of it. Something that did not come out of a can! Miraculously wonderful. Even the kids got excited over it.

Encountered Mrs. Hoverson there and stood around chatting. Mrs. Paul Merculieff and Julia were there watching her work so that they would know how to cope with their cold frame garden that they are starting. Mrs. H. said, "Alexandra is going to have a garden this year." I looked at Alexandra with a smile and said, "Oh, yes, Paul told me about it." Alexandra had enough humor to smile and wink back at me. The cold frame is being made of our borrowed storm windows that Paul is sneaking up surreptitiously from our cellar. Mrs. H.'s sense of decorum would be scandalized at such laxity with government property. So will we be if some kids break the glass and we have no storm windows if we stay another year.

Both were delicious. We only tasted them because they were too rare for mere adults.

As food shortages increased the baby's diet became exotic. To avoid the coarse and very ancient oatmeal from island stocks when her special infant cereal supply was gone, her seabird eggs were stirred into imported whole Irish oatmeal that a doting aunt had sent her.

Many food items were gone by the middle of May. Reindeer meat became monotonous. The sealers suffered most, since both Canteen and government stores were depleted. No one arranged to get them reindeer meat. So the men hunted more assiduously. They went out every dawn to lean over the cliffs with long-handled nets to scoop up the delectable little *choochkies* [*chuuchiix̂*], mere mouthfuls of food when the feathers were removed but the most delicate of all the game birds. It seemed almost cannibalistic to eat the auklets who were so charming and friendly.

On the first of June, Hoverson ordered the hunters to surrender their guns, for the nesting season was under way. The men grumbled and complied. I wondered how long the habits of obedience to officials would survive unless a boat were to bring us food soon.

Chapter 41

Southwest Point lies five or six miles west of Zapadni salt house. *Seethah* [*siitxaaĝux̂*], the Aleuts called the spot, according to Elliott.[1] Seals and sea lions, which had been resorting there, deserted the peninsula after 1884. Approachable only by water or on foot, the land distance depended upon the route chosen. It was much shorter to cut back behind the Zapadni camp house, skirt the loaflike mound of Kleba, and pass across the low inland slope of Ridge Wall. Along this route the tall dark ferns rattled under our feet. When we lifted the dead overgrowth we found the tiny curls of new ferns unfolding.

The more pleasant path was along the cliffs. It meant stout tramping along Antone Lake, jumping from one grass hummock to another, to emerge at Kursoolah to greet the always snarling sea that washed that grim bit of the coast. The narrow path used by fox trappers and bird hunters ran upwards as the land flowed toward the enormous tumulus of a dead volcanic giant prosaically christened Ridge Wall by Elliott. As spring colored the land, the lower portion was painted a light glowing green, the arched lid a stark mahogany brown where no vegetation found root among the coarse reddish brown cinders. From the sea path we ran down into the little dell where Whitney Pond or Botanist Pool lay serenely, nurturing the delicate yellow anemone, two species of *Arenaria,* the mountain goldthread, and the Unalaskan *Arnica,* flowers found nowhere else on the island.

A mile beyond Ridge Wall the landscape altered. Nameless miniature volcanic cones stood like toys along the way. Two vents lay side by side separated by a narrow stone bridge. Their wide mouths were choked with snow when we first saw them. Beyond the craters, a broad strip of loose untidy rock, over half a mile wide, extended inland nearly a mile. Over it one walked as on a bed of spears. No matter how the earth tortured our feet, it was impossible to resist the weird beauty of the spot. Here was the island's face when the last downpour of lava cinders had cooled, the last thunderous note of rock smashing upon rock, splitting and shattering against each other, had been carried far off to sea on the wind. Here was the island before soil was made. The stark bones of the earth, grey, brown, red, and black, were not grim. Even half veiled with lacy fog or blending into the violet

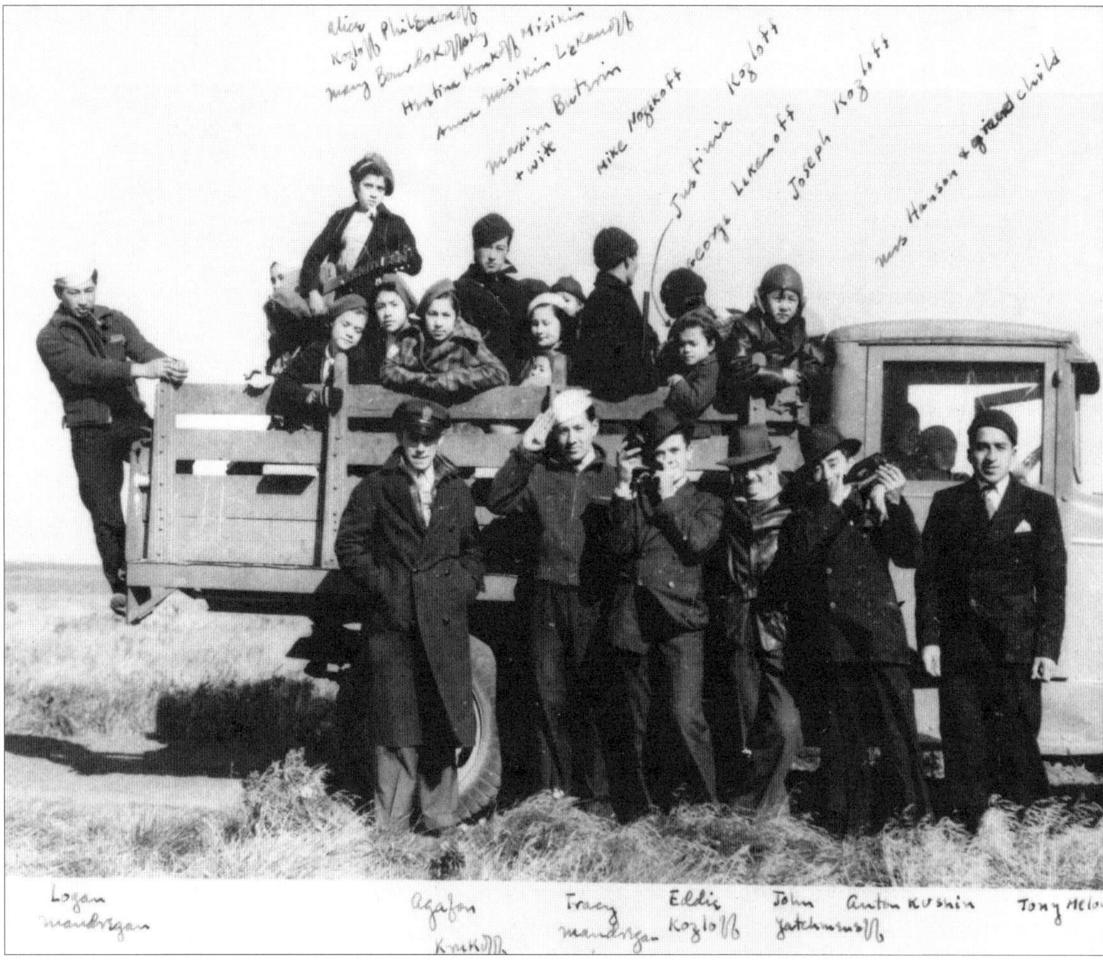

St. Paul people ready for an outing (from the Martin Collection, USUAF210, Archives, Alaska and Polar Regions, Rasmuson Library, University of Alaska Fairbanks).

dusk, as I last saw the field, there was no desolation, no forbidding gloom. The soft whisper of the wind was freshened by the calls of the rosy finches and snow buntings.

The cliff edge at Southwest Point had the ragged serrations of a battered old saw. Its broken face offered thousands of ledges and shelves to the nesting seabirds and housed the largest colony of the island. California murres and red-legged kittiwake shared the region between them. We approached just after dawn on the first of May. At a distance, the projecting seawall was a patchwork of dark rock and unmelted snow. Then the firm wall crumbled into a twirling landslide of black and white fragments. Thousands of murres had followed a leader into the air, leaving the stone cliff grey. They settled in the sea and then as suddenly they began to wheel back. One by one a black and white section was fitted into the pattern until the cliff resumed its bicolored appearance. The murres, called the penguins of the northern seas, are pretentious and comic on land. Standing motionless, staring out to sea, they looked interested in life. But other equally solemn preoccupied fellows gazed into the stone an inch or so from their beaks. The sea viewers were respectable little gentlemen in evening dress with gleaming white shirt fronts. The white rumps of those who turned their backs on the world protruded from under their glossy black coats like disarranged shirttails. I waited expectantly for one of the stuffed shirts to clear his throat and begin, "Ladies and gentlemen."

Murres are skillful divers and swimmers under water. Although their wings beat the air too frantically for graceful flight, they are swift fliers. But on their nesting platforms they are as awkward as sailors fresh from a long voyage. These grave and somber birds create jeweled eggs, marble white, creamy ecru, or aquamarine shell etched with writing scrolls of chocolate brown.

The Kochutin family early staked a claim on the wedge-shaped peninsula of Southwest Point as their own hunting and berrying province. Old Jake, the patriarch of the family, built his barabara so deep underground that the one trapdoor entrance was level with the earth. The barabara, long overgrown and lost, figured in local history because Jake's brother Condrat Kochutin fell and broke his leg near the shore while gathering weed in a fierce snowstorm. Jake carried him to the hut and hurried back to the village for help. When the resources arrived Condrat was dead. During the First World War, a government official recorded the rediscovery of the barabara site with great elation. Once more its location has slipped into obscurity.

Another reputed charm of the neighborhood of Jake's barabara was the waterfall. We heard much from the sealers of its sparkling delicious water that they had always been accustomed to bring back in bottles as a treat for their wives. Elary Gromoff was most lavish in his description of the water "gushing" from the rocky face of a cliff and "dashing" into the sea. Reality was more prosaic: a mediocre little spring oozing from the slope of a hill quite far from shore. When I confronted

Elary with the evidence of my own eyes, he defended his word choice by saying, "Well, it runs. Isn't that so?"

Accidentally, cutting across country to Southwest Point one Sunday morning, we came out to the shore at High Bluffs. We had been led astray by the hide-and-seek antics of a mother reindeer who unwittingly induced us to follow her. We found her velvet black newborn fawn curled in a nest of grass. Even his large brilliant liquid eyes remained still. We took a hasty photograph and hurried away before we gave his mother too much anxiety. We scurried up a hill and looked back to see her rejoin her baby. When we were tired of watching her nuzzle the fawn, we started on heedlessly and there we were at the brink of the highest cliffs looking at the sea 380 feet below. Elliott's maps called the bluffs *Einahnuhto,* and later mapmakers repeated the spelling; actually the Aleut word meaning "the place of bluffs" is *iganatok.*[2] Elliott translated his phrase incorrectly as the three mammae [breasts].[3] The islanders must have been playing tricks on him.

May 16, 1942
We followed the rim of the second crater until we came to the old wooden Russian cross, which is supposed to be placed on the highest point. I secured a lichen from the cross, a pretty lichen-covered stone from its foundation, and dug up a lovely *Pedicularis arctica* to give Father Baranoff from that site. On the inner side of the crater the wind was very sharp but on the eastern outer slope we stepped into a warm world. The sun was tantalizing us by showing its shape clearly in the sky and diffusing a yellow glow to the sky and the fog but it refused to come out and lay the world beneath our feet bare to our curious gaze. We sat down on the soft mats of *Empetrum nigrum* and moss and relaxed above the clouds as it were.

Both of us feel that this morning was not only the most thrilling experience on the island of its kind, but one of the finest spiritual and poetic moods we have known. It is impossible to recapture the magic in this diary.

On the abrupt cruel face of Einahnuhto the red-legged kittiwakes were courting. On even the very tiniest grass-covered projections a loving couple nestled side by side, caressing each other with dainty yellow bills. The murmurs of love from the multitude blended sweetly with the sea song at the cliff's feet. The crimson splendor of their legs and feet lent a piquant gypsy note to their delicate grey Quaker garb.

We left the kittiwake to their lovemaking and crossed the lower rolling ridges of Rush Hill, named for the old revenue cutter. The island's tallest cone, it is only about 655 feet high. The Aleuts call it *Iganatok Kaya* or "hill of the bluff place." Halfway up its slope we rested and looked down upon the camp house and lake of the broad plain called Tsammana, once the hunting domain of the Hanson family.

The origin of the name Tsammana has been a puzzle for many years. Attempts to anglicize the word into "Tasmania" were ridiculed by the native Aleuts although they could not interpret the mutilated word in their own speech. The combined study of Nekifer Mandregan and John Yatchmeneff was able to produce a likely etymology because Nekifer had retained the memory of a more understandable Aleut version of the name, roughly transliterated as *Chmanangan*. The phrase depicted the chase by baidarka after a sea animal endeavoring to keep up with him. The name may stem from a hunter's account of an exciting sea pursuit of an animal from the early village at Zapadni to what is at present best known as Tsammana.

Over the fields hundreds of reindeer accompanied by their fawns were grazing among the dry grasses. The air was filled with their maternal conversation. The fathers were absent, traveling in small groups in search of richer feeding grounds. From Zapadni Headland to Northeast Point the land belongs to itself except during foxing season and brief visits of hunters and, very rarely, a sightseeing official. The reindeer mother feels confident and at ease in the loneliness.

Between Tsammana and Marunich the shores curve into the daintiest sand coves, encircled by sickles of bright jet walls wondrously ornamented. Caves and graceful small arches are frequent. Small headlands built up of blocks of various colored basalt afford good nesting platforms for the cormorants. Near Marunich the hair seals breed in May in the kelp beds among the reefs. Huge colonies of mussels cling to the tide-deserted rocks.

On the maps, Lake Hill seemed a single summit, mounting up gradually from a very broad base. We climbed the cross-crowned slope that faced Little Polovina Hill one morning, treading carefully over the mats of magenta saxifrage, the red and green leafed *Chrysosplenium beringianum* and the opening eyes of the dwarf forget-me-not. On the rocky escarpment we realized that we had merely topped a ridge that spread out into a region filled with hollows and rises until it joined the low spurs of Bogoslof. Wandering among the hillocks we found numerous lakes left by the snows, insignificant pools to inspire the hill's name.

Climbing Bogoslof was bracing and provocative. The litter of boulders offered the least stable footing we had encountered. Every few moments the *kugans* [demons] of the place threatened to tip us back down the hill, straight to the hospital. Not only the earth was hostile. The sky seemed bent on annoying us. Most of the island was drenched in sunlight. One large purple cloud, propelled by a wind paced to match our strides, pursued us. Hurry as we would to get from under it and reach the sun-warmed air ahead, the wind outwitted us. The rim of the cloud kept just ahead of us and spat down a fine chilling rain, the more chilling because we were lightly clad. Up to the very coronet of the summit the cloud accompanied us. Then it withdrew to the west and left us to dry on our high rocky perch.

Bogoslof is holy ground because the seismic powers thrust it first above the seas. From it burst the floods of lava on which the island rested. Its sides are scarred with more open fissures and cracks than other hills as a result of its creative efforts. *Bogoslof* means literally "word of God," but in Russian the term is used only as a name for St. John the Evangelist. A favorite saint of the Russians, they dedicated many Alaskan place names to him, including the newest island in

May 16, 1942
We followed the rim of the second crater until we came to the old wooden Russian cross, which is supposed to be placed on the highest point. I secured a lichen from the cross, a pretty lichen-covered stone from its foundation, and dug up a lovely *Pedicularis arctica* to give Father Baranoff from that site. On the inner side of the crater the wind was very sharp but on the eastern outer slope we stepped into a warm world. The sun was tantalizing us by showing its shape clearly in the sky and diffusing a yellow glow to the sky and the fog but it refused to come out and lay the world beneath our feet bare to our curious gaze. We sat down on the soft mats of *Empetrum nigrum* and moss and relaxed above the clouds as it were.

Both of us feel that this morning was not only the most thrilling experience on the island of its kind, but one of the finest spiritual and poetic moods we have known. It is impossible to recapture the magic in this diary.

May 16, 1942
Vikenty Melovidoff (*Kawah* [*qawax̌*], or Sea Lion to his friends) is the fat, jovial bachelor (which makes him conspicuous around here) who drives the village truck (ashes, garbage, coal, etc.) and when the Canteen has supplies keeps the dashboard case and his pockets stuffed with candy bars and carries a few dozen bottles of pop beside him. He had been hunting at Southwest Point since yesterday afternoon and came home

cont.

the Bering, the quietest, safest refuge of the sea lions.

The Bogoslof of St. Paul, with its two stately coronets encircling the two central craters, deserves the appellation. Simeon Nozekoff, a charming old gentleman from his picture, had told Father Baranoff an interesting legend about the old hill. His story had a definite aroma of a Russian missionary's exhortation. In the beginning when God created the world, he decided to reserve one small portion of it as a gift for the people who proved most devoted to him and faithful in performing religious duties. So, up from the bottom of the sea God lifted the Pribilof Islands, first St. Paul and then St. George. The first land that emerged above the water was the hill named Bogoslof because it rose in response to the word of God.

Then God sent the fur seals to the islands. The English, the Dutch, and the Spaniards sent exploring parties north in search of the fur seal's home. Whenever their boats neared the islands God drew veils of fog around them and the seekers passed by. At last came the Russians. God reached out and pulled aside the fog veils and permitted them to land because of all the people of the earth the Russians were the most devout and obedient children of God. It hardly seems credible that the enslaved Aleuts considered their masters so worthy of God's gift.

The Aleuts called the peak *Machdasuk* or the "hill of the two breasts." I checked and rechecked all possible informants lest I repeat Elliott's error.[4] It seems a most befitting term to be applied to the matrix of the island.

The snow clung late to the hollows on Bogoslof, hiding the entrance to the underground chambers that have won undue repute because they form the only sizable cave on the whole island. The cavern is dangerous to invade. Its walls are not hollowed out of some immense sedimentary stable rock. It is an accidental arrangement of space left open when the mighty basalt blocks toppled down upon one another from their brief skyward flight. The ceilings of the compartments are composed of loosely piled, easily dislodged slabs.

On our first trip to Bogoslof the coarse cinders teemed with crowds of passing green and gold armored beetles, glittering magnificently in the sun. Snow buntings and rosy finches were singing courtship melodies. Their mating calls and the wooing entreaties of the Pribilof sandpipers down the slope trilled liltingly above the deep grumble of herds of reindeer strung along the lower reaches of the hill.

Long ago Elary's foster parents, Julia Gromoff and her husband Nicolai, who came from Attu, had set up a cross on the crest. Nicolai was famed for finding a real mastodon tusk on North Point, although he brought home only a fragment of it that the family lost long ago. He had been dead for years but Julia, old but hale, owning the solemnest face in the village, seemed almost as ageless as the rocks. Yet it is inevitable that the weathered old cross, tipped to one side but still wedged in its rocky crevice, will survive more winters than she.

From Telegraph Hill almost to Lake Hill the long red and grey stone barricade of Kamenisti sweeps in a gradual curve. The series of walls and narrow glens were formed when the arching roofs of huge volcanic tunnels collapsed. The lava segments of the roofs sprawled down the sides of the gorges in bewildering complex compositions. Rock poised on rock in haphazard design. It seemed as if a breath could topple the perilously poised boulders that weighed hundreds of pounds.

In the crannies the flowers had settled. Mosses and mantles of *Empetrum* softened the sharp edges of rough scoria chunks. The ferns loved the cool damp clefts. In the winding alleys it was possible only to look upward at the face of the sky. Even the wind could not steal along the passages. I think I learned in the heart of Kamenisti what the phrase "absolute quiet" means.

with lots of Pacific and red-legged kittiwakes. He stopped by to show them to us. Sam asked him for the skin to a Pacific one and wings and feet of the red-legged. He brought the former and the legs of the latter while we were at the fire [in the machine shop].
I am disappointed because I wanted to compare the wings of the two close at hand but I think we may be able to get a hunter to give us wings of the latter yet, before the season is over. He did not remove the contents of the head so John Hanson can do that for us Monday. He is scheduled to come and skin *Nictea nictea* [*scandiaca*], the large white owl that Dan Krukoff shot on Reef night before last and that some kids brought us.
He is certainly a magnificent animal. It is hard to think of the dead mass of soft fuzzy, almost furry, feathers as belonging to a creature of the sky. I would certainly like to see one in flight.

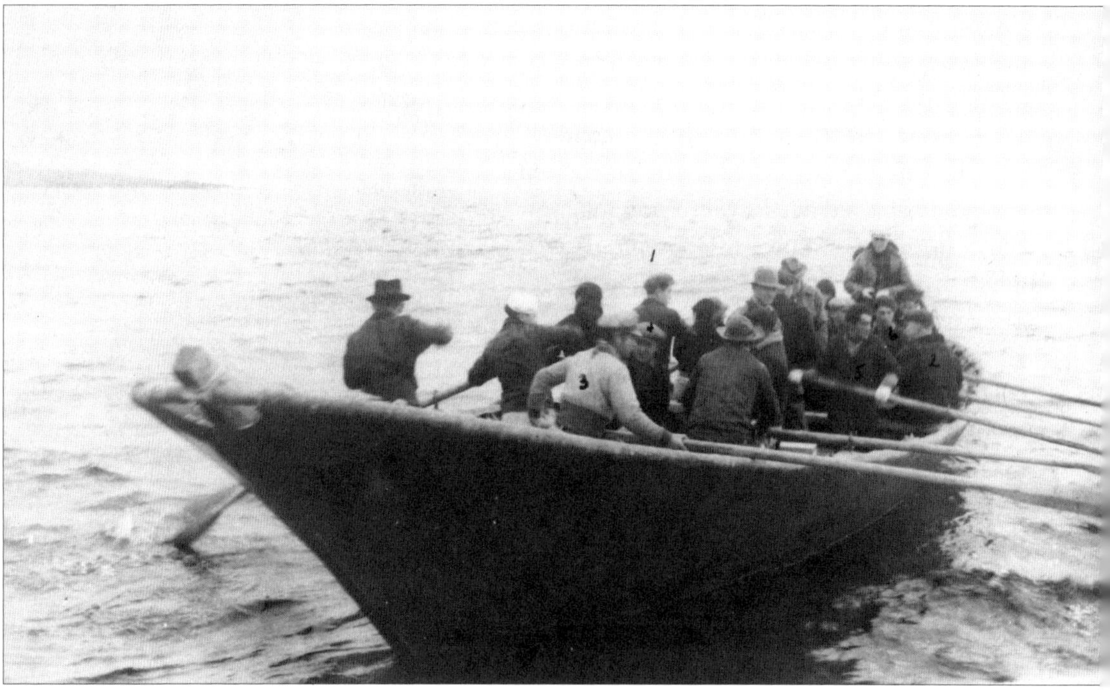

A St. Paul baidar (from the Martin Collection, USUAF210, Archives, Alaska and Polar Regions, Rasmuson Library, University of Alaska Fairbanks).

Chapter 42

May 20 passed but no *Penguin* came with the other returning birds. Only a telegram arrived ordering Hoverson to start sealing at the usual time with knives. Interpreted, the order meant, since no outside workmen will be there to blubber skins, kill only as many seals as the local men can flense each day.

The loss of a date to expect the outside world to end our six months' complete isolation aroused a wave of superstition in the village. One woman, perhaps merely furnishing her husband an island version of being kept late at the office, came home at dawn with a tale of a woman dressed in flowing blue draperies walking the waters of the lagoon. Overcome by her vision, the stay-out had fallen to the ground and lain unconscious nearly the night through. Some believed her tale and forecast dire events. Others scoffed at her attempts to hoodwink her husband. Children dreaded evenings. Even the dark shadows in the cellars concealed lurking ghosts. Just after the day Japan announced the abrogation of the sealing treaty, wakeful folk heard the thrum of motor launches in Zolotoi Bay.[1] One wishful thinker, shortly before the twentieth, had excited the village by declaring he had heard the *Penguin* offshore during the night and had heard familiar voices, such as Stitt's deep-throated cursing, and the rattling of pots and pans in the

May 19, 1942
No walk today. I tried to waken Sam but he couldn't make it. I have nothing fresh to recount but I thought I might as well jot down a few notes about a couple of conversations I had recently–if I can remember any of the quirks.

The first was with George Lekanof, the carpenter. He was repairing the bed in the upstairs room while I was attending to my flowers. I mean he was repairing the window. I asked him whether the old man whom Baranoff had been telling me about as the best character on St. George who died last year, a man who never drank, was a good influence in the community, etc., of whom there are no duplicates on either island. I had come across documents pertaining to the man, Stephan Lekanof, last week. He was first mentioned when the agent of St. George wrote his chief on St. Paul announcing the arrival of Fr. [Innokentii]

cont.

Lestenkof and family and a male servant. A few years later there is a request to the St. Paul agent to confirm the servant's appointment as sealer and in parentheses is the phrase "priest's slave." At one other time Father L. was fined fifty dollars for not reporting the fact that this Stephan Lekanof had killed a seal pup and brought it to the priest's house where he was living. Stephan got off with a light punishment. George said his father had been that famous man, that he thought his father's father had been a ship captain, that his mother had married and come to St. George . . . and that he had come as a servant of the priest in order to get on the island and eventually gain permission to be a permanent resident. I do not know just when or by what means that exceedingly rare privilege was given him.

May 22, 1942

I completed a great deal of proofreading, particularly the notes of Elliott and some flower notes. In the afternoon I tended our garden, planted some more seeds, cabbage and spinach, and gathered a lot of Swiss chard and French chicory for supper.

To bed rather late and I could not rouse Sam at five when the alarm went off. So it was after six of a brilliant sunshiny day when we started out. We drove down the Marunich Road. Almost to the end. We loitered along, getting out to examine any suspicious bit of color that might be budding flowers or blossoms but we found nothing but two

cont.

galley. Stories after the *Penguin* failed to arrive were more gloomy, vague yarns about ghosts and Devil's Fires flickering over the land and sea.

Elary had been nervous and depressed for several weeks, seeking medical advice frequently and finally requesting Sam to sanction his absence from church services. Evidently he felt a doctor's permission might not be sufficiently holy, for Father Baranoff told us the ending of the story. Elary asked to be excused from church because his sister-in-law had "looked at him funny" during choir practice. Elary felt he could not remain in the choir stall near her and permit her to harm him with the "Evil Eye." Father knew the woman had been admitted to the hospital that morning for treatment of an infection involving one side of her face. One eye had been nearly swollen shut before she came to the dispensary and undoubtedly she did wear a menacing leer. Father handled Elary firmly. "Nonsense," he had informed him, "You cannot stay away from the church when you are well. You are not in the choir anyway. You are the psalm reader. The choir stands here. You stand there. You just sing your psalms and nothing will happen to you." Elary meekly surrendered.

The villagers busied themselves practically, despite natural anxieties and fears. Almost every household started a cold-frame garden. Every removable storm window frame was commandeered for them.

On the last day of May we took Vikenty Melovidoff, nicknamed *Kawah,* the "sea lion," because of his bulky body nourished in ordinary times with an enormous number of candy bars, on our outing to Marunich. The Gromoffs, John Hapoff and his wife, and some young boys were camping in the cottage. Their game bags were full, principally of red-legged kittiwakes. The ban against shooting birds was to go into effect at midnight and almost everyone able to stand up straight was out hunting.

We drove through the old car ruts that skirted Marunich Hill toward Tsammana until we tired of being bruised in the rough tracks. We loitered on the beach collecting pumice chips and shells and teasing some foxes who were yelping at us to leave and permit them to continue their feast of bloated sea lion carcasses. We went inland and began to climb Crater Hill. Halfway up the slope, Sam asked me whether I saw something unusual in the water off Tsammana. I thought I saw a dark vertical line like a mast but I could not be certain. We lamented the glasses that we had forgotten. We watched a long time but the line remained so motionless that we decided the impression of a ship offshore was an illusion due to our war-fevered imaginations. I still thank the afternoon fog that saved me from a terrified race back to the village to Tobyanne. We climbed to the top, fighting the wind. A wall of haphazard blocks encircled the rim of the very deep crater. An arched opening, as symmetrical as a cathedral window, strengthened the impression that man and not nature had assembled the rampart unlike the crest of any other island.

While we had rambled on Crater Hill, Vikenty had slain twenty-five kittiwakes. Our only trophy was the first spring bloom of saxifrage. As we drove into the main street children ran to us calling, "Ship. Ship." It had just pulled into Zolotoi and Hoverson and some sealers were just drawing alongside as we reached the brow of the cliff. Our dark mast had been no phantom. It was an American patrol boat putting in for repairs. Its crew were just as nervous about approaching land

tiny lupine with a few flowers opening through their thick wooly veils. Reindeer were scattered all over the landscape and we sat in the car and watched them. . . .

The landscape of the island is peculiarly shaded just now. There is but an occasional patch of moss or foliage that is a real vivid triumphant green of spring. But underneath the sere, recumbent grasses of last year, there is the faint glimmer of struggling grasses reaching up to the air. Close to such grassy areas the new blades are visible, a good hearty green piercing the mat of dead grass . . .

Rumors about the *Penguin* fill the air. Half a dozen people have heard the engines. One person heard the clatter of pots and pans in the galley. But nothing has been heard over the air. So the imaginations of the villagers run riot while we all wait tensely for visitors, mail, and more food.

May 27, 1942
Monday afternoon I went upstairs with *The Timeless Land* to read and rest. . . . Gradually I felt myself falling asleep. But before I could slide away into complete unconsciousness, I heard Sam's hasty feet on the stairs. He looked fairly normal when he entered, just the faintest tinge of excitement. "Sorry to wake you up, but I thought you would like to know the worst."

Carl had just received a wire from Seattle signed by Johnston that began with orders for sealing to commence at the regular time, that the

cont.

seals were to be skinned with a knife instead of the instrument pullers. (The instruments pull off so much fat that such skins must be blubbered on the islands but those removed by knife leave enough blubber on to ensure saving them by salting so that they can be shipped without spoiling.) The final order of the telegram read, "Repair damaged scow at first opportunity."

Translated into reality that fatal line reads—"Something has happened to the *Penguin*. It is safely back in Seattle and as soon as we can get space in the shipyard we will get it repaired and try to get up there by the end of the sealing season at least to pick up the skins."

Maybe. So, no food, no mail, no visitors, no fresh contact with the outside world. The war has made us prisoners at last. Until now we have had hopes, but we dare not hope longer. If the *Penguin* gets into the harbor we shall believe it but not before.

The worse immediate scarcity is the lack of tobacco. The few fragments of tobacco for pipes disappeared from the Canteen before yesterday noon. But I had Sam there before anyone else and he got five packages of pipe tobacco and I am smoking a pipe mainly myself and hoarding every crumb of my Target. Butts are carefully treasured for rerolling. It will be more wearing here to be without smokes than in Spain because of the emptiness of things. Tension over nothing. Petty discomfort. Reindeer meat and seal meat and our own vegetables. And then what next? No

cont.

as shore watchers were at its appearance. Hoverson asked the captain why the crew met him bristling with weapons and why the cannon was pointed toward the island boat. "How the hell did I know if the Japs had landed here or not?" the captain retorted.

In vain the Aleut Village Committee had pleaded with the acting agent to permit evacuation of women and children from the [immediate vicinity of the] village until we knew more of the military situation to the south of us. In vain they pleaded with him to remove stores of food and gasoline from the conspicuous storage depots. He was too timid to act without orders from Washington. But he permitted the men to remove a few barrels of gasoline.

We had begun to dig a deep cave in the scoria bank behind the house, between the hospital and our residence, as a shelter for the patients. At our written request Hoverson, who considered us overanxious, assigned workmen to help finish it. Tempers might have flared nastily but we joked about "Berenberg's Folly" and maintained surface affability.

The Village Committee, perturbed by Hoverson's seemingly casual assumption that nothing could possibly happen, held an unsupervised meeting. They decided to post guards that very night before securing Hoverson's approval at the formal meeting the next evening. At dawn the guards woke Hoverson to report a ship in the distance. His waking reaction was that the men had been on the cliffs netting auklets out of season and began to berate them. The guards answered his accusations with the announcement that they were watchmen appointed by the committee. Hoverson accepted the fait accompli very gracefully for which I admired him. At the official meeting that night he agreed to let night guards have time off from work to sleep in the morning.

Most of the uneasiness arose, not from the reports of the Aleutian raids,[2] but principally from the manner in which the news was handled by the American radio commentators. One day an unnamed spokesman in the nation's capital announced that the Japanese did not possess even a barren rock off the coast of Alaska. The next came news of Attu's seizure. The villagers of Attu were friends and relatives of the sealers. Most of the Attu men came each summer to St. Paul. We knew them, too. The war became too horribly real as we worried about them.

On the afternoon of June 10 we listened to a rationalization of the situation in Lavrenty Sedick's hospital room. Workmen from all nearby jobs had sneaked in to listen. We heard the speaker belittle the loss of Attu, just a barren island, the loneliest place this side of hell and inhabited by only about seventy-five Eskimos. Lavrenty finally voiced the thought in every mind: "If they don't even know in the States what kind of people live in this part of the world, I guess they'll never get here in time to save us."

As danger seemed closer, the Aleut morale became better. Fewer ghosts were seen. No phantom boats were heard. Everyone realized the possible threat, our helplessness in case of either an air raid or a landing party. They were calm with the quietude of people who can expect the worst and be brave in accepting the unavoidable. They wanted only one thing from befuddled officials, the maximum protective measures against air-raid damage. They reasoned that if people in the Middle West were having air-raid practice, a small island neighboring an active military zone should certainly take precautions to prevent casualties. The responsible officials were unable to give leadership and confidence. They comforted themselves, even after Dutch Harbor, that Japan had too much to do in the south Pacific to continue attacking Alaska.

It seemed sensible to us as well as to the Aleuts to prepare against the one chance that a stray Japanese bomber might slip past the American patrol planes

chance to get new clothes for Tobyanne for the winter. She needs vitamin C we can't get here. And her pills are nearly gone. A multitude of minor complaints.

But we are wasting no time on regrets.

May 31, 1942

Nikifer told me that a few years ago when a naval vessel was here that carried a seaplane, the officer in charge came out and rowed about Big Lake and said it would be excellent for landings. That the largest sea planes could make it. How many individuals have taken soundings there and yet the legend persists that no planes could land here, which is nonsense and ordinary planes could even land on our road out along Polovina flats very easily. But still we are isolated from the world by bureaucratic stupidity and inertia and indifference. If the Japs come near, the overlords of our destiny will sit back and wring their hands and shed crocodile tears over our fate when they might have taken the whole damn population off by plane—from both islands, in less than twenty-four hours.

June 4, 1942
The cheerful sound of picks and shovels blends with the tapping of my keys. Three workmen and Sam and Moran Kochergin are delving into the scoria bank outside the window. Part of the deep trench they are digging extends behind our house, with more than two-thirds of it extending over toward the hospital. The first and only air-raid shelter is being erected on St. Paul. Sam's hands are blistered and taped and yet he swings with a hearty rhythm that tends to melt some of the habitual resistance of the workmen to rapid labor. So in a couple of days we ought to have a very good shelter dug into the hill. . . .

The boys of the village are most interested. The crowd of youthful spectators keeps growing and Sam finds errands and tasks for them. Such occupation has dampened the enthusiasm of some of the spectators already but fresh victims keep coming.

Yesterday when the news about Dutch Harbor's being bombed at six a.m. reached us we appealed once more to Carl Hoverson to take some action for the community's safety. We begged him to evacuate the women and children at least if only to the watch houses on the various sealing grounds and hunting points. He said there was not enough room, being fussy about overcrowding suddenly. And said despairingly that there was not even a place to take the food. But he stubbornly insisted that he did not think they would ever come here. Hellbaum came in as we were talking to him and

cont.

and spitefully wreck our exposed village. The calm, reasonable proposals of the Aleut men, their initiative, and their composure when they realized their appointed leaders were weak and irresolute made us feel more keenly the tragedy of their lives. We acquired a new admiration for the people whose inner spirit was so valiantly indestructible. Members of the Service colony spoke romantically of dying for their country if the Japanese bombed the village. I contrasted their maudlin fatalism with the more vigorous attitude of the sealers who said, "It ain't being killed but I'd like to take a Jap with me." I had no difficulty in deciding who were the best Americans.

Meanwhile, as tense days dragged by, with officials' tempers fraying rapidly, we went ahead with our preparations for the people directly under our care in the hospital. We drilled our patients, making them march out to the shelter when a plane was heard. Hoverson, as a sop to the committee, offered sacks for sand that each family might build its own shelters. Evlampia Bourdukofsky, so anxious to emulate a naval man that he wore a sailor hat constantly and always led the other boys in military games, built his personal shelter near a road and asked a chauffeur to drive a heavy truck over it to test its strength. He even ran an electric cord from his house, providing a real touch of luxury. Others began to seriously dig their foxholes.

June 13 the whole family and Alice went to Marunich. Sam spent the morning nailing bars across a bunk to make a crib for the baby. The bombing of Dutch Harbor, the exposed location of the village, the lack of local preparations for safety had influenced us to make our own refuge for the baby. The next morning I planned to return with the baby, Alice, and Heretina and cleaning supplies, bedding, and food. We were going to camp out cozily in the little cottage so inconspicuous among the grassy knolls.

We were sharing the small car with Stacy. Sam was supposed to drive them back to the village at five. In the afternoon he accompanied me almost to Tsammana. I hated to turn back and suggested he take the Stacys to the village, return for Alice and the baby, and pick me up at Zapadni instead of Marunich.

After he left I prowled along the shore, roamed through the fields of Tsammana, peeking into the little hunting shacks there. The multiple peaks of Rush or *Iganatok,* bare and clear in the evening sunshine, tempted me. We had never climbed to the summit. I decided to scale it alone. I raced over the rough meadows, leaping madly from one hummock to the next to reach the top before the sunlight vanished. There was no time to waste looking for the easiest ascent. I started right up the nearest and steepest slope of cinders. Chunks of tuff flew like frightened birds from under my feet. I started hundreds of minor landslides. The closer I came to the top the more insecure the footing. Behind me, out of nowhere a legion of dark clouds was massing. The winds began to gather for an attack. The clouds and I reached the narrow rim of the summit together. The wind nearly threw me right over the edge. The cold rain and wind pushed and pummeled me. At times as I fought my way around the edges of the craters, I knelt and crawled to avoid being toppled down the hill. There were gaps in the clouds though which I could catch glimpses of the island in many directions. Each hill reminded me of a pleasant outing. The landscape had never seemed more beautiful. I loved the island more intensely than ever, every spiny rock that pricked my feet when I explored its reaches, every muddy flat as well as its lovely stone hills, its flowering extravagance, its great animal and bird pageant, and its people.

When I finally tore myself unwillingly from the hilltop I came down to a lovely meadow spangled with primroses and buttercups. I hurried, for dusk was coming swiftly from the water. Midway across the stony meadow I saw a figure

became very belligerent about his viewpoint that this is the safest place in the world to be, and even safer in the afternoon of June 3 because there had been the attack on Dutch Harbor, which would have the naval and Army commanders aroused and their attention drawn to such forgotten arrears as ours. I was so nauseated by his pigheaded insistence that I wanted to get away. "The Japs have been very logical up to now and have never bombed a place unnecessarily," he declared. "Show me a place they have bombed that has not been of importance to their plans."

I mentioned the hundreds of Chinese mud-housed villages and he brushed that away: "Oh, maybe once." He, of course, has a complete understanding of Japan's intentions, objectives, etc. His ridiculous cocksureness bolsters up Carl's inertia although Carl was willing to admit that he would not go so far as to say that they would not come here. They might but it is not likely. And so the normal precautions that are being carried on in most inland parts of America are ignored here.

June 4, 1942
Peter told us this morning that the Aleuts had been watching all night and we supposed that Carl had succumbed enough to our sensible request that at least a watch be kept for planes, that a signal warning be devised, and that people should be told how to act. But after I started typing this, Gabe came over and informed us that he was the one who utilized his police force for the night watch. He is a man. He feels responsible for his people and while he has not enough strong men to back him up in getting action, he and a few others on their own will do what they can. At one thirty they roused him to report the boat and he was up for over an hour. We might have slept had we known it. That he has posted guards. Furthermore, he offered to cooperate with us in any way we asked as far as the village committee can.

Carl has assigned four men for hospital aides when a plane comes. They are to come for instructions later this afternoon. Andronik Oustigoff came in to get a cut hand dressed this afternoon and when I went in to take care of him, he remarked that it was awful lonesome around here at night with the radio cut off. But KGEI came back on the air a little after one so maybe he will have company tonight.

Stacy came over to inspect what was going on. I asked him whether he had come to take a picture of Berenberg's Folly. . . . The pit is finished. Dorofey Merculieff has the measurements for the lumber

cont.

standing on the center of Ridge Wall, a tiny figure that began to descend in my direction, waving. I waved back. Then I caught the outline of a visored cap so I ceased to wave so enthusiastically. Sam wore nothing but a stocking cap. The Aleuts who wore such hats came rarely so far from the village once hunting was over.

Then I was stupefied with bewilderment because the figure that was blending with the dark background of the hill began to signal. Blocks of white appeared and disappeared. I could just get the suggestion of moving arms. Too much war thought made melodrama natural. Who could behave so peculiarly, wigwagging in the Pribilof dusk, but an enemy intruder? I slowed my pace and began to walk more and more toward my left, inland. The figure changed direction, too, and wigwagged more frantically. If, I thought, two landing parties have come in, one at Zapadni and one on the deserted coast somewhere behind me, the scouts might plan to meet midway.

It was silly to try to run away. The ground was too uneven for speed, the nearest hill too far to hide my flight. I assumed if a Japanese scout found he faced a woman, he might be scornful and off guard long enough to permit me to kick him in a vulnerable spot and then knock him in the head with a rock. Rehearsing my little drama, I kept trudging forward. The gathering darkness delayed recognition as we neared each other. Then the man took off his cap and I saw Sam's face and heard him shout, "The Navy is going to evacuate us tomorrow. Hurry up. We have to pack." And then he added crossly, "Why the hell were you trying to run away? I nearly broke my arms signaling." For a long while I could only laugh with relief. The cap that had inspired my fears belonged to Peter, waiting in the car at Zapadni.[3]

My next reaction was to thank the *kugans* who had lured me to *Iganatok*'s summit before the war expelled us from the island.

and knows where some good stuff is out near the Point that would be excellent. I have been out to test the sitting qualities of the place. It should hold thirty sitting, a few less if some are laid out straight . . .

About one o'clock Vivian Oberg heard a listening-post voice saying, "Six bombers coming north. Six bombers coming north. Six bombers coming north. Go up and meet them, boys." Or, "Six bombers from the north." Alice delivered the message and we are not sure of her memory.

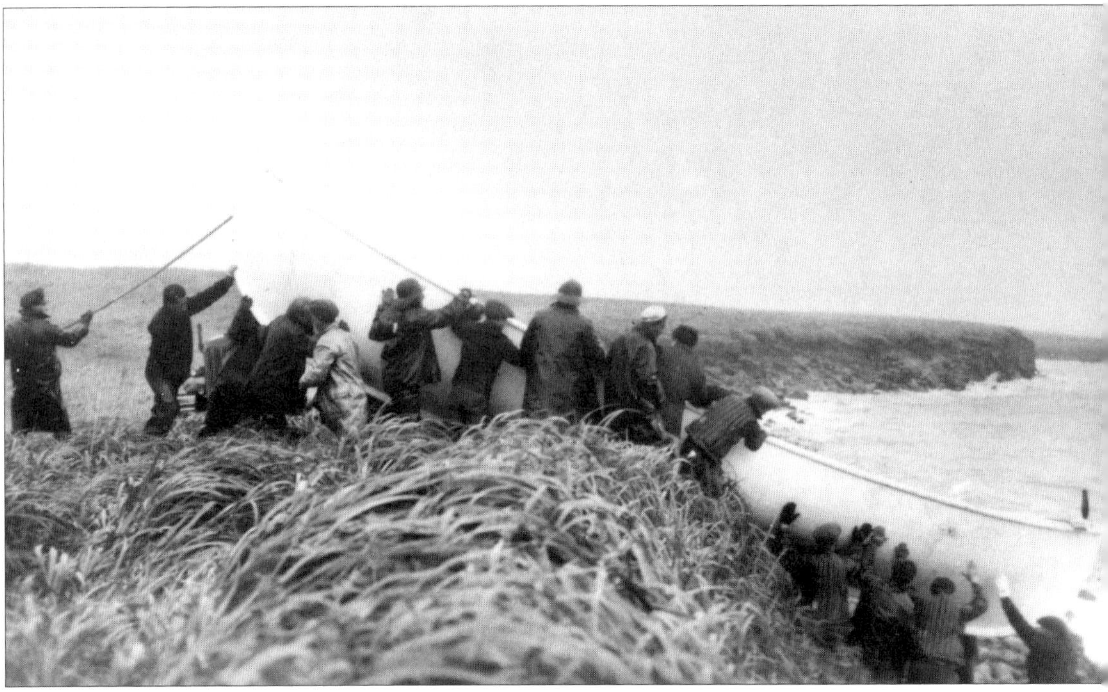

Launching a baidar during the June 1942 evacuation (from the Martin Collection, USUAF210, Archives, Alaska and Polar Regions, Rasmuson Library, University of Alaska Fairbanks).

Chapter 43

If this were my story alone, it would end here, for the evacuation was merely a more dramatic version of the exodus we had intended to make that spring back to Greenbelt, back to familiar faces, streets, and activities. For my Aleut friends, the ship that anchored off East Landing the next afternoon was the herald of the unknown.[1] The people of the Pribilofs were picked up like baggage, torn from the familiar and known, and thrust into a strange world for which they were wholly unprepared. From St. Paul the families packed and moved like travelers. Nearly forty electric washers went into the boat's hold. Most of them took a large share of their belongings.[2] To most the knowledge that they were not to share the fate of their cousins on Attu, that their American brothers had come to help them, was so welcome that sorrow at leaving their world had no chance to enter their thoughts. Spokesmen asked Father Baranoff to hold a service to ask God's blessing on their journey. The women took their houseplants to the cemetery with dignity, bestowing a parting gift on their dead. A thrill of hope ran through their hearts for perhaps the undisclosed destination might be the States. Men who came to help us pack hospital equipment spoke in broken phrases of obtaining work in the States, of joining the Army to fight the Japanese, and securing a complete education for their children.

The orders received by the community of St. George limited baggage to one suitcase to a person. For a day and a half while they waited for the boat, the officials and sealers of St. George sorted and re-sorted their belongings trying to choose the most important and precious articles. St. Paul's cows were let out to graze. The St. George schoolteacher walked between the stalls, shot the cattle one by one, and left them to rot. The long wait, the strict orders, drove home the fact that their homes were being broken up. The future was an anxious question mark.

We arrived at St. George about six o'clock in the morning. No one was on deck to assist the baidar passengers swing from the boats tossing in the rough seas and mount the slippery swinging ladder. Each individual was red eyed, anxious, and on edge. Each person grasped a tiny parcel, an extra treasure.[3] Many carried their holy pictures carefully. One small wooden box contained a fat cat that protruded through the slats alarmingly. I was helping people at the top of the gangplank, reaching down to take their bundles since no one else was around. I grasped a shining nickel coal scuttle with a piece of cloth tied over its mouth. Jerking it upward a cascade of fresh milk poured over my shoes. I never learned which harried mind thought it necessary to bring nourishment aboard. The scuttle stood on a hatch for days unclaimed. Just before we arrived in Seattle it reappeared as a paint bucket used by the sailors.

The grief of the St. George people reminded the St. Paul islanders that they had left behind all the certainties of their experience. Tears mingled with warm greetings. As the ship pointed out toward the open sea, the people massed at the railing facing the town. Old Father Theodosia, clad in his church vestments, his venerable voluminous white beard fluttering in the wind, led them in prayers. Old and young, their trembling lips repeating the words of hymns, gazed landward tragically. Unheeded tears rolled down the singers' cheeks. Mothers held up their tiny infants as if to imprint the image of their birthplace on their young unconscious minds. As we watched from an upper deck our hearts and eyes were filled with sorrow and tears, too.

Once more the Aleuts were adrift. The third alien invader of the island archipelago was the most hostile. From the cauldron of the island war to the southwest, the wind of life had escaped to blow them from the harsh unhappy ruts of sealing and to waft them toward a destination no one dared predict.

I bade them farewell at a hastily selected and unprepared evacuation camp on Admiralty Island in southeast Alaska. I felt as the sealers did surveying the narrow beach and the impenetrable somber green forests stretching up to the naked peaks of mountains: "Too many trees." I knew how they missed the gracious space of their home islands, the sweep of the eternal winds, and the smoky wash of the Bering on the lava shores.

Strange new hopes filtered through official silence in the camp. *We are not imprisoned wards but free citizens.*[4] Men, inexperienced in the ways of the world and frightened, braved the agent's disapproval and found jobs in canneries, on boats, and in Juneau. The men were at last registered for Army service like other Americans. They missed, because of confusion over their rightful voting district, the opportunity to inscribe their votes on absentee ballots.

Life is harsher in the improvised camp than on the Seal Islands. Distraught officials hampered by the fear that the Aleuts may desert the Service completely lack the insight and training to help the Aleuts adjust to temporary or permanent jobs. Even Mr. Bower wrote me that he had to consult legal advice about the Pribilof Aleuts' legal status and seemed stunned to realize that the Fish and Wildlife Service could not forbid the families to leave the evacuation camp.

The remnant of the proud Aleut seal hunters, except for the inhabitants of Attu, the small colony on the Russian Seal Islands, and a few able-bodied men working on Aleutian fortifications, are scattered now in camps along the Inland

Passage. It is possible that none of them will want to return north. If the war drags on for years the last illusive tie that bound them into unity may snap.

Whatever happens to the sealers today, tomorrow, or next year, they can never be completely isolated and insulated from American life again. Unconsciously they have breathed in some of the sweet true breath of democracy. They have been affected by meeting men and women who did not look upon them as natural inferiors because of their ancestry. I dare predict that no government agent will ever again be able to pen in his report that the Aleuts are a docile people. From Russian serfdom and American oversight they have suffered too long. The bombs that dropped on Dutch Harbor have broken the walls that hid the islands where feudalism has reigned for seventy years under the Stars and Stripes. Attempts may be made to rebuild those walls but they will never be reared so high again that the sealers cannot look beyond them. The burning spirit of democracy, which flamed anew in the hearts of all Americans to challenge the invaders, will destroy the vestiges of old wrongs on the Seal Islands.

"The wind is no river," wisely philosophized the ancient Aleut hunter, waiting in his underground home for the storm to break. Democracy, too, has no fetters, no constricted channel. Its wind will invade at last the four corners of the earth. The Aleuts will one day speak its language, live by its precepts, and become a vital part of the great community of America.

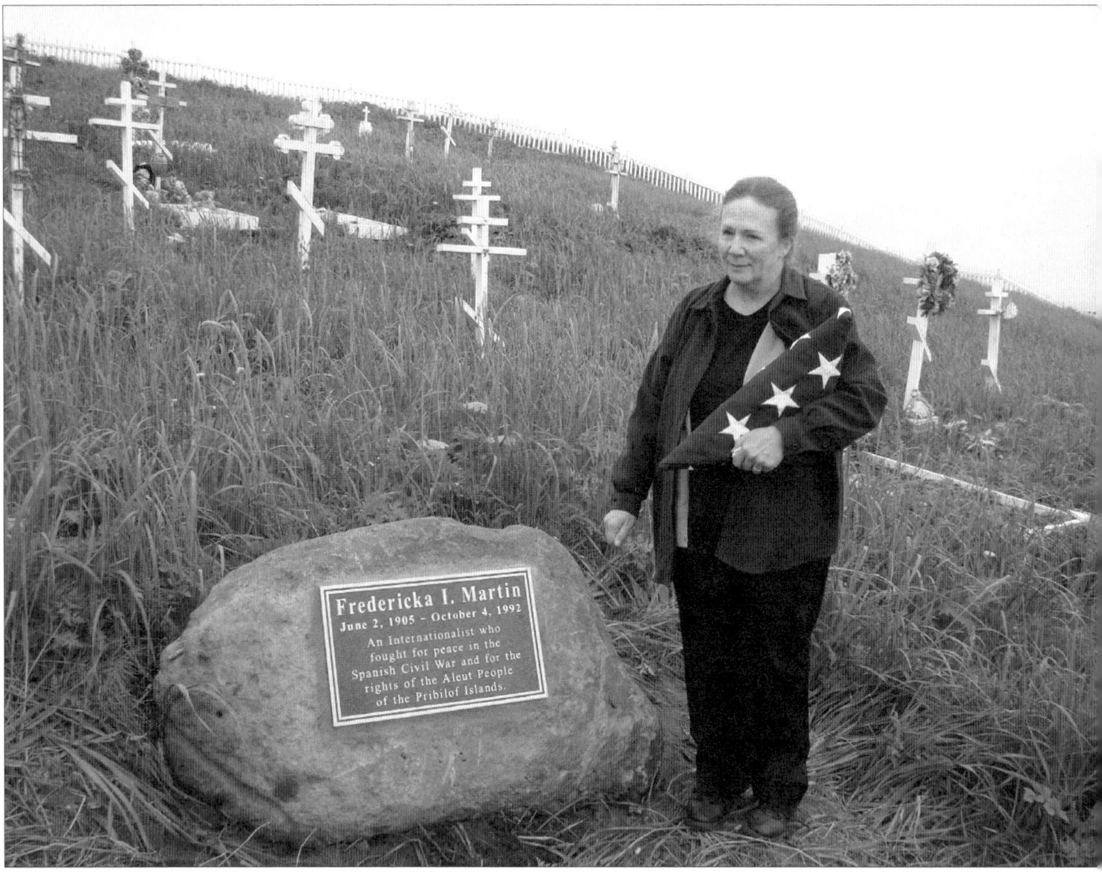
Fredericka I. Martin
June 2, 1905 - October 4, 1992
An Internationalist who
fought for peace in the
Spanish Civil War and for the
rights of the Aleut People
of the Pribilof Islands.

Fredericka Martin's daughter, Tobyanne Berenberg, at Martin's grave, holding a flag presented by the Coast Guard commander during the memorial service in 2008 when Martin's ashes were interred in the St. Paul cemetery. The wording on the grave marker was approved by the people of St. Paul Island. (Photo by Mario Berenberg).

Afterword

Raymond Hudson

The guarded optimism with which Fredericka Martin ended her manuscript was eventually mirrored in the lives of the Pribilof people. However, their emancipation from "a century of servitude," from years as "slaves of the harvest," would take decades of work. Martin played a significant role in encouraging individuals to persevere in their efforts. She championed their endeavors and helped them make significant contacts with experts in the field of Indian law. In addition to her two books, published in 1946 and 1960, she brought living conditions on St. Paul and St. George to public attention through published articles and innumerable letters to government officials. People at St. Paul knew her as a tireless promoter of Pribilof independence.

The 477 Aleuts from St. Paul and St. George arrived at Unalaska on June 17, 1942, having traveled all night on the U.S. army transport *Delarof.* The next day, the ship's crowded conditions were intensified when eighty-three residents from Atka Village in the central Aleutians came aboard. Immediately following the Japanese occupation of Kiska and Attu on June 7, American forces had begun extensive bombing raids over Kiska. Navy PBY patrol planes had used Nazan Bay on Atka for refueling. This was the site of Atka Village and the residents were ordered to disperse to fish camps in outlying bays. After a Japanese plane was sighted over the island on June 12, men from the USS *Gillis* and the USS *Hulbert,* seaplane tenders, were ordered to raze the village and evacuate the residents. By ten thirty that night, the village was in flames. Consequently, the Atkans had arrived at Unalaska with only the clothes on their back and a foretaste of what was in store for Aleut communities.

While Fredericka Martin waited on the *Delarof* for departure from Unalaska, John Yatchmeneff came aboard with a set of church books published in Aleut. He had inscribed each and "positively refused any payment" for them. She was deeply touched.[1] John Harrington had been won over by Yatchmeneff and planned to use his photograph as a frontispiece in his anticipated Aleut publication. He wrote:

> I was very fortunate securing the service of John A. Yatchminoff, son of the late Unalaska chief who died some four years ago. The Yatchminoff material covers every corner of the Aleutian ethnology from the names of the various Aleutian islands to names of plants and animals and minerals, including names of the various species of whale, with many curious bits of information to which the naturalists on the island, Banner and Wilke, contributed. The stuff is really fine and will interest anybody . . . Yatchminoff writes the language the way all of the Aleuts who know how to write do, using Russian letters, and in a beautiful clear hand.[2]

Harrington further wrote, "He and I saw everything through the same eyes, he caught on instantly to grammatical terminology. He was quick as a cat, and most accurate."[3] To Yatchmeneff himself he had written, "You and I saw things through the same eyes, and were just like one person. You can be sure that I shall be back at Unalaska at the earliest possible opportunity, and that all our plans will be realized to fullest glory."[4] A month after giving Martin the Aleut texts, John Yatchmeneff drowned in a boating accident on July 15 while crossing the narrow channel between Amaknak Island, in Unalaska Bay, and the village. Martin and Harrington felt his loss deeply.

The *Delarof* departed Unalaska on June 19 with 560 evacuees.[5] Neither they nor any employee of the government knew where they were headed. "The frantic search for a destination was still under way," wrote Kohlhoff in his history of the debacle.[6] Inadequate planning, the precipitous orders for departure, the failure to anticipate the most fundamental human needs, resulted in a disaster that Congress would eventually address. The evacuation, however, had not been unexpected to authorities. The mayor and the nurse at the Bureau of Indian Affairs hospital at Unalaska had been agitating for evacuation since shortly after the attack on Pearl Harbor. In late December and early January, John Harrington had warned both John Yatchmeneff and Archimandrite Dionisiy, the priest at Unalaska, of an impending evacuation. "Everything not needed by the Defense has been ordered out of Unalaska," he wrote the priest. "If hostilities continue, the civilian population of Unalaska will be forcibly removed, probably to several points, and ships will be allowed to come to Dutch Harbor only if bonded and bringing Navy supplies. The [sand]bar where Unalaska [village] stands will be needed for storage, and a civilian population in the midst of a fort will be removed since it would be undesirable."[7] To his Aleut collaborator he wrote, "I hear horrible stories of how all the civilian population of Unalaska is about to be removed."[8]

The Atkan people were set ashore at an abandoned herring cannery on tiny Killisnoo Island. Incredulous at the total lack of facilities or supplies, the captain of the *Delarof* provided food for four days, along with cooking supplies and a mattress and blankets for each adult. The destinations for the St. Paul and St. George people were an abandoned fish cannery and an abandoned gold mine in Funter

Bay, on the west coast of Admiralty Island, about sixty miles from Juneau. The Fish and Wildlife Service (F&WS) was nominally in charge, and agent McMillin described conditions for the 294 St. Paul people: "The only buildings that are capable of fixing is [*sic*] the two large places where the natives are sleeping. All other houses are absolutely gone from rot. It will be almost impossible to put toilet and bath into any of them except this one we are using as a mess hall and it leaks in thirty places."[9] He went on to describe how people fell through rotten floors and how a single toilet, poised above the low water mark on the beach and with an elevated wooden walkway leading to it, served ninety percent of the evacuees. The 183 St. George residents met equally repugnant conditions at the former gold mine. The St. George camp was supervised by the agent Daniel Benson and his wife. Father Baranoff and Father Theodosia remained with their respective parishes.

For both groups of Pribilof people, the immediate and overwhelming needs were food, water, shelter, and medical care. It was "a God-forsaken place," recalled Flore Lekanoff. "I mean, the place was not fit for even animals to live in."[10] The people got to work "constructing bunks, making beds from chicken wire, repairing walks to facilitate traffic, installing electric wiring in various dwellings, repairing leaking roofs, broken windows, rotten flooring, dilapidated outhouses."[11] Their efforts were hampered by a lack of food. "The native gang was worked every day same as on the Island," wrote the agent. "It all depended on the supplies available for food whether we worked five or six hours. When the food was low we were only able to give one good meal per day and of course the working hours were not so long."[12]

Having seen their friends put ashore, the Berenbergs remained on the *Delarof* and continued south to Seattle, arriving on June 26. Fredericka made arrangements to travel to New York City with Tobyanne. Sam, on the other hand, prepared to return to Funter Bay until his replacement could arrive. He reached the camp on July 13 and remained until late September. Before leaving St. Paul, he and a group of Aleut men had packed medical supplies and equipment into eight sealskin barrels. The X-ray machine was also carried aboard. Without his knowledge, the eight barrels of supplies, along with a package of X-ray film, were transferred to the military hospital at Dutch Harbor by the medical officer aboard the *Delarof.*

A few days after the *Delarof* had left Unalaska with the Pribilof and Atkan people, the 160 residents of Nikolski, Makushin, Kashega, Biorka, and Akutan villages were brought into Unalaska. On July 6 they left aboard the SS *Columbia,* an Alaska Steamship Company vessel. On July 16, anticipating their own evacuation, people at Unalaska inventoried and packed the church belongings for safekeeping and three days later the 111 residents boarded the SS *Alaska.* People from the smaller villages were housed at Ward Lake, an old Civilian Conservation Camp eight miles from Ketchikan, following a brief stay at Wrangell Institute. The Unalaska people were placed at Burnett Inlet, an abandoned cannery site on Etolin Island.

During the weeks he lived at Funter Bay, Berenberg wrote down impressions in a sort of diary.[13] In no sense a systematic log, these jottings convey the enormity of the situation facing people suddenly uprooted, transported, and confined in an environment of utter strangeness. By the time he returned, Berenberg found that the summer heat and the lack of food had sapped the initiative of almost everyone.

[July 20] Sanitary—privy facilities especially—very bad—& the Aleuts moving so slowly, stubbornly & sullenly that it'll be a long time before anything is accomplished. Gabriel Stepetin complaining @ their inefficiency. . . .

[July 22] Water is dark brown with the vegetation just washed down by all recent rains. Less rain today. Stove installed in disp. yest. heats the place very well. Having movable screens made to insure some privacy in hosp. Will be ready for pat'ts in a few days. . . . One wk. here has seemed like a life sentence. . . . Everything proceeds @ snail's pace. Workmen scarcely move. . . . Whole Bay filled with brown fresh water. Many new streams on hillsides. St. G. a morass & utterly depressing. Health hazards terrific.

[July 27] Fr. Baranoff . . . [is] very depressed by his outlook—wants to return to Seattle for work; the canteen has adequate funds, but at Mac's insistence refuses to pay him even a reduced Salary. He & mother both want to return to Russia to fight the Japs whom they wholeheartedly loathe . . . Several Juneau people stopped in today on their vacation cruise. They'd been to Sitka—one woman said the people there were very "jittery." And "Time" says that Army & Navy expect Japs to go from Kiska to Pribilofs . . . Peter [Kochergin] continues to handle most first aid & nuisance calls during office hrs. & at other times. Saving me many, many steps.

Baranoffs both want to be remembered to Freddie ("Freda") "From de bottom of de hearts"—with significant and meaningful gestures—indicating real, & not simulated, affection.

[July 28] The women went clamming early this A.M. & brought back enough to literally feed the village. Horseshoe clams—6"–8" long—& very tough. Not like fried clams . . . Mac, as do all the others, waver[s] between stupid tyranny & complete lack of intelligent discipline. In general the Aleut mood continues to be one of indifference, apathy & lack of appreciation of both what is & is not being done for them. Re. hosp. laundry—Mac refused to allow anyone to do it as a regular hosp. task. Ergo—Mary will lysolize it & give it to the relatives to wash.

Not long after his arrival, Berenberg listed the needs of the community:

Present lacks here are:

(1) Housing—i.e. shelter—space

(2) Sanitary Facilities

a. laundry

b. toilet
c. washing & bathing
d. sewage disposal
e. adequate water supply
(3) Heating
(4) Beds
(5) Hospital.
Present arrangements utterly mediaeval & unworthy of U.S. potentialities.
Human Lacks:
(1) Democracy, citizenship rights, freedom
(2) Education
(3) Opportunity
(4) Discriminatory perception
(5) Responsibility, Duty
Replaced by
(1) Pseudo-feudalism
(2) Exploitation
(3) Demoralization
(4) Restriction of opportunity & of responsibility

Dr. Berenberg's fury at what he called the vicious, mean, and amoral attitude of the whites in charge of the camp grew daily. Near the end of his stay he wrote:

> Mac's personal views & authority are of course most dangerous since he uses them to warp the lives of these 300 people. He refused today to allow them to register for absentee voting, as the Attg. Gov. of Alaska had decided they might do. "Where are they absentee from?" says Mac. "They never voted up there." Which, acc. to Johnston himself is untrue. The people are so completely cowed that they refuse to fight back & to leave here for work or otherwise.
>
> Mac says they must be kept here because (1) They must be a unit—to return to the islands (2) They'd get drunk (e.g. look at the 16 people fr. Atka (Killisnoo) now in jail—Juneau for drinking, & they can & even [do] pay their fines.) (3) Can't care for themselves (4) They got no brains (5) Mac says so. Most important reason.
>
> The administrative set up is minor fascist repression + slight benevolence provided by meals—inadequate salaries $20, 17.50, 15, 10/mo.—sub-slum quarters; nor will there be any place for a school—despite the 2 sch. teachers who return next wk. or so.
>
> The repression stands forth in bolder relief now than on the Pribilofs because there they had no immediate contact with the outside whereas here they have immediate access to Juneau (3–6 hrs. away)—& there is a

> great demand for all classes of workers. Mac. has lied to all manner of people who have come in offering jobs—temporary & permanent to the Aleuts.

The damp soaked into people's bones. On September 17 Berenberg wrote about "frost, dampness, cold, sleeping with a bathrobe & flannel pajamas & all windows closed—& freezing all day." Despite their strong differences, Berenberg and McMillin were alike in their assessment of the situation. "Mac most insistent," the doctor wrote in his diary, "that I tell Bower [in Washington, D.C.] the true story of what is happening here."

After Dr. Berenberg left, the community that had depended on a resident physician now found itself with a single nurse to serve the two camps. The "hospital" was a room about twenty feet square, heated by a small stove. Peter Kochergin continued to render his services efficiently. The director of the Division of Maternal and Child Health and Crippled Children's Services visited in October 1943. She described him as "the night man 'Peter' who had been helping the physician on the Pribilofs before they were evacuated. He had a good understanding of the routine for taking temperatures, forcing fluids and the general care of patients."[14] A physician assigned to the camps arrived on December 29, 1943.

In October 1943, after hearing about deaths at Funter Bay, Martin wrote to Charles Ralph and Ruby Magee, teachers who had accompanied the Atka people. "The list of those Aleuts who have died in the camps is horrifying and heart breaking," she wrote. "I do not know about your people but many deaths at Funter or in Juneau were avoidable had they had better housing, sanitary facilities and medical care. The Hellbaums, the teachers from St. Paul, have recently quit the Service, thoroughly disgusted at the inhuman conditions there and the letters from the Hoversons are truly most discouraging and unhappy in tone."[15]

The first task Fredericka Martin set for herself was publication of Richard Henry Geoghegan's translation of Veniaminov's grammar and vocabulary in 1944. Geoghegan encouraged her and sent her directives from his hospital bed in Fairbanks, where he died in October 1943. Martin enlisted the help of Ruth Gruber, still with the Department of the Interior. Secretary Harold L. Ickes and the Commissioner of Indian Affairs, John Collier, supported the project. "Today when fewer Aleuts read and write their own language fluently and wartime evacuation to southeastern Alaska has widened their horizons," she wrote in the introduction, "the Aleut people will welcome this first overt proof of genuine American interest in their existence and culture."[16] Although several divisions of the Department of the Interior supported the publication, the F&WS did not. Martin caustically remarked, "The fur seals have no need for a dictionary and grammar."[17]

For many young Aleuts from the Pribilof Islands, the evacuation became a door of opportunity. "It struck me as a great adventure," recalled Flore Lekanoff, who left Funter Bay to attend school at Wrangell Institute. Jake Lestenkof transferred from Wrangell Institute to the Mt. Edgecumbe boarding school before

TABLE 1: Population figures for the Pribilof Islands, 1942–1944.

	St. Paul Deaths	St. Paul Births	Pop. of St. Paul	St. George Deaths	St. George Births	Pop. of St. George	Total Population
1942	1	9	295	1	5	185	480
1943	14	10	291	2	5	179	469
1944	8	7	289	6	9	176	465
	23	26		9	19		

embarking on a long and distinguished military career.[18] Gabriel Stepetin, whose activism had been encouraged by the Berenbergs, did not stay long at Funter Bay.

His wife, Zenia, gave birth to a son five days after their arrival. As soon as possible, Gabe and his family stole aboard a fishing boat headed to Juneau. "They wanted to keep us in one place so that we wouldn't go out and learn how other people were living," he said in 1979, referring to F&WS supervisors. "They didn't even allow fishing boats to dock at Funter Bay. There used to be a watchman with a sidearm." In Juneau, Stepetin, along with a few other Pribilof men and women, found employment until the return to the islands. "I think if it wasn't for the War and the evacuation," he continued, "we would still be behind in getting our independence. We got out and saw how other people thought."[19]

Men began to volunteer for service in the army and navy. The F&WS, however, stridently opposed both volunteer enlistment and the inclusion of Pribilof men in the draft. This was, needless to say, a battle the F&WS lost (see appendix 3). In the summer of 1943, men from the islands, including many who were in military service, were taken back to harvest seals.

The deplorable conditions of all the evacuation sites have been documented in numerous studies and will not be repeated here.[20] Population statistics published in the annual Alaska Fishery and Fur-Seal Industries reports were misleading and reflected only a slight decrease from December 1941 through December 1944, from 482 to 465, a difference of seventeen. Death rates, however, were high even though they were offset by birth rates.

Edward C. Johnston noted that during the calendar year 1943 there had been twenty-five deaths, not the sixteen in Bower's report.[21] At the beginning of May 1944, the residents of St. Paul and St. George, along with sealers from other relocation camps, left southeast Alaska for good. During the return trip, influenza spread aboard the ship and lasted for two weeks following their arrival home. Dr. Will F. Speers, the physician on St. Paul, summarized the evacuation when introducing his report covering the first year back on the island:

> This community, while not actually in the war zone, experienced all the horrors of war for about 2 years by comparison of their unsanitary living conditions there and what they had been accustomed to on this island.

> While at Funter the congested living quarters, lack of sanitation and medical care resulted in almost constant epidemics of Influenza or Measles with such a resulting increase in the death rate that should the same conditions have been allowed to exist much longer, they doubtless would have wiped out a large proportion of the population.[22]

He continued by describing what the people discovered upon returning:

> A decent home life was still a problem due to the condition of their homes as a result of occupation by the Army. A great portion of their personal belongings had disappeared, furniture and other household equipment destroyed or missing and their houses in general left in a filthy condition. To get their homes in a livable condition with 2 or 3 or more of the family ill with Influenza required the supreme effort on the part of some.

A different federal agency was now in charge of the islands. After Japan had abrogated its participation in the fur seal treaty of 1911, a conservation measure was reached in 1942 with Canada to protect the seals. Two years later the Fur Seal Act transferred control of the fur seals to the secretary of the interior acting through the Bureau of Commercial Fisheries. Several former F&WS employees transferred to the new bureau, bringing the attitudes and policies that had long been standard. In 1945 the agent at St. Paul, Daniel Benson (formerly agent at St. George), was relieved that the people were showing "every sign of returning to normal." He referred to "a very few who are still a bit restless or who haven't worked out all the ideas accumulated down there." Guardedly optimistic that pre-war patterns would be reestablished, he conceded that there were a few "who continue to be a bit troublesome in some respects . . . and [that] even some of the employees . . . seem to believe that 'the natives are being held down.'"[23] The bureau did its best to reassert its authority. There were Unangan, however, who were determined to upset the status quo and to liberate the islands.

In 1946 Martin's "Wanted: A Pribilof Bill of Rights" was published in *The American Indian.* She continued to voice her outrage. "They are not supervised by administrators," she wrote, contrasting residents of the Aleutian chain with those on the Pribilof Islands, "who try to forbid or hamper either their education or their freedom to move from one place to another to seek new jobs." She called for the obliteration of "social caste barriers" between islanders and white employees, for "just cash wages for all their work," and for "the sealers' right to a voice in settling their own community problems and casting their votes as citizens."[24]

By 1947 some of the men in the armed services had returned home. To the agent's relief, he found these men "aided greatly in satisfying the community that their lot here is quite all right. It was feared for a while that such contacts with the 'outside' would create more dissatisfaction with life on the Island, but the opposite is definitely true." The following year, the agent grew even more optimistic following several investigations. "Even satisfaction with conditions in general by the natives themselves," he wrote, "was established quite definitely."

The agent's sanguine assessment testifies to the effectiveness of those who worked for independence and stayed below his radar. His optimism belied the unrest within the community, but it was necessary for those most active in bringing about change to do it as surreptitiously as possible or to risk expulsion from the island. Martin continued to encourage action. Gabe Stepetin, Elary Gromoff, and others held meetings, organized a chapter of the Alaska Native Brotherhood, and worked with attorneys who had been drawn to their cause through the National Congress of American Indians. Martin acknowledged their sacrifices: "But what comes out of all those struggles is the phenomenal event that a group of men, thrown back into isolation, harassed in countless petty ways continually and threatened with worse, had the courage to stand firm and feed ammunition to people many of whom they never saw but to whom they gave their trust . . . how brave Gabe and Elary were, how much harder it was for them—how easy it was for me."[25]

Jones summarized the gradually increasing momentum:

> The interaction between these actors—the Aleuts, their attorneys, Fredericka Martin, and Indian Rights organizations—had a snowball effect as each group drew encouragement and inspiration from the support of the others; in the process, they merged themselves into a relatively cohesive force for change, a force that posed a powerful challenge to the Pribilof management bureaucracy.[26]

In 1948 Martin testified before a subcommittee on Interior Affairs and Insular Possessions against proposed legislation (Senate Joint Resolution 162 and Senate Bill 2037) that would have radically reduced federal support for Native institutions. Martin said, "[T]hese measures would destroy every means by which the Aleuts hope to obtain economic and social security and self-government." She concluded, "Do not deny them their opportunity to obtain self-government. Do not jeopardize their title to their home islands. Do not condemn them to remain . . . practically serfs of a government bureau, the Fish & Wildlife Service."[27]

In 1949 a study of living conditions on St. Paul and St. George was part of a wider study of villages around the Bering Sea. One outcome was a job classification and wage-based compensation system for the Pribilofs although food, housing, health, and education costs were still the responsibility of the federal government. Martin had submitted a wage plan to the director of the F&WS and the Labor and Interior secretaries in 1949 and this "proposal was the basis for the 1950 wage plan and subsequent revisions to it."[28]

In 1950 St. Paul received a charter, constitution, and by-laws under the 1934 Indian Reorganization Act (IRA). A year later, the St. Paul IRA council filed a claim for land and compensation for past injustices. The land issues would not be resolved for twenty years. Compensation for past injustices would take even longer. In 1976 this claim was settled through the Fair and Honorable Dealings Act and resulted in what was known as the "corn-beef settlement." In 1957, the United States, Japan, the Soviet Union, and Canada entered into a new agreement to protect fur seals, the Interim North Pacific Fur Seal Convention. In 1959, the Bureau of Commercial Fisheries recommended that sealing become strictly a seasonal activity and that the people on the Pribilof Islands be relocated and given job training. There was great opposition to this and so the bureau encouraged St. George people to move to St. Paul in the hopes of consolidating the two villages into one. Vacated St. George houses were destroyed. This program ended in 1965.

In 1962 the Berenberg's former student Ishmael "Smile" Gromoff began writing for the *Tundra Times*, a Native newspaper published in Fairbanks. In 1964 this newspaper championed independence for the islands in a number of articles. "We are in a state of servitude," Gromoff declared in a letter to the editor, Howard Rock. The paper covered the story of how in October 1964 Carl E. Moses, running for the state House of Representatives (and soon to be elected), was denied permission to visit constituents after he and his wife had flown to St. Paul.[29]

Following hearings held in 1965 by the Senate Commerce Committee, Congress adopted the Fur Seal Act of 1966. Provisions were made for a town site to be conveyed to a local self-governing community. In 1971 St. Paul became a fourth-class Alaskan city. However, the entire question of land ownership changed when in December of that year the Alaska Native Claims Settlement Act (ANCSA) was passed. Under ANCSA, St. Paul residents established the Tanadgusix Corporation (TDX) and people on St. George formed the Tanaq Corporation. (In 1983 St. George became a second-class city.) Conflicts between the 1966 Fur Seal Act and ANCSA were resolved in favor of ANCSA. "By 1983, each Island was home to an IRA tribal council, a municipal government, and a village corporation," summarized the Pribilof Islands Transition Act of 2000. "TDX received the right to select 138,240 acres of land in the Aleutians, on the Alaska Peninsula and on St. Paul. Ultimately, 113,000 acres have been conveyed to TDX. Tanaq received an entitlement of 115,200 acres, of which 106,000 acres were ultimately conveyed."[30]

Management of the fur seals once again changed hands. In 1970 the Bureau of Commercial Fisheries merged with the newly created National Oceanic and Atmospheric Administration (NOAA) within the Department of Commerce. Control of the fur seals devolved on the National Marine Fisheries Service. NOAA began an active withdrawal from the islands under the Fur Seal Act Amendments of 1983. Funds of twelve million dollars for St. Paul and eight million dollars for

St. George were established in 1984 "to promote the development of a stable, self-sufficient enduring and diversified economy not dependent on sealing."

The transfer of authority over the islands from federal to civilian administration has been fraught with difficulties.[31] Commercial harvesting of fur seals ceased on St. George in 1973, and in 1985 it terminated on St. Paul. (A limited number can be harvested for subsistence.) There was, consequently, no income available to the island from sealing. A successful transition from a fur seal–based economy to one centered on commercial fisheries required the construction of breakwaters and docks. Storms and funding questions, however, delayed their timely construction. Development of an infrastructure necessary for a successful municipal government also lagged behind the arrival of the severe economic crisis precipitated by the end of sealing. There were serious concerns over the pace of the required cleanup of contaminated property resulting from a century of federal management. In December 2000 Congress extended the government's commitment to establishing successful independent communities in the Pribilofs with passage of the Pribilof Islands Transition Act (Public Law 106-562.)

In 1984 Larry Merculieff, then president of TDX, testified before the Alaska Native Review Commission, headed by Thomas R. Berger.

> You probably have researched our history, which is unique, to say the least. You can see that despite genocide, slavery, internment, cultural and economic upheavals and just generally a history of major uphill struggles and domination by outside forces, we are still here, still fighting for what we believe in, still a proud people. . . . We are the Aleut capital of the world, with a deep culture still intact, despite what was done to us.[32]

Merculieff interviewed Fredericka Martin in 1986 when she visited St. Paul after receiving an honorary doctorate from the University of Alaska. "There are Aleuts on St. Paul today who remember and were part of the struggle for Pribilof reform," he said in 1991, "people who were in constant contact with Fredericka."[33]

Today St. Paul is the home base for the Central Bering Sea fishing fleet. A local halibut fishery has developed. Shore-based and offshore commercial processors have been drawn to the island. With the fur seal rookeries and more than 210 species of nesting seabirds, the community is working to develop eco-tourism. Residents of the island continue their struggle to preserve a viable community within the Aleutian region. Many of those involved are the children and grandchildren of people whom Fredericka Martin knew. They have become administrators and teachers. They serve on local and regional governing and corporation boards. They promote an enduring Unangan culture.

Appendix I

Foreword by Fredericka Martin, c. 1943

An Explanation for Tobyanne to Whom This Book Is Dedicated

Someday Tobyanne is going to ask her parents, "Why was I born on St. Paul Island? Where is it? Who lives there? What happens there?"

This book is her mother's attempt to answer such questions. It is also an attempt to describe fully the physical character of the island, to relate the manner of existence and habits of plant, animal, and human life, and to collect within one volume the meager scraps of history now hidden away in old government reports, in forgotten scientific papers.

Many facts that had never been written for the public I learned from the Aleut people but, as my narrative makes clear, their memories were limited because they had become a despoiled people without group pride, lacking a past because they possessed no future. If others had written of the Pribilof Islands I should not try to combine personal experience, the history of the Aleut people, a few hints about their shrinking language, an account of the fur seals, a synopsis of the tangled political scandals over the fur seal, and diverse other matters into one harmonious structure of words. These topics are too widely variant to string together neatly. Yet after all how could I write a book for Tobyanne and not include them all? For the gathering of information was our life on St. Paul and to omit one feature would be to overlook a large piece of our life. Whether it were the dry statistics of the diet code or the detection of the true form of the alleged Aleut word *Ardiguen;* whether it were the sound of Russian church bells or the long tramp to Whitney Pond in search of a flower reported seen there fifty years before; whether it were the cry of a woman in labor in the hospital or the ugly spectacle of seal killing, each event, each fact, each truth, oral or written, concerned us. I have tried to keep out unessentials.

After I made my first outline for this book I discovered that Robert Marshall had used that method for his wonderful *Arctic Village.* So I chose the more commonplace way of telling events rather than follow unworthily in his wake. I have maintained as nearly as possible the chronological order of happenings, inserting certain information at a point as faithfully close to the moment I began to study the subject as possible. Of course I have utilized material in certain chapters that I did not know at the time the principal events of the chapter occurred. For instance, facts about the old village sites of St. Paul I did not make sure of until a few weeks before I left the island. There were gaps in the library of St. Paul that I had to fill in when I was able to visit the Library of Congress and the National Archives. But the general continuity of the way circumstances directed my studies I have conscientiously adhered to.

Our personal experiences were happy. Near the end of a year's sojourn we emerged safely from a geographic area that had grown perilous during our stay laden with bright memories that increased our hatred of the predatory warlords of Nippon who drove us too soon from our personal northern Eden. Always our hearts will ache with homesickness for the silvery dunes of Vesolia Mista, the poetry of Lukanin Sands, the coroneted crests of Bogoslof, the bird-thronged cliffs of Iganatok, the dignity of the little red volcanic hills, the flower-spangled lowlands, the great throbbing seal beaches, the gentle mists, and the wild winds. If these writings convey only a faint impression of the beauty of St. Paul the fault is the writer's for the beauty and the wonder exist in abundance for the skilled author to capture.

To love a particular piece of one's country with intense devotion is good, stabilizing, and comforting but it is not enough if we lose our identity with our fellows who share that piece of land, who are part of the social pattern whether their skins be black, brown, or white. Our joys on St. Paul were accompanied by the nagging sense of our own inadequacy to help the Aleut people beyond caring for their bodies when they were ill.

The world forces that sent us homeward to the cluttered ways of twentieth-century life, to the complexities and difficulties of our great nation protecting its existence against the attacks of unscrupulous strong foes, were only hastening our inevitable journey back, terminating an experience we knew must be temporary. But those forces uprooted the Aleuts from their known, and therefore endurable, ruts and transported them to another island, to new problems, anxieties, and insecurities. As I write I must leave them midway between their old life and an unpredictable future. Will they return to the dehumanizing unwise paternalism of a government agency on the Pribilof Islands? Will they lose the last shreds of their identity as a tribal group and be absorbed as individuals into the life stream of America? No one can foresee their next destination.

If this book arouses in Tobyanne and a few other Americans an indignant pity for an unfortunate group of descendants of early Americans, it fulfills the most earnest desire of the writer. That pity must inevitably help to strike off the chains of ignorance and official oversight that have fettered the Pribilof sealers for generations.

The Aleuts have been a patient people. They have retained their capability for full American rights through many bitter years. Since they know, as their forefathers knew, "the wind is no river," they hope ever for that moment when the currents of history will permit them to regain their dignity as men among men, as citizens among Americans. They long to be an active part of that great adventure, the American Way of Life.

I hope, Tobyanne, that this book answers your questions and that you are not disappointed either in your parents or your birthplace on that lovely island in the Bering Sea. And if others forget as soon as they close this volume I ask you to remember forever the kindly island people, young and old, who came bearing homely and simple gifts to you on the day of your birth.

Appendix 2

Excerpts and Synopsis of Samuel R. Berenberg's Annual Medical Report, 1941–1942

March 31, 1942

[If for nothing else, this report would have been notable for its length, sixty-eight typed pages.[1] Berenberg's holistic approach to health resulted in a report that covered a spectrum of concerns, often mirroring those in Martin's book. He introduced procedures and expectations that he saw as a foundation for future medical services. These became all the more futile and poignant with the removal of the citizenry to the sordid camps in southeastern Alaska. Editorial comments are bracketed. Berenberg's own sources and asides are in parentheses.]

Introduction

It has been traditional for many years to begin the annual report with the comment that "the health of the Natives has been generally good." Since our physician wishes to submit the medical and medical-social problems of the community to an objective analysis he will omit this euphemism. Good health, after all, is something more than the absence of sickness. "A healthy individual is a man who is well-balanced bodily and mentally, and well adjusted to his physical and social environment. He is in full control of his physical and mental faculties, can adapt to environmental changes, so long as they do not exceed normal limits, and contributes to the welfare of society according to his ability. Health is, therefore, . . . something positive, a joyful attitude toward life and a cheerful acceptance of the responsibilities that life puts upon the individual." (Dr. Henry Sigerist, *Medicine and Human Welfare.* Yale University Press. 1941, page 100) Medical care can no longer be discussed as an isolated activity; adequate medical care and good health should be an accepted part of the fabric of living.

Aristotle's statement that "the unexamined life is not worth living" suggests the paraphrase that the unexamined community is not worth living in. There is ample precedent for your physician to discuss the social aspects of the community. As long ago as 1848 Virchow, the father of modern pathology, said, "The physicians are the natural attorneys of the poor, and social problems fall to a large extent within their jurisdiction." The physician should understand the community as a whole if he is to understand the individual patient as a total personality. He must know all the external stimuli that determine the patient's reactions in health and disease. It is not enough to view the patient as a series of biochemical processes occurring within an anatomical structure of skin and bones and muscles. His reaction to health and diseases is governed by his responses to the dynamics of his environment and ultimately the environment determines his mode of reaction. In other words his total personality depends not only on his heredity, but also, and perhaps largely, on the kind of life and the opportunities and responsibilities that his community, or, more broadly, his society offer him.

We are living in an age when the people have a fundamental right to, and will demand, all the fruits of our most modern preventive and therapeutic medical techniques. But to fully benefit from these advantages, these aids to a fuller life, the people must have an educational background broad enough to understand and to accept the newer health measures. Health education must be continuous; beginning with the preschool child it should accompany the student through all his school years and become part of the daily routine of the adult in his personal and family life.

The medical department has sought, for many years, to inculcate some health education into the community, with minor degrees of success. It appears that the principal obstacle to greater success has been and still is the community's poor comprehension of the English language and low educational status. Since health education must be carried on with English as the medium, and since, except in the rare instance, a really useful command of English is sadly lacking, the immediate problem becomes one of instituting a modern educational setup. Such a change, however, will not solve the problem permanently. For education in itself, unless it can be socially useful, becomes eventually a sterile, empty effort—meaningless and, perhaps, even demoralizing to both the giver and receiver. We have abundant examples of the failure of education per se—without concomitant responsibilities and opportunities; we need but examine the history of the past fifteen years to find college graduates, skilled workers, scientists, teachers, linguists, physicians, lawyers forced to accept work for which they were not trained, while years of specialized study in their own fields were too often partially or totally wasted. So then it becomes clearer that the problem of health education at St. Paul becomes one of a far better general education and this, in turn, resolves itself into the necessity for offering to all our people here a way of life that will stimulate them to seek it and accept it. Such an interest in education, however, can be heightened only by broadened economic and social opportunities, involving full democratic rights and responsibilities for all the community. The solution of the problem in its entire aspect involves a fundamental change in its attitude to the people here by the Department of the Interior. But unless the change is truly basic, with the full imposition of rights and responsibilities—as well as an education equal to that in the States—it can be expected that any compromise measures will result in no permanent improvement.

One of the reasons given for continuing the present setup is that "the Natives here are so much better off than in the rest of Alaska." If this be true then it is indeed a sad reflection on our entire national policy toward the original inhabitants of Alaska; and the magnification of an unprogressive policy does not lead to ultimately positive or beneficial results. Another assumption is sometimes proffered: "The Natives are not intelligent enough to partake of community responsibility. They are not bright enough to absorb any more education than they get, and if they could, and did, they'd be unhappy with their lot." To the physician and the social scientist this is specious and reactionary reasoning, all the more so because it is utterly false. By all the standard psychometric measurements these people are as intelligent as any cross section of the population in the States. To deny them every opportunity is to deny them their basic rights; to refuse to accept their potential contributions to our commonweal is to degrade them and to nullify the aspirations, the hopes, the ideals of men.

The legal responsibility of the government is clear from the original treaty of cession. . . . [Berenberg quotes from the 1867 treaty and from a statement by W. S. Dodge on the educated status of Aleuts.]

The anomalies that constantly present themselves to the physician are startling and discouraging. For example, many of the hospital patients have provided themselves with the most modern radio receiving sets with which to while away the tedium of convalescence. But their comprehension of a news broadcast is so limited as to be virtually useless. And they listen with almost as great interest to broadcasts spoken in Spanish, Japanese, or Italian. This is true of both old and young patients alike. It is true also of most of the community, startling though it may sound. Twentieth-century American science has given them a magic toy, but twentieth-century America has not supplied them with the tools of language with which to understand its progress. (Unfortunately Sears Roebuck can't supply these necessary tools of language.)

How can a patient with pulmonary tuberculosis learn all about himself—the nature of his disease, its cure, its prevention, how to control its epidemic spread—when his education has not taught him how to speak his native tongue—English—sufficiently well so that he can absorb more than a smattering of any printed literature or oral instruction given him?

Let us examine more minutely some of the chronic ulcers on the body of our social group. We have spoken generally of education and so can begin to particularize by studying the school since it is the center of a large part of the local educational program; and we shall see how ineffective it is as presently organized.

School

The school population of eighty pupils presents an impossible physical and mental challenge to its two teachers. Two teachers may have been a sufficient number when the school census was lower, in years long past. A teaching load of forty students per teacher is too great and is completely out of line with modern pedagogy. Since this would be even true in a classroom devoted to pupils all of whom are in the same grade, how much worse does the picture become when we find that our two teachers must cope with the problem of instructing eight grades of pupils. And in addition to teaching the three *R*s, they must supervise manual training, cooking, and sewing classes. Their duties do not even seem to end there! The teachers are also responsible for supervising semiweekly showers for the schoolchildren; treating their heads for lice, maintaining a daily tooth-brushing routine, and dispensing cod liver oil. Splendid projects, all of them, but what time is left for teaching the three *R*s? In the hugger-mugger of such an "educational" program it is remarkable that the teachers remain sane or that the pupils learn anything. Little wonder is it that the most advanced senior student, who will have to leave school in a few months, because of the sixteen-year age limit, didn't know when Columbus discovered America or what the Civil War was about.

On examination of the facts, how futile are the repeated official communications through the years urging that English be spoken more by the Aleuts, when the provisions for teaching it have been so inadequate.

Constructive suggestions to remedy this particular ulcer are in order and their attainment is possible without introducing any radical changes. Obviously a long overdue increase in the teaching staff is immediately necessary. Such activities as school showers, dispensing cod liver oil, tooth brushing, etc., should be assigned to a committee of mothers who would perform these tasks during nonteaching hours. There is a number of mothers sufficient to do this, so that they could rotate their duties among themselves without encroaching unduly on their leisure or their housework. It would not only give the teacher more teaching time but equally important it would place the responsibility for these tasks where it belongs—with the parents. Since the need for personal hygiene doesn't begin and end with the opening and closing of the school term, this mothers' committee should function throughout the year. Of course, at such a time as there is running water in all the houses personal hygiene will be wholly effected where it should be—in the home.

With the number of preschool children increasing it is necessary that a kindergarten program be started for the four- to six-year-old group. At the other end of the age group further facilities for study must be made available for those students who reach sixteen years and now find themselves with one choice per sex—marriage for females, perhaps preceded by an all-out effort at thumb twiddling for a year or two, and the sealing gang for the males.

The school year should be lengthened by adding another month to the present school year. Provisions for installing modern, visual teaching aids should be made.

Several structural changes are at present necessary: an improved method of ventilation in the building is needed so that those pupils sitting near the cold air intakes are not subjected to sudden and frequent changes in temperature. The chairs and desks do not conform to standards permitting good posture and minimal eye strain. The technical specifications necessary for correcting these deficiencies are readily available in any standard work on school health.

School Health

Physical examinations on all the schoolchildren have been conducted. Previous medical files have not recorded data on school examinations in such form that they would be of any value to future physicians in following the children through their school years. Accordingly a standard school health card has been devised, similar to those recommended by the American School Health Association; this card will carry the pupil's health record throughout his entire school career. Its simplicity alone should encourage future physicians to do careful work and enable them more easily to detect new or progressing pathologic processes. . . . [Berenberg provides examples of students who would have benefited from regular checkups.]

Diphtheria Immunization

As one phase of a preventive health program, the entire school population was Schick-tested to discover those susceptible to diphtheria so that they could be immunized against it. Of eighty pupils examined seventy-five (94 percent) were Schick positive (susceptibles)—an astoundingly high figure . . . All susceptibles have been given two 1-cc doses of Ramon's yellow diphtheria toxoid (anatoxin). The third and final injection will be given directly a fresh supply of the toxoid arrives. The value of diphtheria immunization is so widely recognized that it needs no further comment here.

Tuberculin Tests

Tuberculin testing was done on the school population by means of the Vollmer patch test, a simple test whose results correlate closely with the older tuberculin testing methods—the Von Pirquet and the Mantoux. The following table shows the results:

TABLE 2: Tuberculin test results for school students, ages 6 – 15.

Age	Percent of positive reactors
6	50
7	29
8	43
9	63
10	56
11	57
12	50
13	100
14	100
15	83

These figures take on greater significance when compared with those of studies done elsewhere, in the States . . . A positive tuberculin reaction does not mean, of course, that the reactor necessarily has active tuberculosis; it does mean that the reactor has, at some time in his life history, been exposed to and been host to tubercle bacilli. Since we have here such a high percentage of positive reactors it follows that the exposure opportunities have been great, which means that the island has been up to the recent past rampant with active and "open" cases of tuberculosis . . .

Smallpox Vaccinations
Most of the schoolchildren have in the past been immunized against smallpox. It had been hoped to vaccinate the remainder, as well as every child over eight months of age. However, the requisitioned vaccine arriving on the November supply ship was so old that it would have been unwise to use it and accordingly it was returned. A new supply has been ordered and on its arrival the smallpox prophylaxis will be effected. One hopes that the McKesson Company will henceforth have the good grace to refrain from sending unusable medical supplies, as was true in this case.

Teeth
[Berenberg summarizes the result of dental inspections.] This means that the coming generation of adults is going to endure the same unspeakably poor state of oral hygiene as the present one. Inquiry into preventive dental care for children in the past uncovers the sad fact that extraction of teeth has been the principal method used. "An extracted tooth won't decay," seems to have been the dental slogan. Methods of correcting this local scourge will be discussed later.

Movies—Effect on Children
[Berenberg objects to children attending movies that last until nine or nine thirty at night as it seriously reduces their hours of rest.]

Infants and Preschool Children
[Berenberg reviews recent studies on the need for monitoring health throughout childhood. He quotes the U.S. Children's Bureau motto, "The health of the child is the power of the nation."]

Let us examine the situation at St. Paul and see how closely such precepts have been followed. The past records do show that there have not been periodic examinations of this age group. True a newborn infant was usually seen once or twice during his first six months of life. Thereafter, the indications are that he was seen at infrequent intervals, if at all, unless some disaster befell him—burns or boils or colds or diarrhoea, etc. . . . Nor are previous physicians to be personally blamed or criticized for such attitudes toward medical care. Indeed this Service has been generally fortunate in the choice of its past physicians. These attitudes are a carry-over from the earlier traditions of American medicine; the sick patient represents the doctor's livelihood; preventive care of healthy citizens is, unfortunately, all too new an idea.

Periodic Examinations

During the past nine months a system of regular examinations has been inaugurated for the zero to five-year group. Children under the age of one year are seen at monthly intervals. During the second year they are examined every two months. Between the ages of three and five years they are seen every four months. Only by rigidly following such procedure can developmental defects be discovered in their incipiency; only in such fashion can the physician fully learn to know the child as a growing organism. . . .

No child has escaped the present routine. Following each examination the mother is given a card stating the time and date of the next appointment for her child, a copy being kept in the dispensary files. The response has been excellent . . .

Health Advice

[Berenberg describes several publications of the U.S. Children's Bureau, Department of Labor, that were available. This literature, however, was not distributed widely because of the lack of reading ability. Those "who do comprehend some of the material find that there are too many suggestions that are difficult or impossible of fulfillment." He provides numerous examples, including eating fresh vegetables, fruits, a daily egg, bread, and butter.]

This is a good, well-rounded children's diet, conforming to our newer knowledge of nutritional requirements. But what can the St. Paul mother do after she reads it? Not much. First because the "Native Rations Code Sheet—weekly supply" contains no provision for doling out food to anyone under four years of age. Second, although the Canteen carries some infant foods, the community may not have the wages to buy them, or, as is too often the case, the stocks have been wholly depleted long before a supply ship comes in. Even now such vital necessities as eggs and milk have been out of Canteen stock for many weeks, and it will be two months at least before the new supplies arrive.

What is this same literate mother to do when she reads . . . the following: "Each child should sleep in a bed alone, and if space permits, in a room alone . . ." Here again such health advice cannot be and is not followed. In many of the homes the limitation of space necessitates one or more children sharing the parents' bedroom. In some cases a young child sleeps in the same bed as the parents, in others two children may be sleeping in a bassinet, if they are small enough to fit into it; two larger children sleeping in one cot is not uncommon; three children in a three-quarters or full-sized bed is all too frequent and four children in one bed is the lot of one family. If the health of these children is to be truly "the power of the nation" changes must be effected so as to provide living quarters adequate to allow the accomplishment of the teachings of our own U.S. Children's Bureau. Indeed these teachings articulate the minimal, not the maximal requirements.

Immunization

[Berenberg summarizes the status of childhood vaccinations against diphtheria and smallpox.]

Adults

[Berenberg discusses adult physical examinations and the low state of dental health.]

In passing, your physician would like to record that his experience with the "dependability" of our citizens here in following medical instructions is not one whit worse than with patients in Boston, New York, Greenbelt, or Washington, D.C.; if anything, when one realizes the deplorable sanitary facilities here, they may be said to be somewhat more attentive to suggested treatment, when instructions are clearly given and understood.

Tuberculosis

To discuss tuberculosis is to venture into territory where even angels fear to tread. A comprehensive treatise on this Pribilof plague since 1870 would require a tome of no mean size. The objective historian would conclude that it is truly remarkable that anyone survived the ravages of this deadly but preventable scourge. Bitter words on the subject have been spoken by agents, physicians, investigators. Some physicians have overdramatized the tuberculosis story (if a fatal disease can be overdramatized), others whether in ignorance or indifference have belittled it. The true story of tuberculosis is best learned from the unnumbered graves on Cemetery Hill. Even the death records have concealed the facts, for many deaths attributed to bronchitis, meningitis, grippe, pneumonia, malnutrition, etc. were most clearly tuberculous deaths. From these unnecessary tragedies of the past we may draw the obvious moral: tuberculosis is preventable, it is curable, it is unnecessary, and, laying humane considerations aside, it involves tremendous economic waste. The past is our heritage, the present our problem, and the future our challenge.

To clarify the present status of the tuberculosis question certain studies were undertaken. Every adult, except a few visiting at St. George, was tuberculin-tested, with the following results:

Females, positive reactors	39
" negative "	20
Males, positive reactors	65
" negative "	8

Old records were surveyed to find the names of any patients previously listed as having tuberculosis or designated as suspects. Each of these people was studied fluoroscopically and roentgenographically one or more times; x-ray films previously taken were compared (if they were found) with the newer ones; previous suspects have been clinically checked up from time to time. The full story still cannot be told, for a longer period of time is necessary to show whether every case of tuberculosis has been uncovered. A study of "tuberculous" x-ray films taken in 1938 shows that some of them reveal no evidence of tuberculosis and some were so poorly taken that they could really have been of no diagnostic assistance whatsoever.

To date four cases of active tuberculosis have been isolated in the hospital, where they may no longer spread the tubercle bacilli about the community . . . [He describes the four men with active TB.] These patients shall remain in the hospital, where they cannot infect others, until they are cured, die, or, preferably, are removed to a tuberculosis sanitorium in the States. Only by such continued isolation can the rest of the population be protected and the eradication of the disease effected in the near future. It is clear that no other therapy than bed rest can be afforded here. Not even a pneumothorax outfit is available to collapse tuberculous cavities and thereby accelerate healing. In 1870 bed rest was the only treatment available anywhere to these patients—in 1942 modern medicine affords surer and earlier recovery . . .

Hospital

Progress has been made in converting the hospital from a forbidding, dirty bedlam into a structure where the sick patient may convalesce in relatively pleasant surroundings. The formerly dark rooms are now bright and cheerful and clean. The painting has been done principally by Peter and Victor Kochergin, both of whom were hospital patients when the work was started. . . . No remote corner of the building has escaped the paintbrush or the scrub brush. . . . [He describes several renovations.]

Beds have been made more comfortable by replacing mattresses and springs. The results hardly represent the zenith of comfort but are a slight improvement. Ventilation can now be obtained by opening the windows. Ordinarily it would seem superfluous to mention so prosaic an activity as window opening, yet not within the memory of any patient or attendant had it been possible to open a single hospital window—they had been painted shut and no attempt had been made to excavate them.

The previous lack of hot water has been corrected. Under the genial guidance of Jack Eggis several of our local plumbers not only installed large coils in the furnace but for good measure concocted a fine shower for the first floor out of stray bits of pipe.

[The school sewing class under Mrs. Hellbaum made curtains, and Mr. Hellbaum's manual training class made bed stands. A buzzer system was installed. "No longer is it necessary for the patient to expend energy shouting for some needed attention hoping he will be heard."]

Attendants
[He describes the difficulties in finding good help in the hospital until a patient, Peter Kochergin, began working for them.]

Nursing Care?? [question marks in the original]
[Of the three who nursed patients, only Peter Kochergin proved satisfactory but he was "often forced to bed by his own illness."]

In fact the nursing arrangements are so deficient that your physician would have left on the September 1941 boat were the skilled nursing services of his wife not available. If this word picture of "nursing" sounds discouraging, the actuality is even more disheartening . . . What does this mean in terms of health? It means that the patient suffers unnecessary discomfort and pain and that his recovery is prolonged, in direct proportion to the extent of the lack of modern nursing care. And that lack is and has been great.

[He recommends hiring a competent nurse through the U.S. Public Health Service or budgeting for the training of some local girls.]

Girls can hardly be expected to work at the present scale of four cents per hour. So the request is made that a wage of fifty dollars per month be provided in the future (about fourteen cents per hour) for three hospital attendants.

Miscellaneous

[Berenberg describes instituting strict regular visiting hours and how the entire hospital has been kept awake at night by cows released from the nearby barn because there was insufficient hay to feed them. He introduced regular change of linen for bed patients.]

Obstetrics
All obstetrical patients have spent at least two weeks in bed before discharge to their homes where they are allowed slowly increasing activity over a two- or three-week period. To date no patient has had a postpartum temperature over 100 degrees Fahrenheit, and that, in only one case, the temperatures of all other patients remaining below 99 degrees.

With a few exceptions, prenatal care has been sought early in pregnancy. The exceptions were women who have had so many previous pregnancies that they felt it unnecessary to "bother" the doctor. All patients are examined monthly for seven months, twice in the eighth month, and weekly in the last month. . . . [He describes various recommendations made to the women.]

A postpartum examination of the patient is done at six weeks and three months. At these times any pathology can be corrected—this has consisted largely of minor cervical tears that have been electrically cauterized. The former practice of delivering women in their beds has been discontinued; all are now delivered in the Delivery (Operating) Room, providing better facilities for patient and physician, allowing semi-aseptic deliveries and greater obstetrical efficiency.

[He lists the seven women who gave birth, the names of each child, sex, and birth date. One child died shortly after birth and he describes the cause.]

At present there are nine patients receiving prenatal care. [They are named along with approximate delivery dates.] This list was longer by four names several weeks ago. The decrease has been due to an epidemic of four spontaneous miscarriages, all within a week of one another.

Deaths

[There were two deaths: Metrofan Krukoff, age fifty-nine, on November 25, 1941, and John H. Emanoff, one day old, on December 18, 1941.]

Number of Patient Days

[Berenberg lists all hospital patients by name and diagnosis from July 1, 1941. He provides a breakdown of the 1,829 patient hospital days by disease:

traumatic surgery	57
skin	85
medical	348
surgical	453
obstetrical	88
newborn	72
eye	9
tuberculosis	717

He adds the note, "The days spent in jail during its use as a contagious disease hospital for German measles are not included in these figures."]

Hospital Diet

Meals have been supplied to patients from the Company House kitchen . . . In studying these sickbed menus one need not be highly trained in dietetics to understand their deficiencies. Several of the lacks are readily comprehended:

1. Restricted variety.
2. Insufficiency of vegetables—fresh or otherwise.
3. Excess of starch foods.
4. Almost complete absence of fruits or desserts.

One need not even consider the aesthetics of serving food so that it will be tempting and appetizing to the sick patient. Simply on the basis of its lack of nutritional rationale such diets stand condemned. Nor can it be argued that any great improvement should have been made locally in this matter. Unless the Service's policy is changed in regard to such matters as providing decent hospital fare one may expect the sick to get nothing more than minor menu variations on a theme of reindeer, canned beef, and potatoes.

In passing, reference should be made to a former custom of requiring each family to bring meals to their hospitalized relatives. The village diet is even worse than that supplied by the Company House; great confusion results from people running in and out of the hospital at all times; and the patient's convalescence is retarded. It is hoped that there will be no reversion to this policy in the future and that some arrangement will always obtain for supplying hospital meals from a single kitchen.

[He provides a table of "Typical Hospital Menus" for January 3 through January 15, 1942, and for March 10 and 11. "Succeeding days are simply mirror images of the preceding ones."]

Equipment

The following should be added to the hospital equipment at the earliest possible moment.

1. An automatic electric autoclave.
2. An automatic refrigerator.
3. Electrolux-type vacuum cleaner.

All pieces of equipment have been previously requested. The present method of "sterilizing" instruments, gloves, surgical linen, packings, rubber tubing, etc. in a small pressure cooker is archaic, unscientific, and completely unsatisfactory. Twentieth-century medicine cannot be practiced by nineteenth-century methods. Airplanes will not run on kerosene, and neither can hospital goods be sterilized in a pressure cooker . . .

As to the refrigerator. The present method of using a cabinet with a few wall slots exposed to the outside world as a refrigerator is unquestionably unique in contemporary American hospital practice . . .

Janitor

A full-time janitor is needed, his time to be divided between the dispensary and the hospital . . . [He provides a table of dispensary and hospital duties for a janitor.]

Dispensary

A regular schedule of office hours has been adhered to since July 1, 1941.

8:00 a.m. to 9:00 a.m.
5:00 p.m. to 6:00 p.m.

During December and January these were temporarily changed to

9:00 a.m. to 10:00 a.m.
4:00 p.m. to 5:00 p.m.

because of the shorter days, which, because of their darkness, made it difficult for patients to come to the office. Emergency and accident cases are seen at any time. . . .

The total number of calls made from June 25, 1941, to March 31, 1942—a nine-month interval: 2,055.

Office—1,983

Home—72

Individuals examined or treated in any of the mass surveys have not been included under "total calls." Also not listed are many calls for bandages, tooth powder, cod liver oil, etc., which have in other years been recorded as office calls. Patients under treatment at home, if seen at time of village inspections, are likewise not included as "house calls." This procedure was followed simply to eliminate much fruitless bookkeeping. Also not included in "office calls" were the follow-up surgical dressings and treatments carried out by Mrs. Berenberg. These would ordinarily have been the physician's duties.

[Berenberg includes a four-page table of "Summary of Diagnoses."]

Renovation

[He describes the work done at the dispensary.]

Journals

[Two journals are received: *Surgery, Gynecology & Obstetrics* and *The Journal of the American Medical Association*. He recommends that the *American Journal of the Diseases of Children* be added.]

Books

Most of the books now carried on the inventory represent the medical thinking of one, two, or even three generations ago. As reference works they are of value only as historic documents. Mention is made of this lest anyone examining the inventory be impressed by the size of our medical library. The total worth of the useful books here does not greatly exceed fifty or seventy-five dollars—the value of the eight or ten books that are recent enough to warrant study.

Inventory

In regard to the inventory as a whole it should be stated that the figures given present an exaggerated picture as to the value of the equipment and drug supplies. Some of the instruments are unusable; several of the sets of instruments (given by the Navy) are not complete; some drugs are listed that have long outlived their expiration dates, others are museum specimens and worthy of retention only as such.

Purchasing
It has been your physician's policy to purchase medications that are of proven value. [He elaborates with reference to specific drugs.]

Methods of Purchasing
[Because of the cost of purchasing small amounts of drugs, "It is suggested that some arrangement be made with the Army or Navy—or other governmental bureau for joint purchasing—a matter that should not be difficult to arrange."]

Weekly Inspection

This peripatetic practice of many years has been continued on Wednesday afternoons. The ostensible reason for doing so is to encourage good hygiene and sanitation, in itself a worthy project. It would seem wiser, if this procedure must continue (and there is doubt of this), to inspect the houses at unannounced times, rather than at a fixed, expected hour. Only in such a way can any valid idea be gotten of the state of the local housekeeping. If this arrangement would seem to be not quite cricket, then it would follow that intrusion into the sanctity of one's home by a landlord or his representatives is unfair at any time—including Wednesday afternoons. The fact of the matter is that, with two or three exceptions, the houses are well kept, by any standards, and, considering the meager sanitation facilities available in them, they are in remarkably good order.

Communicable Diseases (Other than Those Mentioned)

During late June and early July 1941, there was a minor epidemic of German measles (rubella)—principally confined to workmen from the Aleutian chain. Recovery was complete, without sequelae, in every case.

[Berenberg considers a diagnosis of measles by the previous doctor possibly erroneous. He lists the "outside workmen" who were isolated in the jail during their illness with rubella.]

This jail is a modern version of the Black Hole of Calcutta and should never again be used as an isolation quarters for sick patients. With a little ingenuity more suitable quarters can be found should the necessity for quarantine again arise.

[There was a moderately severe epidemic of "acute tonsillopharyngitis" in August and September, with about seventy-five people so affected. "No cases of gonorrhea or syphilis have been clinically detected among the local population . . ."]

Clinical Pathological Studies
[He lists the laboratory examinations conducted.]

Roentgenographic Examinations
X-ray films were made in sixty-nine cases. As previously noted all of these films are on permanent file in the dispensary office.

Fluoroscopic studies, principally of the heart and lungs, were done in a great many cases . . .

Eye Refraction
Eyeglasses were prescribed for fifteen patients during the summer. This group included local people and outside workmen—from the Aleutians and from the States. No glasses were necessary in the case of twelve others examined.

Dentist

Earlier pages of this report indicate the great need for a dentist for the island (probably for St. George, too, judging by the dozen or so St. George mouths seen here). It is fully realized that the problem of finding a qualified and competent dentist at this time of international strife is not easily solvable. However, dental care for the Pribilofs should be given a high "priority" rating and every attempt made to provide a dentist immediately . . .

Village Rations and Diet

At present food is dispensed to the local population on the basis of a code sheet made some years ago. Ostensibly the Service is responsible for the full feeding of the people here, and it is with this in mind that inquiry into the food question should be made. This is best done by studying the code sheet itself. Having heard many complaints about the food issues, your physician decided to restrict his family's meals to a duplicate of the general village diet for a period of one week. However, after examining the code sheet and endeavoring to plan a menu that would be both edible and provide food sufficient to avert hunger, he decided to abandon this dietary adventure. For to err may be human but to make the mistake of voluntarily living on such a diet would be psychotic.

[He discusses recommended daily diets for good nutrition by reference to the National Nutrition Conference of May 1941 and to the surgeon general of the U.S. Public Health Service.]

In what way, then are the findings of the National Nutrition Council for Defense locally relevant? They mean that the present code sheet must be revised immediately to conform to decent, humane living standards. They mean that when people work for their daily bread the people should receive this bread and not a few crumbs.

[Berenberg then discusses the food allotments in detail.]

It is easy enough to minimize the necessity for change, when reading this discussion, after a good full meal topped off by a flavorsome cigar. Yes, at a distance of five thousand miles the reader may say the indictment is too severe, based on emotional reformism, steeped in academic irrelevancies, and therefore worthy of little more than casual study. Here, in this community, however, remains the actuality—the daily problem of seeking one's daily bread and not finding enough.

Here we know the actuality of children who are hungry because your physician has seen and fed such children on numerous occasions; he has seen them lurking about the Company House kitchen in the hopes of getting a few extra bits of food to allay hunger pains—both in summer and winter. However, personal observations aside, the code sheet figures speak for themselves.

Let us further study the actualities, by examining the complaints at their source. Let us ask the people who live their lives on the prescribed rations: it is they who eat the food; they who, in a democracy, should be the final judges of its sufficiencies and insufficiencies.

Questionnaire

Several weeks ago your physician, in anticipation of this report, released to the head of each family (forty-nine) a questionnaire seeking information on general household facilities. [The questionnaire is too light to read in the copy available.]

As can be seen not a single question was asked concerning food. Despite this intentional omission, thirty-eight of the forty written replies contained some comment on food or matters pertaining to food. Here are some of the replies—those omitted are in a similar vein. These are direct quotes, the spelling, words, punctuations being exactly reproduced. Each is from a different family. [He quotes seventeen, of which only five follow.]

"we don't have enough Grub to last us a week and sometimes when we get home the table is bare (otherwise empty), just bread and coffee without any milk and butter of course, breakfast without any eggs, ham or bacon and cereals of different kinds"

"we want shot gun shells to be issued to us from store, as we have to buy them from Canteen ourselves to go out hunting for food to eat, I remember they used to get them from store"

"during winters we want breakfast cerals beside oats form store also shotgun shells for hunting Ducks for food and yeast cake for Bread"

"not enough cream for our kids" ("cream" means "evaporated milk." SRB)

"what we eat up here is caned goods most of time, seal meat in summer time and salted meat in winter. Some people up here I see have tea or coffee for their dinner and supper"

Not a single request for any luxuries: no demand for black caviar, sturgeon, artichokes, brook trout, filet mignon, or chartreuse! One simple refrain—"Enough food for three nourishing, appetizing meals a day—for seven days a week."

Diet Discussion Continued

The deficiency in fresh vegetables, eggs, and meat products could be partly met by encouraging the local cultivation of truck gardens, the raising of chickens and pigs.

[Berenberg then quotes Geoghegan's translation of Veniaminov on the Pribilof Islands related to gardens.]

To sum up, then, the Service must either improve and increase the present food allotment, thus eliminating the present necessity for a family to purchase basic foods from the Canteen, or it should stop supplying any foods and, paying an equitable weekly wage, require all foods to be purchased from the Canteen—which could easily be run on a cooperative basis, selling at slightly above wholesale prices.

Sanitation and Housing Facilities

[Berenberg addresses accusations that the local people are "naturally dirty" and that they would waste running water if they had it. He writes that "such statements as this are discussed, not because they are historically interesting, but because some of them have become part of the folklore of the Service and color its relations with the community in matters pertaining to health as well as other things."]

Having condemned attitudes such as these that have hindered progress, let us seek the facts. We do know that no water is wasted from the several village faucets that now serve to provide water for the community . . . If, because of the war crisis, enough metal pipe cannot be obtained to tap all the necessary additional lake reservoirs, then water for toilets could be piped a short distance from the Bering Sea—as it is for the Fouke washhouse—and the drinking water led in from the nearer lakes. The technical details are readily solved by the sanitation engineer.

With the installation of water, there must be provision for toilets and baths and sewage disposal facilities in each house. In twentieth-century America it would seem unnecessary to point out that running water in homes, toilets, baths, drain pipes are not luxuries but the most elemental accompaniments of living. The provision of these facilities for the Service employees throughout the year and for the temporary government employees and Fouke workmen in summer, while the permanent residents of the island are denied them, reveals an example of flagrant disregard for scientific sanitation—for disease beginning in an outside toilet will not necessarily be stopped by the fences of the Service employees' yards . . . Certainly on moral grounds alone it would seem unfair to provide a minority of St. Paul's population with sanitary facilities and condemn the majority to a Neo-Stone Age civilization. . . .

Although not a single question was included concerning water, thirty-nine of the forty families replying to the aforementioned questionnaire spontaneously urged the installation of running water. And of these, thirty-seven requested both water and toilets. . . .

[Berenberg included thirteen excerpts from the questionnaire requesting water and toilets. He then included a "breakdown of figures on thirty-five typical local houses, giving number of persons occupying each house and number of rooms in each house studied."]

Deducting two rooms (kitchen and living room) from each house will give the number of bedrooms available for sleeping quarters in each case. Taken in sum the results show much overcrowding and insufficient cubic footage per adult, per child, and per infant in the cases cited, which are typical of the village as a whole. Increases recently (births) in the size of several of the families cited above and anticipated increases during the next six months will overburden the houses even more. In certain cases several families occupy one house, a condition that usually results in familial tensions and difficulties in social relations. The overcrowding of individual beds as a result of the lack of sleeping quarters has been previously mentioned.

The solution lies, of course, in the enlargement of some houses and the building of new ones. Modern housing standards, specifications for heating, ventilation, sleeping quarters, living quarters, etc., are easily available from any of the federal housing bureaus.

Typical of comments on the warmth of the houses are the following:

"need more coal to keep warm in winter"
"kitchen stove not enough for our families"
"would appreciate heating system"

Summer Quarters

Before concluding these notes on housing, mention should be made of the quarters furnished in summer months to outside workmen from the Aleutian chain. The men sleep on sheetless mattresses arranged bunk style. Bathing, toilet, and laundry facilities are unspeakably bad. The old-type dwelling house, a museum relic of St. Paul housing of the 1880s, which is used by some of these men should be condemned immediately.

Arrangements should be made to provide restful sleep; last summer men working on different shifts occupied the same rooms—so that, with some men up and about, continuous rest periods were impossible for the men trying to sleep. The contrast between the better quarters provided for the temporary "white" employees and those supplied the "native" temporary employees, is obvious enough; the reasons for this great discrepancy are not only not obvious but are incomprehensible. The results in health, however, are a matter of medical record: the sickness rate of "outside" Aleuts was, last summer, 5.3 times greater than that of the "outside" non-Aleuts.

Barn

So much should be said about the setup in the dairy barn that this will be left for the future. A great immediate need is the installation of hot water as a first step to attempting cleanliness there.

Theatre

[He describes the ventilation needed in the theater.]

The Canteen and Health

At certain times in the past the Canteen has found itself acting as a competing medical department, selling much highly advertised patent medicines as Lysol, Castoria, Alka-Seltzer, Unguentine, etc. Several patients have suffered vaginal pathology from using Lysol as a contraceptive; four patients have neglected to seek medical attention for severe burns, thinking that their home treatment with Unguentine would suffice, thereby delaying healing and encouraging infection. As the self-use of these and other such substances may lead to more disastrous results it is urged that the sale of any drugs be permanently forbidden.

There are other ways in which the Canteen can contribute to the health of the community. The partial or complete discontinuance of the sale of enormous quantities of such valueless beverages as Coca-Cola and Fox's ginger ale (at twice the sale price in the States) would allow the purchasing of nourishing foods (such as evaporated milk). Nor would anyone suffer from a wiser selection of confections; your physician has found candy bars that could compete with concrete for hardness and digestibility.

The greatest contribution of the Canteen to the local health would result from a lowering of all its prices, allowing the community's dollars to buy more food and clothing than at present. Such a reduction in prices can be effected if the Canteen will buy its wares at truly wholesale prices or will submit its requisitions for competitive bidding.

Alcoholism

The Eighteenth Constitutional amendment, of tender memory, proved quite conclusively that drinking cannot be legislated out of existence. Drinking and drunkenness have been problems confronting Pribilof authorities since the 1870s—in varying degrees at various times. Regulations have been passed, wages reduced, sermons preached, jail sentences meted out—all to no avail.

Kvass manufacturing and imbibition still continue and will continue as long as the community is denied the opportunity to seek a fuller life and so long as it is so poorly educated that it is unable to enjoy even such simple cultural activities as reading and understanding the radio. Difficult it is to answer the person who wrote at the bottom of his questionnaire: "I admit I like to drink. I also make my own drink. But my Doctor tells me it's very bad for me. Still I make my own homemade, after all I'm human, like to celebrate once in awhile on holidays. For this reason why can't I have a real beer up here? As I know and we know they are drinking all over the world and telling me and us not to drink. Again there is nothing going on on this lonely island anyway."

When the horizons of the St. Paul inhabitant are lifted beyond the confines of the seal rookeries and the scoria pit, then, and only then, will the problem of alcoholism vanish.

Auxiliary Nonmedical Health-Related Activities

[Berenberg praises the Girl Scouts and the Woman's Club, both organized by Geneva Hoverson.]

The Case of the Incompetent Mother

[Berenberg discusses a mother whom he thinks is a bad influence on the community and a danger to her children.]

Patients (Other than Tuberculous) Recommended for Seattle Care

[He lists four patients needing in-depth medical care or diagnostic treatment.]

Potential Use of Seal Carcasses as Source of Vitamin D

[He suggests fur seal flesh may be a high source of vitamin D and, if so, could prove to be a profitable source of income.]

Cooperation of Personnel

[Berenberg expresses appreciation for assistance and cooperation from members of the Service staff: Ed Johnston, Lee McMillin, Carl Hoverson, Thelma Hellbaum, Richard Hellbaum, Earl Oberg, John Stacy, Elvin Elliott, Mrs. Oberg, and Mrs. Elliott.]

Summary of Recommendations

[Berenberg lists his recommendations in a table covering three pages.]

Conclusion

A valid picture of the state of the community's health has been attempted. The approach to the problem of medical care has been socio-medical with the intention of showing that the Pribilof educational and cultural fogs will not be lifted until the winds of progress blow northward to sweep away the encompassing bonds of paternalism and feudalistic communism inherited from czarist Russia.

Economic and social opportunities and responsibilities must be made available to the people of the Pribilofs as they are to the rest of the millions living under the American flag. Education worthy of a twentieth-century American community must be provided. Until the people are paid a weekly wage commensurate with their skills, allowing them to support themselves and to worthily make their contributions to society—until that time—they must be given certain things already mentioned and summarized in the recommendations. We hope that this time is near at hand; then, trained and skilled in their chosen fields, these people will assume the stature of men among men. Then will the physician of tomorrow truthfully record, "The health of our people has been generally good."

Appendix 3

Pribilof Island Men Who Served in the Military During World War II

As of December 31, 1944, there were eighteen men from St. Paul and seventeen from St. George who were serving in the military. Their names were included in the Alaska Fishery and Fur-Seal Industries annual report for 1944. In the subsequent report, dated April 5, 1945, Daniel Benson noted that during the past year nine more men had joined the army, one was at Dutch Harbor awaiting induction, and two others had registered and would probably be enlisted during the coming summer. Their names were not recorded.

Bourdukofsky, George
Bourdukofsky, Victor*
Galanin, Ferman
Galanin, Laurence
Galanin, Martin*
Galanin, Moses
Gromoff, Smile*
Hanson, John Jr.*
Hapoff, Arthur*
Kochergin, Victor*
Kochtin, Andrey
Kozloff, Christopher*
Kozloff, John*
Krukoff, Agafon
Lekanof, Ermogen
Malavansky, Daniel
Mandregon, Tracy
Melovidov, Alexander
Merculief, Alexay
Merculief, Andrine
Merculief, Daniel
Merculief, Innokenty

Merculief, Isiah
Merculief, Nicolai S.
Merculief, Terenty
Merculieff, Nicander*
Nozekof, Gregory
Oustigoff, Peter
Philemonoff, Terenty
Prokopiof, Alexay
Prokopiof, Michael
Stepetin, Alexey
Stepetin, Nicolai
Swetzof, Ferapont
Swetzoff, Simeon

*Men who were given leave from military service to participate in the 1943 seal harvest on St. Paul. Information from *St. Paul Island Logbook*, June 14, 1943. (U.S. Fish and Wildlife Service, Records, 1868–2008, National Archives and Records Administration, Pacific Alaska Region, Record Group 22, including Pribilof Island Logbooks, compiled 1870–1961, Record Group 56, Alaska File of the Office of the Secretary of the Treasury 1868–1903 [M720]).

Source: Ward T. Bower, *Alaska Fishery and Fur-Seal Industries: 1944*, U.S. Fish and Wildlife Service, U.S. Department of the Interior (Washington, DC: GPO, 1946), 58–59. For information on Aleut military service during the war, see Raymond Hudson, "Aleuts in Defense of Their Homeland," in *Alaska at War, 1941–1945* (ed. Fern Chandonnet, Anchorage: Alaska at War Committee, 1995).

Notes

Introduction

1. These two books concern the mid-1970s. *Slaves of the Harvest,* by Barbara Boyle Torrey, was published by the TDX Corporation (St. Paul Island, AK) in 1978. She began the book in 1975–1976 while living on St. Paul. The last chapter was drafted by Agafon Krukoff (email from Torrey, May 8, 2007). *A Century of Servitude: Pribilof Aleuts Under U.S. Rule,* by Dorothy Knee Jones (Washington, DC: University Press of America, 1980), was the result of a study of the islands prompted by a 1975 suit the islanders filed against the United States.
2. The consolidation was part of President Roosevelt's Reorganization Plan No. 3, Public Resolution 75, 76th Congress.
3. Fredericka Martin's typed journal, April 17, 1942 (Fredericka I. Martin Collection, 1890–1969, USUAF210, University Archives, Alaska and Polar Regions Collections, University of Alaska Fairbanks). Because of books published since 1942 (Arnold Griese, *The Wind Is Not a River* [New York: Thomas Y. Crowell, 1978]; Dean Kohlhoff, *When the Wind Was a River* [Seattle: University of Washington Press, 1995]), it has seemed propitious to change Martin's proposed title. Martin considered using *Fog, Wind and Ice* because, during the months leading to the Japanese invasion of Alaska, they were the "only three friends to count on to protect us" (typed journal, Jan. 31, 1942). *Before the Storm* is taken from the final paragraph of her manuscript.
4. Martin to Harrington, May 18, 1942 (John Peabody Harrington Papers, National Anthropological Archives, Department of Anthropology, National Museum of Natural History, Smithsonian Institution, Washington, DC).
5. Martin's typed journal, July 9, 1941.
6. In 1964–1965 and again in 1976 Martin donated historical documents from St. Paul to the University of Alaska archives and manuscript collections. Her removal of the documents was fortuitous because during the World War II evacuation all Aleutian and Pribilof villages were ransacked and virtually every document of significance was lost.
7. This biographical material is from the guide to the Fredericka Martin Papers written by Jessica Weglein and Jennifer Waxman, Tamiment Library, Robert F. Wagner Labor Archives, Elmer Holmes Bobst Library, New York City.
8. "Seven American Nurses Survive Rebel Air Raids in Year's Service," *New York Times,* Feb. 6, 1938, p. 85. This article is entirely about Martin and features a photograph of her.
9. In 1967 Martin began assembling extensive material for a history of the Medical Bureau volunteers. This is now in the Tamiment Library, Robert F. Wagner Labor Archives, Elmer Holmes Bobst Library, New York City.

Chapter 1

1. This sentence comes from a July 24, 1941, letter to "Dearest Carl and the gang" (Fredericka I. Martin Collection, 1890–1969).
2. Rudyard Kipling, "The White Seal," in *The Jungle Book* (London: Macmillan, 1894). This is a story about Kotick, a white seal born on St. Paul Island.
3. The power vessel *Penguin* was launched at Seattle on Jan. 8, 1930. She was 129.6 feet long with a breadth of 27.7 feet and drew 17.1 feet. Registered at 394 gross tons, she had 268 net tons and carried a complement of four officers and seven men.
4. When the *Penguin* anchored at St. Paul she carried forty-one passengers plus the crew.
5. Johnston had succeeded Harry J. Christoffers, who had died in September 1939.
6. The 1939 population for St. Paul was 299 and for St. George, 183. The largest city in the territory was Juneau with 5,729 residents; Ketchikan had 4,695; Anchorage had 3,495; and Fairbanks had 3,455.
7. The city was named after Ketchikan Creek: "It has been suggested that the name means `eagle wing river' derived from the fact that `a boulder in the stream of the falls broke the water giving the appearance of the spread wings of an eagle.' This suffused meaning has not been verified and may be a form of folklore." Donald J. Orth, *Dictionary of Alaska Place Names* (Washington, DC: GPO, 1967), 511.
8. The ship anchored at 9:00 p.m. on June 24, 1941.

Chapter 2

1. "He has been coming to the island since 1928 and is an old inhabitant." Martin's typed journal, part 1, page 22.

Chapter 3

1. *Anilgux̂* in Knut Bergsland, *Aleut Dictionary, Unangam Tunudgusii* (Alaska Native Language Center, University of Alaska Fairbanks, 1994).

Chapter 4

1. The navy transferred the radio station to the Bureau of Fisheries on Aug. 10, 1937. Ward T. Bower, *Alaska Fisheries and Fur Seal Industries in 1937,* 1938, 127–128 (reference courtesy of John A. Lindsay).
2. Henry W. Elliott, *Our Arctic Province: Alaska and the Seal Islands* (New York: Charles Scribner's Sons, 1886), 347. See also the eyewitness account by Vincent Colyer, *Fur-Seal Fisheries of Alaska* (41st Cong., 2d sess., H. Ex. Doc. 144 [Feb. 9, 1870], serial 1418, 1870), 2–3.
3. Henry W. Elliott, *Report on the Seal Islands of Alaska* (47th Cong., 2d sess., H. Misc. Doc. 42, pt. 8, 1884), 48–49.
4. Elliott, *Our Arctic Province,* 235.
5. Ibid., 230–231.
6. As noted in the introduction, translations from Veniaminov were made by Richard H. Geoghegan and sent to Martin. For a published translation, see Ivan Veniaminov, *Notes on the Islands of the Unalashka District* (ed. Richard A. Pierce, trans. Lydia T. Black and R. H. Geoghegan, Fairbanks: The Elmer E. Rasmuson Library Translation Program, University of Alaska Fairbanks / Kingston, Ontario: Limestone Press, 1984; distributed by University of Alaska Press), 48–49.

7. Rev. Makary Baranoff was the resident priest on St. Paul. The spelling is that used by the priest himself in a letter to John P. Harrington, Aug. 4, 1942 (Smithsonian Institution, Natural History Archives, Washington, DC).
8. See Jones, *A Century of Servitude,* 19–20, for an account of Charles Bryant's attempts to help Aleuts secure title to their homes.
9. Elliott decided *Nah Speel* was a corruption of the Russian phrase *Nah Speetsah,* "on the point," but he could not understand the process of the spelling change [Elliott, *Report on the Seal Islands of Alaska,* 164]. Other recorders refer to "Spilki" or "Naspilki," "sharp points" or "on sharp points." Father Baranoff and I wrangled cheerfully for months about the meaning, the exact location of the sharp points and what they actually were. Father protested that Russians employed "spilki" principally for high pointed objects like flagpoles. He concluded that the Americans had copied Russian precedent in erecting a flagpole on the top of the hill. Therefore there had always existed a valid reason for using the term. I argued that the cliff's face bristled with spears of rock that fitted the plural form of the word perfectly. Also a seal rookery atop a flagpole was absurd. Neither of us convinced the other but we had lots of fun. When Dr. Harrington arrived I had an authoritative ally to back me up. (F.M.)
10. Elliott, *Report on the Seal Islands of Alaska,* 52.

Chapter 5

1. Elliott, *Our Arctic Province,* 137.
2. *Iĝadagax̂.* See Knut Bergsland, *Ancient Aleut Personal Names* (Alaska Native Language Center, University of Alaska Fairbanks, 1998), 200.
3. Veniaminov, *Notes on the Islands of the Unalashka District,* 134–135.
4. Ibid., 135. Elliott, *Our Arctic Province,* 194; *Report on the Seal Islands of Alaska,* 146.
5. Martin used Veniaminov's account of the discovery. Pierce says Pribylov was gone from Unalaska only twenty-four hours before discovering St. George. Richard Pierce, *Russian America: A Biographical Dictionary* (Kingston, Ontario: Limestone Press, 1990; distributed by University of Alaska Press), 412.
6. Elliott, *Our Arctic Province,* 193.
7. Veniaminov, *Notes on the Islands of the Unalashka District,* 135.
8. Pierce (*Russian America: A Biographical Dictionary,* 413) says Pribylov died in April 1796, probably at Okhotsk.

Chapter 8

1. Elliott, *Our Arctic Province,* 317.

Chapter 9

1. Joseph DeLee (1869–1942) was an influential obstetrician in the early twentieth century.
2. Veniaminov, *Notes on the Islands of the Unalashka District,* 140.
3. Ibid., 141.
4. Actually the temperature never dropped below twenty degrees above zero Fahrenheit. The bite of the winds did demand clothing suitable for withstanding a much colder temperature. The thermometer registered between thirty and fifty degrees above zero all winter. (F.M.)
5. Petroff used *parka* his reports, but when the census report was republished in 1900, the spelling was changed to *parkee.* Ivan Petroff, "Report on the Population, Resources, etc. of Alaska," in *Compilation of Narratives* (U.S. Senate, Committee on Military Affairs, 1900), 230.

Chapter 10

1. Elliott, *Report on the Seal Islands of Alaska,* 158. *St. Paul Island Logbook,* Oct. 22, 1876, described the gale as "a gale blowing with a force of sixty miles per hour accompanied with sleet and rain" (National Archives and Records Administration, Pacific Alaska Region, U.S. Fish and Wildlife Service, Records, 1868–2008, Record Group 22, including Pribilof Island Logbooks, compiled 1870–1961). The two Aleut companions were Anton Melovedoff and Ivan Galonin.

Chapter 11

1. "USCGC *Atlanta* anchored off East Landing at 4:00 A.M. Liberty party came ashore at 9:30 A.M. and visited a rookery; vessel left at 11:30 P.M. Among those who came ashore was Dr. Ruth Gruber of the Department of Interior who is making a survey of social conditions of Alaska natives." *St. Paul Island Logbook,* July 28, 1941.
2. On May 15, 1941, the House of Representatives had voted sixty-four to forty-nine to remove Gruber from the payroll of the Interior Department because of her book *I Went to the Soviet Arctic* (New York: Simon and Schuster, 1939). The department had announced that she was to conduct a survey of economic conditions in Alaska. The closing sentence of her book was read as an example of her "communistic philosophy." It said, "But I know that some day I shall go back, and bathe again in the Yenisei at Molokov Island, take midnight walks in Igarka, work with its newspaper people and pioneers, get up at dawn at a polar station, swim in the Arctic Ocean and rush back to a steaming breakfast shouting 'Zdravstvuitye' until that full-mouthed greeting seems to ring across the Arctic." Representative Mason of Illinois declared, "That's enough [proof] for me." Representative Bulwinkle of North Carolina retorted, "The only thing she said is she wants to take a bath." *New York Times,* May 15, 1941, p. 16.
3. The Battle of Madrid was a major engagement of the Spanish Civil War.
4. The *Penguin* left at 2:00 p.m., July 29, 1941. Born in 1911, Ruth Gruber was a journalist for the *New York Herald Tribune* and the *New York Post.* In 1944 she was asked to escort a thousand Jewish refugees from Italy to the United States. Following this experience, she worked tirelessly on behalf of Jewish refugees. In 2001 CBS featured this period of her life in the miniseries *Haven.* She has written fifteen books. The second volume of her autobiography, *Inside of Time: My Journey from Alaska to Israel,* was published in 2004 (New York: Carroll and Graf.) In June 2005 her 1931 doctoral thesis on Virginia Woolf was published for the first time in the United States. At the age of ninety-four, she celebrated this event with two parties and continued to work on the third volume of her life's story (Myrna Blyth, "A Woman of Substance," *National Review Online,* July 2, 2005). Gruber described Fredericka Martin in her autobiography: "Mrs. Berenberg was a large, handsome woman dressed in bright green slacks and a matching shirt, which brought out the reddish color of her hair. She was to have a baby in a month, but she joined us on our excursions around the island, doing whatever it took to keep up with the group. Without being paid for it, she was helping her husband run the hospital, using the experience she had gained as a trained hospital organizer. The two of them had determined to make the most of their stay on the island. They were studying the Aleut language, which few people ever learned, and reading everything they could get their hands on about the people, the islands, and the fur seals." Gruber, *Inside of Time,* 84–85.

Chapter 12

1. Elliott, *Our Arctic Province,* 313.

2. Here Martin is using Veniaminov's nineteenth-century definition of an amphibian as an aquatic animal that has the ability to live or remain a long time in water.
3. Martin found much of her information about sea lions in Edward A. Preble, *A Biological Survey of the Pribilof Islands* (North American Fauna No. 46, U.S. Department of Agriculture, Washington, DC: GPO, 1923). Martin's typed journal, July 8, 1941.
4. See Georg Wilhelm Steller, *Journal of a Voyage with Bering, 1741–1742* (ed. with an introduction by O. W. Frost, trans. by Margritt A. Engel and O. W. Frost, Stanford, CA: Stanford University Press, 1988), 150, for an account of sea lion meat.
5. Elliott, *Our Arctic Province,* 363.
6. William J. McIntyre was not related to the brothers Dr. H. H. McIntyre and Hamden McIntyre, both of whom were employed by the Alaska Commercial Company.
7. Elliott, *Report on the Seal Islands of Alaska,* 89n; *Our Arctic Province,* 365n.
8. Elliott, *Report on the Seal Islands of Alaska,* 91; *Our Arctic Province,* 369–370.

Chapter 14

1. This was true for the Pribilof Islands but not for the Aleutian Islands as a whole. See William Laughlin, *Aleuts: Survivors of the Bering Land Bridge* (New York: Holt, Rinehart and Winston, 1980), 10–15.
2. William Byrd Hunter was the physician on St. Paul from July 1914 to October 1916 and again from November 1917 to August 1918. He left the island on Dec. 10, 1918. See his eighteen-page report covering Sept. 1, 1917, to Nov. 1, 1918, for details of his work. National Archives and Records Administration, Pacific Alaska Region, Record Group 22 (hereafter NARA), Box 25 (U.S. Fish and Wildlife Service, Records, 1868–2008).
3. George and Cora Giles Haley were teachers at St. George from 1914 to 1915 and at St. Paul from 1915 to 1916.
4. Ward T. Bower and Henry D. Aller, *Alaska Fisheries and Fur Industries in 1917* (Appendix II to the Report of the U.S. Commissioner of Fisheries for 1917, U.S. Department of Commerce, Washington, DC: GPO, 1918), 74.

Chapter 15

1. Nov. 25, 1941.

Chapter 17

1. *St. Paul Island Logbook* for Aug. 14, 1876, notes that the old surgery, built in 1869 by Captain Pomeroy, agent of Hutchinson and Kohl, was torn down. It was said to have been the first wooden building built after the transfer and was still in good condition. This is one more example of Martin's use of primary source material, however lacking her manuscript is in documentation.
2. Aug. 8, 1877.
3. An epidemic of influenza, measles, and smallpox swept across Alaska in 1900. "The Great Sickness," as it was called, "struck with lightning force and within days whole villages were sick or dying." Robert Fortuine, *Chills and Fever: Health and Disease in the Early History of Alaska* (Fairbanks: University of Alaska Press, 1992), 215–226. It reached Unalaska in late August. Mortality records are scant, but informal reports say thirty residents died. Smaller villages across the Aleutian chain were similarly struck, with a third of the population of Kashega Village dying.

Chapter 18

1. George M. Bowers to Walter I. Lembkey, March 31, 1909, in U.S. Congress, *Seal Islands of Alaska, Letter from the Secretary of Commerce and Labor Transmitting in Response to House Resolution No 73, Information Relating to the Seal Islands of Alaska* (62d Cong., 1st sess., H. Doc. 93, 1911), 706–709.
2. Walter L. Hahn had arrived on St. Paul on Aug. 23, 1910. The day described was May 31, 1911. John Hanson left the island in July to attend the Salem Indian Training School at Chemawa, Oregon, until 1915.
3. Walter I. Lembkey, "Fur-Seal Service in 1911," in *Alaska Fisheries and Fur Industries in 1911*, by Barton Warren Evermann (Bureau of Fisheries Doc. 766, Washington, DC: GPO, 1912), 90.
4. Bower and Aller, *Alaska Fisheries and Fur Industries in 1917*, 74.
5. Robert E. Davis began work on St. Paul in October 1922.
6. Passed by Congress in 1919, the National Prohibition Act was known as the Volstead Act after its author, Representative Andrew Volstead. It was repealed in 1933 by the adoption of the Twenty-first Amendment.
7. See appendix 2 for excerpts from Berenberg's annual report.
8. Seventeen cases in all were treated. The Coast Guard cutter *Alert* rushed antitoxin from Unalaska to St. Paul. This helped to check the spread of the disease. Ward T. Bower, *Alaska Fishery and Fur-Seal Industries in 1936* (Administrative Report No. 28, Bureau of Fisheries, U.S. Department of Commerce, Washington, DC: GPO, 1937), 329.

Chapter 19

1. Ben East, "Baldy of the Aleutians" *(American Forests* 48, no. 10 [October], 1942); "The Aleutians . . . Rocky Bridge to Tokyo . . ." (*American Forests* 49, no. 12 [December], 1943).
2. Expedition Island with its grove of Sitka spruce.

Chapter 20

1. July 30, 1941, 7:30 a.m.
2. This is an error. The priest in 1894 was Nikolai Rysev, who served St. Paul from 1893 until 1901.
3. Aug. 17, 1941.

Chapter 21

1. Map: The Zapadnie Rookeries, in Henry W. Elliott, *Report Upon the Present Condition of the Fur-Seal Rookeries of the Pribilof Islands of Alaska* (54th Cong., H. Doc. 175, 1896), opposite p. 39.
2. The name was first reported in 1891 by Joseph Stanley-Brown, U.S. Geological Survey. He was soon to become the North American Commercial Company's agent at Unalaska. Stanley-Brown's rookery surveys were included in Vol. 3 (1893) of *Fur Seal Arbitration, Proceedings of the Tribunal of Arbitration, Convened at Paris, etc.*, 13 vols. (Washington, DC: GPO, 1895).
3. Bergsland translates *Maanam Anii* as "steambath's lake," from *maanax̂*, "steambath." *Aleut Dictionary*, 273h.
4. Both lupine and monkshood were termed bumblebee's house by Aleut speakers. See Bergsland, *Aleut Dictionary*, 71, and Suzi Golodoff, *Wildflowers of Unalaska Island: A Guide to the Flowering Plants of an Aleutian Island* (Fairbanks: University of Alaska Press, 2003), 74.

Chapter 22

1. "Two planes of bomber design displaying U.S. markings surveyed the island, arriving at 2:35 P.M. Left in a northerly direction a quarter of an hour later." *St. Paul Island Logbook*, Aug. 14, 1941.

Chapter 23

1. Later finds were made at Einahnuhto Bluffs, on the west coast under Rush Hill. Tom F. W. Barth, *Geology and Petrology of the Pribilof Islands, Alaska* (Geological Survey 1956, Bulletin 1028-F, Washington, DC: GPO, 1956), 118–119.
2. Voznesenskii was at St. Paul briefly in June 1843 when he left Filat Druzhinin to make collections. He returned in September for a short stay. A. I. Alekseev, *The Odyssey of a Russian Scientist: I. G. Voznesenskii in Alaska, California and Siberia 1839–1849* (ed. by Richard A. Pierce, trans. by Wilma C. Follette, Kingston, Ontario: Limestone Press, 1987; distributed by University of Alaska Press), 39–45.
3. Veniaminov, *Notes on the Islands of the Unalashka District,* 139.

Chapter 24

1. "This is reported as the first live walrus seen on St. Paul since 1924." Statement by Ford Wilke, assistant biologist, *St. Paul Island Logbook*, Aug. 24, 1941.

Chapter 27

1. For the Whitneys' role in exposing mistreatment of St. Paul residents, see Jones, *A Century of Servitude,* 55–56.
2. Martin generalizes here, as can be seen in the next paragraph where she places Whitneys' comments "two decades" after 1890. In fact, as John A. Lindsay has pointed out, the Whitneys arrived shortly after the termination of four decades of government leasing to private companies.
3. "Report of Assistant Agent Joseph Murray, inclosure with Goff's Annual Report for 1890," in Vol. 1 of *Seal and Salmon Fisheries and General Resources of Alaska* (U.S. Department of the Treasury, Special Agents Division, 4 vols., serial 3576, Washington, DC: GPO, 1898), 236.
4. This was probably *Flora of the Aleutian Islands and Westernmost Alaska Peninsula with Notes on the Flora of Commander Islands* (Stockholm: Bokförlags Aktiebolaget Thule), published in 1937. Hultén began work in the Aleutians in 1932.
5. Martin is incorrect regarding the year Shayashnikoff [Shaiashnikov] and the government agent were at odds. He was not ordained until 1877. It was in 1887 that the agent referred in his log to the priest as "un-American" and "a notable instance of . . . clerical cussedness" (*St. Paul Island Logbook*, June 10, 1887). Her general description of education during the late 1800s is accurate.
6. Educated in San Francisco, Melovidov began teaching around 1889 and continued until approximately 1910. The earliest schoolteachers on St. Paul were S. N. Buynitsky (1870), Mrs. C. P. Fish (1873–1876), Juniatte B. Pierce (1876–1877), James Buterin (1878–1882), "Professor Atkans" (1882–1883), Nicholas Gray (1883–c. 1889), and Simeon Melovidov (c. 1889–1911).
7. Simeon Melovidov's salary changed over the years. For a number of seasons, he worked as "an able sealer" during the summer and was paid under one of the categorized "shares" that laborers received.
8. Martin's source for this report has not been located and requires confirmation.

9. The report by the agent in charge, Walter I. Lembkey, for 1913 omitted any reference to education. The report for 1914 raised several objections to the relocation suggestion. See Wilfred H. Osgood, Edward A. Preble, and George H. Parker, *The Fur Seals and Other Life of the Pribilof Islands, Alaska, in 1914* (63rd Cong., 3rd sess., S. Doc. 980, Washington, DC: GPO, 1915), 140–141.

Chapter 28

1. Attendance at Chemawa began in 1911 and continued until 1921 or possibly later. For details see Jones, *A Century of Servitude,* 59–61, and Torrey, *Slaves of the Harvest,* 121–122.
2. For another account of an Aleut at Chemawa, see Henry Swanson, *The Unknown Islands: Life and Tales of Henry Swanson* (ed. by Raymond Hudson, Unalaska, AK: Cuttlefish VI, Unalaska City School District, 1982), 34–38.

Chapter 29

1. Harrington arrived on the *Penguin* on Sept. 18 and remained until Dec. 11, 1941.
2. The reference may be to Barton Warren Evermann, a noted ichthyologist, who collaborated with Jordan on various projects.
3. Eric Hultén, *Flora of the Aleutian Islands* (Weinheim/Bergstr., Germany: J. Cramer / New York: Hafner, 1960), 68.
4. Martin spelled the name "Yatchmenoff." Harrington used "Yatchmenev," "Yatchmenoff," and "Yatchmeneff." Both Alexei and John signed their surname "Yatchmeneff." This spelling was used to distinguish their family from the Yatchmenoff family based in Kashega Village on Unalaska Island.
5. The minutes of the Unalaska Panteleimon Brotherhood meeting of Oct. 1, 1928 (Russian Church Collection, Library of Congress, Washington, DC), noted that John Yatchmenev had been elected vice-chairman because he could speak English.
6. David Starr Jordan and George Archibald Clark, "The History, Condition, and Needs of the Herd of Fur Seals Resorting to the Pribilof Islands," in Part I of *The Fur Seal and Fur-Seal Islands of the North Pacific Ocean,* by David Starr Jordan (Washington, DC: GPO, 1898), 39.
7. See Bergsland, *Aleut Dictionary,* 13, for *adgu-n* under *hadgu-lix,* "pile of rocks heaped up by hunters on their trail."
8. See Bergsland, *Aleut Dictionary,* 567.
9. See Bergsland, *Aleut Dictionary,* xxxvii–xliv, for a listing of published and manuscript material in Aleut.

Chapter 30

1. Tobyanne Berenberg informed the editor that her mother kept a framed photograph of Geoghegan on her desk until the end of her life.

Chapter 31

1. Michael Oleksa, ed., *Alaskan Missionary Spirituality* (Mahwah, NJ: Paulist Press, 1987), 306–307. See also Lydia T. Black, trans. and ed., *The Round the World Voyage of Heiromonk Gideon 1803–1809* (Kingston, Ontario: Limestone Press, 1989; distributed by University of Alaska Press).
2. Veniaminov sought and received linguistic help from several Aleuts, most importantly from the chief Ivan Pan'kov.

3. Martin's source for this driftwood chapel is unknown. Information from Veniaminov on the St. Paul church is found in *Notes on the Islands of the Unalashka District,* 140 and 238.
4. This church was built in 1840. Barbara Sweetland Smith, *A Sure Foundation: Aleut Churches in World War II* (with Patricia J. Petrivell, Anchorage: Aleutian/Pribilof Islands Association, 1994), 61–62. For a history of the St. Paul church, see Smith, *The Church of the Holy Apostles Saints Peter and Paul on Saint Paul Island, Pribilof Islands: A History—1821–2001* (Anchorage: Aleutian/Pribilof Islands Restitution Trust, 2007).
5. He served from 1936 to 1960.
6. When the agent was upset over a domestic dispute caused by the abuse of alcohol, he threatened to withhold the use of any government services in the construction of the church if the people did not comply with his dictates: "It might be herewith stated that they are trying to build a new church, and as this is not a Government building, they were told they would not have the use of this office for any business connected with the building of the church. They were given a few days to think this over before any definite steps are to be taken." *St. Paul Island Logbook*, Oct. 27, 1941.
7. This is an error. The central and western islands were served by a priest resident at Atka.
8. Several Aleut priests served the Pribilof Islands, the Aleutians, and Kodiak during the twentieth century. See Smith, *A Sure Foundation.*
9. The treasury agent, George R. Tingle, wrote to Rev. Paul Shayashnikoff on Aug. 18, 1885. Tingle, in the log, states that he issued this order "in the absence of any provision of law" and he concluded his letter to the priest with the words, "Neglect or refusal to comply with this order will render any Will null and void." *St. Paul Island Logbook*, Aug. 18, 1885.
10. St. Paul Log, June 10, 1887. In this entry, Tingle writes about Shayashnikoff's "clerical cussedness."
11. In 1889 H. H. McIntyre, superintendent of the Alaska Commercial Company operations in the islands, answered the question, "Who appoints the chief?" in this way: "The chief at the present time is appointed by the Government agent in charge. Formerly the people elected him; but such abuses arose under that system that the Government assumed the authority several years ago, and have since continued to exercise it." U.S. Congress, *Fur-Seal Fisheries of Alaska* (50th Cong., 2d sess., H. Rep. 3883, serial 2674 and 2675, 1889), 335.
12. In 1895 the secretary of the interior directed that "There should be no interference by the Agents of the United States, or by the North American Commercial Company [the successor to the Alaska Commercial Company as lessee of the Pribilofs] or any of its agents or employes [*sic*], or other persons, with the inhabitants of the Seal Islands in the selection of their chiefs." Nevertheless, he went on to say, "The Government Agent in charge of the Islands may, if in his opinion the interests of the United States requires such action, refuse to recognize the chiefs selected by the native inhabitants, and may call upon them to elect new chiefs." J. G. Carlisle, Secretary of the Interior, to J. B. Crowley, Special Agent on the Seal Islands, May 9, 1895. U.S. Department of the Treasury. Alaska File of the Office of the Secretary of the Treasury 1868–1903, National Archives and Records Administration, Record Group 56 (M720).
13. *St. Paul Island Logbook*, Oct. 12–15, 1888.
14. Murray, "Report of Assistant Agent Joseph Murray," Nov. 1, 1891, Exhibit R, vol. 1, 293–295.
15. The history of the Jesse Lee Home is complex. There were periods, primarily before 1900, when children from the Pribilof Islands and elsewhere were not permitted to attend the Orthodox church and active attempts were made to proselytize them. For details, see Raymond Hudson, *Family After All: Alaska's Jesse Lee Home*, Vol. 1, *Unalaska 1889–1925* (Walnut Grove, CA: Hardscratch Press, 2007).

Chapter 32

1. Elliott, *Report on the Seal Islands of Alaska,* 55.
2. Ibid., 55–56.
3. The original intention in introducing reindeer was to supply "food for the inhabitants of the islands [and] . . . for use in transportation." Evermann, *Fishery and Fur Industries of Alaska in 1912* (Bureau of Fisheries Doc. 780, Washington, DC: GPO,1913), 12.
4. The animals did not actually arrive until the end of August 1911. Of the forty head taken at Unalakleet, twenty-one cows and four bulls were left at St. Paul and twelve cows and three bulls at St. George. By the end of 1912, there were sixty-five reindeer on the two islands.

Chapter 33

1. In 1946 Fredericka Martin published *The Hunting of the Silver Fleece: Epic of the Fur Seal* (New York: Greenberg). In 1960 a more condensed form appeared as *Sea Bears: The Story of the Fur Seal* (Philadelphia: Chilton).
2. Martin based much of her history of the early American period on a letter William Healy Dall wrote to B. W. Evermann, U.S. Bureau of Fisheries, Dec. 7, 1910 (William Healey Dall, Papers, c. 1839–1858, 1862–1927, Record Unit 7073, Smithsonian Institution Archives, Washington, DC).
3. "An Act to extend the Laws of the United States relating to Customs and Navigation over the territory ceded to the United States by Russia . . ." Section 6, July 27, 1868. 15 Stat. 241.
4. Elliott, *Report Upon the Present Condition of the Fur-Seal Rookeries,* 158.
5. For a review and critique of Dall's work, see Morgan B. Sherwood, "William Healy Dall, Dean of Alaskan Experts," in *Exploration of Alaska, 1865–1900* (New Haven, CT: Yale University Press, 1965). 36-56.
6. Deposition of John A. Henriques, Tribunal of Arbitration, *Fur Seal Arbitration,* Vol. 3, 31.
7. U.S. Congress, *Fur-Seal Fisheries of Alaska* (41st Cong., 2d sess., H. Ex. Doc. 129, serial 1417, 1869), 2.
8. Charles Bryant was appointed special treasury agent in 1868 and served on the Pribilofs from 1869 to 1877. Hugh Henry McIntyre served as special treasury agent from 1868 to 1870, and in 1871 he became an employee of the Alaska Commercial Company.
9. U.S. Congress, *The Alaska Commercial Company* (44th Cong., 1st sess., H. Rep. 623, serial 1712, 1876).
10. Elliott, *Report on the Seal Islands of Alaska,* 27.
11. He was twenty-five. At the age of eighteen he had been a member of the Collins Overland (Western Union) Telegraphy Expedition for which he did work in British Columbia.
12. For information on her, see Lisa Marie Morris, *Keeper of the Seal: The Art of Henry Wood Elliott and the Salvation of the Alaska Fur Seal* (PhD thesis, University of Alaska Fairbanks, 2001), 35–36. See also Robert L. Shalkoop, *Henry Wood Elliott 1846–1930: A Retrospective Exhibition* (Anchorage: Anchorage Historical and Fine Arts Museum, 1982), 11–12. She had been born in Sitka, but she was only sixteen when she married Elliott. (Note courtesy of John A. Lindsay.)
13. He became chief in 1884 and resigned in 1891. Tribunal of Arbitration, *Fur Seal Arbitration,* Vol. 3.
14. In the acknowledgments to *The Hunting of the Silver Fleece* (p. viii), Martin mentions receiving information from Simeon Melovidov and his niece Grace Elliott.
15. Sherwood, *Exploration of Alaska, 1865–1900,* 50.
16. See Tribunal of Arbitration, *Fur Seal Arbitration,* Vol. 5, 739–747.
17. Jordan, *The Fur Seal and Fur-Seal Islands of the North Pacific Ocean.*
18. Martin had written the visit occurred in 1915 but, as John A. Lindsay pointed out, it occurred in 1913, while the hearings were under way.

19. U.S. Congress, *Minority Report, Fur-Seal Industry of Alaska* (July 27, 1914) (63rd Cong., 2d sess., H. Rep. 500, pt. 2, serial 6559, 1914).
20. G. Dallas Hanna has pointed out that in 1918 there were 34,890 seals taken compared with 8,169 in 1917. Hanna, *The Alaska Fur-Seal Islands* (ed. by John A. Lindsay, U.S. Department of Commerce, NOAA Technical Memorandum NOS ORR 16, 2008), 59. Information courtesy of John A. Lindsay.
21. This was the largest take since 1889. The sales for 1941 totaled $2,343,214. Bower, *Alaska Fishery and Fur-Seal Industries: 1941* (Statistical Digest No. 3, U.S. Fish and Wildlife Service, U.S. Department of the Interior, Washington, DC: GPO, 1943), 47, 55.

Chapter 34

1. U.S. Congress, *Information Relating to Seal Islands of Alaska* (62d Cong., 1st sess., H. Doc. 93, serial 6113, 1911), 387–392, 439–440.
2. Ben East wrote that from 1906 "the Aleuts of St. Paul and St. George dreaded Japanese vengeance." "Uncle Sam's Prize Fur Factory Closes Down" (*Natural History* 51, no. 4 [April], 1943), 189.

Chapter 35

1. Japan gave notice on Oct. 23, 1940, and the treaty terminated one year later. U.S. Fish and Wildlife officials noted in 1940 that "appropriate attention is being given to this matter by the Department of State." Bower, *Alaska Fishery and Fur-Seal Industries: 1940* (Statistical Digest No. 2, U.S. Fish and Wildlife Service, U.S. Department of the Interior, Washington, DC: GPO, 1942), 54.
2. On November 25 Martin had written to Harrington, "Your letter touched us both very deeply. What little we have been able to do to help you has been so very, very little and was selfish because we enjoyed doing it so much. We regret only that some seriously ill, the renovation of the hospital, and a few other tasks stemming from Sam's responsibilities here, prevented us working with you much more." She offered to make further linguistic inquiries for him during the winter. Harrington Papers, Correspondence, reel 1.
3. The visitation to the cemetery during starring continues to be part of the Orthodox Christmas on St. Paul.
4. The St. Paul Log for Jan. 27, 1942, said, "The *Penguin,* formerly painted white, now drafted for naval duty, displayed the official grey black naval color from stem to stern."
5. A letter Harrington wrote from Unalaska to Leonora F. Curtin on Dec. 17, 1941 (Harrington Papers), described his stay on St. Paul.

I have been on St. Paul Island, and had no idea I was going there. With the summer half gone and in a frenzy over the impending death of an old last-speaker, I took the Greyhound out of the bathing Washington heat to Seattle, there to get on the *Penguin,* Government boat[,] to take me to presumably Unalaska sans expenditure. On the boat, which belongs to the Fish and Wild Life, I met three Russian priests, and formed a friendship with one of them—Father Makariy A. Baranoff. This tall priest persuaded me to stay on the *Penguin* to accompany him to his parish, which is at St. Paul Island, the northern and principal one of the Pribiloff group, which group is the famous home of the fur-seal. It takes about a half dozen of the pelts of these seals to make a coat. Well, went ashore on that little island, the shore of which consists of one rookery after another of these marine mammals, and for more than EIGHTY days no ship put in at that island. Of course there were no mails out or in. This is the first chance that I have had to write. 250 Aleuts on the island, all talking the little known Aleutian language. You would have loved it. Seattle prices. They gave me free a big room in the Government House, looking out over the front of the Russian Church. They told me that the most intelligent Aleut in the whole bunch was Johnny Yatchminoff, son of the late Unalaska chief. He proved to be a wonder. He writes the language, using the Russian alphabet as the early missionaries did. He was employed during the day, so I had Father Baranoff during the day and evenings and all Sat. afternoons and Sundays "Yatch" came over. It was ideal. In those 80 odd days I accomplished about a year's work. Got names of the islands, all names of animals, plants. Hundreds of odd items. Yatch wrote the language and I just sat by and popped the questions. All his writings in red ink. It sure was a feast. Yes, and I forgot to mention the place names of the seal islands. At last the boat came—the same boat, the *Penguin*. It took ten days to reach Unalaska, since we lay for days around St. George putting ashore and taking aboard passengers and cargo. And here at Unalaska we have lain for a week. A convoy is being formed. It will take us to Seattle? or part way to Seattle? No one is allowed to say whither or when. The Japs might get wind of it. Unalaska base was to be bombed the same day as Pearl Harbor and the joint bombardment was announced by the Japanese propaganda radio. Those best qualified to judge say that this war will last at least five years, so it has turned out to be a lucky thing that I got the Aleutian while it was gettable and let the Arabic go till later. I have a rich bunch of Aleutian, all ready for the final dictation into form.

Chapter 36

1. U.S. Congress, *Food, Fuel, etc., for Natives of Seal Islands, Alaska* (52d Cong., 1st sess., H. Ex. Doc. 154 [March 5, 1892], serial 2955, 1892).
2. Ward T. Bower, Chief, Division of Alaska Fisheries, to Fredericka Martin, Sept. 29, 1942, in Jones, *A Century of Servitude*, 45–46.

Chapter 37

1. I could not find many instances of this in the logbooks. On Dec. 18, 1873, the government and Alaska Commercial Company agents attended a dinner and dance for Anton Melovedoff's nineteenth birthday at his mother's home.
2. There is little documentation for the ceremony Martin describes. Dall, quoting William Coxe almost word for word without attribution, wrote that in celebrations following the taking of a whale "some of the men were dressed in their most showy attire, and others danced naked in large wooden masks which came down to their shoulders, and represented various sea animals." William H. Dall, *On Masks, Labrets and Certain Aboriginal Customs with an Inquiry into the Bearing of Their Geographic Distribution* (Bureau of American Ethnology, Third Annual Report for 1881–1882, Washington, DC: Smithsonian Institution, 1884), 139. For Coxe, see *Account of the Russian Discoveries Between Asia and America* (London: Readex Microprint Corporation, originally published 1787, 1966), 153–154. Because Dall followed his account with a sentence on festivals held in December, it is sometimes assumed that this was a winter dance. There is little in Coxe to confirm this supposition.
3. *Wind, Sand and Stars*, by Antoine de Saint-Exupéry, was published in 1939.
4. The story grew as it was told to Martin. The St. Paul Log for the day after Russian Christmas, Jan. 8, 1941, states that "thirty quass barrels and metal container that had been used to make quass in" were confiscated.
5. Captain Bryant read the instructions of the secretary of the treasury and Francis Lessen translated them into Russian. St. Paul Log, May 19, 1874.
6. St. Paul Log, Sept. 13, 1885.
7. This list was based on Veniaminov's work in the 1820s.
8. *The Forgotten Village*, by Rosa Harvan Kline and Alexander Hackensmid, story by John Steinbeck (New York: The Viking Press, 1941).

Chapter 39

1. Walter I. Lembkey, "The Fur-Seal Fisheries of Alaska in 1910," in *Seal Islands of Alaska,* 62d Cong., 1st sess., H. Doc. 93:1034, serial 6113, 1911), 29.
2. Ira N. Gabrielson was the director of the U.S. Fish and Wildlife Service. Harold L. Ickes was the secretary of the interior.

Chapter 40

1. Elliott, *Report on the Seal Islands of Alaska,* explanatory note to map of St. Paul.
2. Robert Marshall's *Arctic Village,* published in 1933, was a portrait of Wiseman, Alaska.

Chapter 41

1. Elliott, *Report on the Seal Islands of Alaska,* map of St. Paul.
2. See Bergsland, *Aleut Dictionary,* 1994, 207. *Inganax̂,* "a precipice, steep cliff." He gives the name for Einahnuhto as *Qayalgux̂,* "big hill."
3. Elliott, *Report on the Seal Islands of Alaska,* map of St. Paul.
4. *Maqdusix,* "breasts," is applied to Polovina Hill in Bergsland, *Aleut Dictionary,* 617.

Chapter 42

1. The treaty ended on Oct. 23, 1941.
2. Unalaska had been bombed by the Japanese on June 3 and 4, 1942. The Japanese took Attu on June 7, capturing the village and holding the residents until sending them to Japan on Sept. 17.
3. Alexandra Gromoff recalled that day during a conversation with a reporter in 1944: "I had gone on a picnic with the doctor and his family. I was in one of the shelter houses made for their baby when a messenger came with the terrible news. 'You must hurry back. We are all to be evacuated!' he shouted. We rushed to the village. There everyone was busy packing. To the kids it was fun, but the older people looked very sober. We were allowed to take only what we could put into one suitcase. That meant leaving all our furniture and we had such nice things that we had bought from Sears and Roebuck. Mom did put into her suitcase some cups and saucers that she treasured. I suppose our house is an awful mess now, for some soldiers have been quartered in it for two years." Mary L. Beech, "Refugees from the Pribilofs" (*Alaska Life,* Aug. 18–21, 1944), 18.

Chapter 43

1. St. Paul Log, Monday, June 15: "Received orders yesterday to evacuate the entire population of St. Paul Island. Entire gang turned to at 6:00 A.M. this morning in hauling baggage and freight in preparation for complete evacuation this afternoon." The U.S. Coast Guard cutter *Onandaga* had come in to East Landing on June 14 and had left at 3:55 p.m. At 2:50 on the same afternoon, a U.S. Navy boat M-7 had anchored off East Landing. The U.S. Army transport *Delarof* arrived and this was the vessel on which 294 Aleuts and 15 non-Aleuts departed the island. At St. George they were joined by 183 Aleut residents and 7 non-Aleut Fish and Wildlife employees. The *Delarof* was accompanied by the *Onandaga.*
2. This is an error. Most residents were allowed to depart with only one suitcase of belongings. In 2002 Mary Bourdukofsky recalled receiving orders for evacuation. Her husband, George, had been playing baseball following Sunday church services when a large ship arrived. He ran home to inform his wife: "'What happened?' Mary asked. George excitedly told her how 'a great big

boat' like the annual supply ship had come to the village, flanked by two smaller vessels. 'They want all us men to come down for a meeting,' George answered. He left again and came back angry. Fearing a Japanese invasion, the government had ordered an evacuation, but George said only white employees of the US Fish and Wildlife Service . . . would be taken. 'I was crying,' Bourdukofsky recalls. 'They had already taken the Attu people as prisoners. He said, 'Don't cry. We're having another meeting. The Elders are really mad and they're trying to figure out how they can help the women and children.' When George returned from the second meeting he announced that everyone was going to be evacuated, but no one could bring more than one little suitcase, or one little box." Bill Hess, ed., "Return to Funter Bay," in *Alaska's Village Voices* (Rural Alaska Community Action Program, Inc., Vol. 6, Issue 4 [November], 2002), 13.

3. Father Baranoff wrote that the St. George people were allowed to take only clothing (Baranoff to John P. Harrington, Aug. 5, 1942, Harrington Papers).
4. Writing about Aleut men joining the military, Martin stated, "Only when all citizens were called to arms, the litter of ancient falsehood and current misunderstandings was swept away and the stigmatizing label, 'Government ward,' exposed as legally invalid. Aleut despair, which that degrading label had fostered for decades, evaporated; hope for restoration of their human dignity was kindled." Martin, *Sea Bears*, 173.

Afterword

1. Martin to Harrington, Sept. 21, 1942 (Harrington Papers).
2. Harrington to Leonora Curtin (?), Jan. 2, 1942 (Harrington Papers).
3. Harrington to Dionisiy, Dec. 30, 1941 (Harrington Papers).
4. Harrington to Yatchmenev, Jan. 3, 1942 (Harrington Papers). Harrington lived until 1961 but his Aleut work was never published.
5. Kohlhoff gave both June 17 and 18 as the date the *Delarof* left Unalaska. *When the Wind Was a River*, 74, 72. Kirtland and Coffin provide evidence that the *Delarof* was at Unalaska on June 19. John C. Kirtland and David F. Coffin Jr., *The Relocation and Internment of the Aleuts During World War II* (Anchorage: Aleutian/Pribilof Islands Association, Inc., 1981), 26.
6. Kohlhoff, *When the Wind Was a River*, 74.
7. Harrington to Dionisiy, Dec. 30, 1941 (Harrington Papers).
8. Harrington to Yatchmenev, Jan. 3, 1942 (Harrington Papers).
9. Commission on Wartime Relocation and Internment of Civilians, *Personal Justice Denied: Report of the Commission on Wartime Relocation and Internment of Civilians* (Washington, DC: GPO, 1982), 338.
10. Hess, *Alaska's Village Voices*, 17.
11. St. Paul Island Logbook, June 27–Aug. 2, 1942.
12. St. Paul Island Logbook, June 27–Aug. 2, 1942. There were no individual daily entries for this period.
13. Excerpts from this unpublished diary are used by permission of Tobyanne Berenberg.
14. Report of N. Berneta Block, M.D., in Kirtland and Coffin, *The Relocation and Internment of the Aleuts During World War II*, 45.
15. Fredericka Martin to Charles and Ruby Magee, Oct. 22, 1943, in Kirtland and Coffin, *The Relocation and Internment of the Aleuts During World War II, Index to Evidence, Vol. III, Conditions at the Camps*, 57–58.
16. Richard Henry Geoghegan, *The Aleut Language: The Elements of Aleut Grammar with a Dictionary in Two Parts Containing Basic Vocabularies of Aleut and English* (ed. by Fredericka I. Martin, Washington, DC: U.S. Department of the Interior, 1944), 2.
17. Martin, *The Hunting of the Silver Fleece*, 289.

18. In 1994 he was appointed adjutant general of the Alaska National Guard.
19. "The Aleuts—Past Tense and Future Present: An Interview with Gabe Stepetin." Interview conducted by Thomas Richards Jr., *The Tundra Times* (Fairbanks), Sept. 12, 1979, pp. 7, 10.
20. See testimony from Pribilof residents in material collected for the Commission on Wartime Relocation and Internment of Civilians in 1981 on file at the Aleutian/Pribilof Islands Association, Inc. See Torrey, *Slaves of the Harvest,* Jones, *A Century of Servitude,* and Kohlhoff, *When the Wind Was a River,* along with Commission on Wartime Relocation and Internment of Civilians, *Personal Justice Denied.*
21. "Memorandum, Superintendent Edward C. Johnston, 'Housing and Related Matters at Funter,' Feb. 11, 1944," in Kirtland and Coffin, *The Relocation and Internment of the Aleuts During World War II, Index to Evidence, Vol.III, Conditions at the Camps,* 63.
22. Will F. Speers, "Annual Medical Report for 1945—St. Paul" (March 1, 1944, to March 1, 1945), NARA, Box 1 of 1 (Pribilof Island Program Records, Annual Reports, 1929–1963).
23. Daniel C. R. Benson, "Agents Annual Report" (April 5, 1945). NARA, Box 1 of 1 (Pribilof Island Program Records, Annual Reports, 1929–1963).
24. Fredericka Martin, "Wanted: A Pribilof Bill of Rights" (*The American Indian* 3, no. 4 [Fall], 1946), 15, 24, 26.
25. Fredericka Martin to Dorothy Jones, Jan. 12, 1979, quoted in Jones, *A Century of Servitude,* 125.
26. Jones, *A Century of Servitude,* 120.
27. Hearings before the Subcommittee of the Committee on Interior and Insular Affairs, U.S. Senate, 80th Cong., 2d sess., on Senate 2037, Feb. 24–March 5, 1948.
28. Jones, *A Century of Servitude,* 131.
29. *The Tundra Times,* Nov. 23 and Dec. 7, 1964.
30. Pribilof Islands Transition Act, U.S. Congress (106th Cong., 2d sess., H. Rep. 106–569, April 11, 2000), 7.
31. In addition to the older works by Torrey (*Slaves of the Harvest*) and Jones (*A Century of Servitude*), there have been numerous recent studies by individuals and government agencies. See the work of Helen D. Corbett and Susanne M. Swibold at www.amiq.org/aleuts.html.
32. Alaska Native Review Commission, Transcript of Proceedings, Village Meetings, Vol. 53, St. Paul, Dec. 3, 1984, pp. 15–16.
33. Lisa Marie Short, *Fredericka I. Martin* (Master's thesis, Pacific Rim Master of Arts Program, Alaska Pacific University, Anchorage, 1995), 8.

Appendix 2

1. National Archives and Records Administration, Pacific Alaska Region, U.S. Fish and Wildlife

Bibliography

Unpublished Material

Berenberg, Dr. Samuel R. Diary, 1942. Collection of Tobyanne Berenberg.

Dall, William Healey. Papers, c. 1839–1858, 1862–1927. Record Unit 7073, Smithsonian Institution Archives, Washington, DC.

Harrington, John Peabody. Papers. National Anthropological Archives, Department of Anthropology, National Museum of Natural History, Smithsonian Institution, Washington, DC.

Martin, Fredericka I. Manuscript of *The Wind Is No River,* typed journal, and letters. Fredericka I. Martin Collection, 1890–1969, USUAF210, University Archives, Alaska and Polar Regions Collections, University of Alaska Fairbanks.

Unalaska Panteleimon Brotherhood. Minutes. Russian Church Collection, Library of Congress, Washington, DC.

U.S. Department of the Treasury. Alaska File of the Office of the Secretary of the Treasury 1868–1903, National Archives and Records Administration, Record Group 56 (M720).

U.S. Fish and Wildlife Service. Records, 1868–2008. National Archives and Records Administration, Pacific Alaska Region, Record Group 22, including Pribilof Island Logbooks, compiled 1870–1961.

Published Works

Alekseev, A. I.

1987 *The Odyssey of a Russian Scientist: I. G. Voznesenskii in Alaska, California and Siberia 1839–1849.* Edited by Richard A. Pierce. Translated by Wilma C. Follette. Kingston, Ontario: Limestone Press (distributed by University of Alaska Press).

Barth, Tom F. W.

1956 *Geology and Petrology of the Pribilof Islands, Alaska.* Geological Survey 1956, Bulletin 1028-F. Washington, DC: GPO.

Beech, Mary L.

1944 "Refugees from the Pribilofs." *Alaska Life,* August, 18–21.

Bergsland, Knut

1994 *Aleut Dictionary, Unangam Tunudgusii.* Alaska Native Language Center. University of Alaska Fairbanks.

1998 *Ancient Aleut Personal Names.* Alaska Native Language Center. University of Alaska Fairbanks.

Black, Lydia T., trans. and ed.

1989 *The Round the World Voyage of Heiromonk Gideon 1803–1809.* Kingston, Ontario: Limestone Press (distributed by University of Alaska Press).

Bower, Ward T.

1937 *Alaska Fishery and Fur-Seal Industries in 1936.* Administrative Report No. 28. Bureau of Fisheries. U.S. Department of Commerce. Washington, DC: GPO.

1938 *Alaska Fishery and Fur-Seal Industries in 1937.* Administrative Report No. 31. Bureau of Fisheries. U.S. Department of Commerce. Washington, DC: GPO.

1942 *Alaska Fishery and Fur-Seal Industries: 1940.* Statistical Digest No. 2. U.S. Fish and Wildlife Service. U.S. Department of the Interior. Washington, DC: GPO.

1943 *Alaska Fishery and Fur-Seal Industries:* 1941. Statistical Digest No. 3. U.S. Fish and Wildlife Service. U.S. Department of the Interior. Washington, DC: GPO.

1944 *Alaska Fishery and Fur-Seal Industries:* 1942. Statistical Digest No. 8. U.S. Fish and Wildlife Service. U.S. Department of the Interior. Washington, DC: GPO.

——— *Alaska Fishery and Fur-Seal Industries:* 1943. Statistical Digest No. 10. U.S. Fish and Wildlife Service. U.S. Department of the Interior. Washington, DC: GPO.

1946 *Alaska Fishery and Fur-Seal Industries:* 1944. Statistical Digest No. 13. U.S. Fish and Wildlife Service. U.S. Department of the Interior. Washington, DC: GPO.

Bower, Ward T., and Henry D. Aller

1918 *Alaska Fisheries and Fur Industries in 1917.* Appendix II to the Report of the U.S. Commissioner of Fisheries for 1917. U.S. Department of Commerce. Washington, DC: GPO.

Colyer, Vincent

1870 *Fur-Seal Fisheries of Alaska.* 41st Cong., 2d sess., H. Ex. Doc. 144 (Feb. 9, 1870), serial 1418.

Commission on Wartime Relocation and Internment of Civilians

1982 *Personal Justice Denied: Report of the Commission on Wartime Relocation and Internment of Civilians.* Washington, DC: GPO.

Coxe, William

1966 *Account of the Russian Discoveries Between Asia and America.* London: Great Americana, Readex Microprint Corporation. Originally published 1787.

Dall, William H.

1884 *On Masks, Labrets and Certain Aboriginal Customs with an Inquiry into the Bearing of Their Geographic Distribution.* Bureau of American Ethnology, Third Annual Report for 1881–1882. Washington, DC: Smithsonian Institution.

East, Ben

1942 "Baldy of the Aleutians." *American Forests* 48, no. 10 (October).

1943 "The Aleutians . . . Rocky Bridge to Tokyo . . ." *American Forests* 49, no. 12 (December).

———"Uncle Sam's Prize Fur Factory Closes Down." *Natural History* 51, no. 4 (April).

Elliott, Henry W.

1877 "Ten Years' Acquaintance with Alaska, 1867–1877." *Harper's Magazine,* November.

1884 *Report on the Seal Islands of Alaska.* 47th Cong., 2d sess., H. Misc. Doc. 42, pt. 8.

1886 *Our Arctic Province: Alaska and the Seal Islands.* New York: Charles Scribner's Sons.

1896 *Report Upon the Present Condition of the Fur-Seal Rookeries of the Pribilof Islands of Alaska.* 54th Cong., H. Doc. 175.

Evermann, Barton Warren

1913 *Fishery and Fur Industries of Alaska in 1912.* Bureau of Fisheries Doc. 780. Washington, DC: GPO.

Fortuine, Robert

1992 *Chills and Fever: Health and Disease in the Early History of Alaska.* Fairbanks: University of Alaska Press.

Geoghegan, Richard Henry

1944 *The Aleut Language: The Elements of Aleut Grammar with a Dictionary in Two Parts Containing Basic Vocabularies of Aleut and English.* Edited by Fredericka I. Martin. Washington, DC: U.S. Department of the Interior.

Golodoff, Suzi

2003 *Wildflowers of Unalaska Island: A Guide to the Flowering Plants of an Aleutian Island.* Fairbanks: University of Alaska Press.

Griese, Arnold

1978 *The Wind Is Not a River.* New York: Thomas Y. Crowell.

Gruber, Ruth

1939 *I Went to the Soviet Arctic.* New York: Simon and Schuster.

2004 *Inside of Time: My Journey from Alaska to Israel.* New York: Carroll and Graf.

Hanna, G. Dallas

2008 *The Alaska Fur-Seal Islands.* Edited by John A. Lindsay. U.S. Department of Commerce, NOAA Technical Memorandum NOS ORR 16.Washington, DC: GPO.

Hess, Bill, ed.

2002 *Alaska's Village Voices.* Rural Alaska Community Action Program, Inc. Vol. 6, Issue 4 (November). Special edition featuring several articles on the World War II evacuation of Aleuts.

Hudson, Raymond

1995 Aleuts in Defense of Their Homeland. In *Alaska at War, 1941–1945,* edited by Fern Chandonnet. 161–164. Anchorage: Alaska at War Committee.

2007 *Family After All: Alaska's Jesse Lee Home.* Vol. 1, *Unalaska 1889–1925.* Walnut Grove, CA: Hardscratch Press.

Hultén, Eric

1937 *Flora of the Aleutian Islands and Westernmost Alaska Peninsula with Notes on the Flora of Commander Islands.* Stockholm: Bokförlags Aktiebolaget Thule.

1960 *Flora of the Aleutian Islands.* Weinheim/Bergstr., Germany: J. Cramer / New York: Hafner.

Jones, Dorothy Knee

1980 *A Century of Servitude: Pribilof Aleuts Under U.S. Rule.* Washington, DC: University Press of America.

Jordan, David Starr

1897 *Matka and Kotik: A Tale of the Mist-Islands.* San Francisco: Whitaker and Ray.

1898 *The Fur Seal and Fur-Seal Islands of the North Pacific Ocean.* Washington, DC: GPO.

Jordan, David Starr, and George Archibald Clark

1898 The History, Condition, and Needs of the Herd of Fur Seals Resorting to the Pribilof Islands. Part I of *The Fur Seal and Fur-Seal Islands of the North Pacific Ocean,* by David Starr Jordan. Washington, DC: GPO.

Kipling, Rudyard

1894 The White Seal. In *The Jungle Book.* London: Macmillan.

Kirtland, John C., and David F. Coffin Jr.
1981 *The Relocation and Internment of the Aleuts During World War II.* Anchorage: Aleutian/Pribilof Islands Association, Inc.
1981 *The Relocation and Internment of the Aleuts During World War II. Index to Evidence, Vol.III, Conditions at the Camps.* Anchorage: Aleutian/Pribilof Islands Association, Inc.
Kohlhoff, Dean
1995 *When the Wind Was a River: Aleut Evacuation in World War II.* Seattle: University of Washington Press, in association with Aleutian/Pribilof Islands Association, Anchorage.
Laughlin, William
1980 *Aleuts: Survivors of the Bering Land Bridge.* New York: Holt, Rinehart and Winston.
Lembkey, Walter I.
1911 The Fur-Seal Fisheries of Alaska in 1910. In *Seal Islands of Alaska,* 62d Cong., 1st sess., H. Doc. 93:1034, serial 6113.
1912 Fur-Seal Service in 1911. In *Alaska Fisheries and Fur Industries in 1911,* by Barton Warren Evermann, 89–99. Bureau of Fisheries Doc. 766. Washington, DC: GPO.
1913 Fur-Seal Service. In *Fishery and Fur Industries of Alaska in 1912,* by Barton Warren Evermann, 74–98. Bureau of Fisheries Doc. 780. Washington, DC: GPO.
1914 Fur-Seal Service. In *Alaska Fisheries and Fur Industries in 1913,* by Barton Warren Evermann, 140–172. Bureau of Fisheries Doc. 797. Washington, DC: GPO.
Marshall, Robert
1991 *Arctic Village.* Originally published in 1933. Classic Reprints No. 1. Fairbanks: University of Alaska Press.
Martin, Fredericka
1946 *The Hunting of the Silver Fleece: Epic of the Fur Seal.* New York: Greenberg.
——— "Wanted: A Pribilof Bill of Rights." *The American Indian* 3, no. 4 (Fall).
1960 *Sea Bears: The Story of the Fur Seal.* Philadelphia: Chilton.
Morris, Lisa Marie
2001 *Keeper of the Seal: The Art of Henry Wood Elliott and the Salvation of the Alaska Fur Seal.* PhD thesis. Department of Art, University of Alaska Fairbanks.
Oleksa, Michael, ed.
1987 *Alaskan Missionary Spirituality.* Mahwah, NJ: Paulist Press.
Orth, Donald J.
1967 *Dictionary of Alaska Place Names.* Washington, DC: GPO.

Osgood, Wilfred H., Edward A. Preble, and George H. Parker
1915 *The Fur Seals and Other Life of the Pribilof Islands, Alaska, in 1914.* 63rd Cong., 3rd sess., S. Doc. 980. Washington, DC: GPO.

Petroff, Ivan
1900 Report on the Population, Resources, etc. of Alaska. In *Compilation of Narratives,* U.S. Senate, Committee on Military Affairs, 55–281. Also issued as Senate Report 1023, 56th Cong., 1st sess. Washington, DC: GPO.

Pierce, Richard
1990 *Russian America: A Biographical Dictionary.* Kingston, Ontario: Limestone Press (distributed by University of Alaska Press).

Preble, Edward A.
1923 *A Biological Survey of the Pribilof Islands.* North American Fauna No. 46. U.S. Department of Agriculture. Washington, DC: GPO.

Shalkoop, Robert L.
1982 *Henry Wood Elliott 1846–1930: A Retrospective Exhibition.* Anchorage: Anchorage Historical and Fine Arts Museum.

Sherwood, Morgan B.
1965 *Exploration of Alaska, 1865–1900.* New Haven, CT: Yale University Press.

Short, Lisa Marie
1995 *Fredericka I. Martin.* Master's thesis, Pacific Rim Master of Arts Program, Alaska Pacific University, Anchorage.

Smith, Barbara Sweetland
1994 *A Sure Foundation: Aleut Churches in World War II.* With Patricia J. Petrivell. Anchorage: Aleutian/Pribilof Islands Association.
2007 *The Church of the Holy Apostles Saints Peter and Paul on Saint Paul Island, Pribilof Islands: A History—1821–2001.* Anchorage: Aleutian/Pribilof Islands Restitution Trust.

Steller, Georg Wilhelm
1988 *Journal of a Voyage with Bering, 1741–1742.* Edited with an introduction by O. W. Frost. Translated by Margritt A. Engel and O. W. Frost. Stanford, CA: Stanford University Press.

Swanson, Henry
1982 *The Unknown Islands: Life and Tales of Henry Swanson.* Edited by Ray Hudson. Unalaska, AK: Cuttlefish VI. Unalaska City School District.

Torrey, Barbara Boyle
1978 *Slaves of the Harvest.* St. Paul Island, AK: TDX Corporation.

Tribunal of Arbitration
1895 *Fur Seal Arbitration. Proceedings of the Tribunal of Arbitration, Convened at Paris, etc.* 13 vols. Washington, DC: GPO.

U.S. Congress

1876 *The Alaska Commercial Company.* 44th Cong., 1st sess., H. Rep. 623, serial 1712.

1884 *Fur-Seal Fisheries of Alaska. Letter from the Secretary of the Treasury, etc.* 41st Cong., 2d sess., H. Ex. Doc. 136, serial 1417.

1889 *Fur-Seal Fisheries of Alaska (The Fur-Seal and Other Fisheries of Alaska. Investigation of the Fur-Seal and Other Fisheries of Alaska).* 50th Cong., 2d sess., H. Rep. 3883, serial 2674 and 2675.

1892 *Food, Fuel, etc., for Natives of Seal Islands, Alaska.* 52d Cong., 1st sess., H. Ex. Doc. 154, serial 2955.

1911 *Information Relating to Seal Islands of Alaska.* 62d Cong., 1st sess., H. Doc. 93, serial 6113.

——— *Seal Islands of Alaska, Letter from the Secretary of Commerce and Labor Transmitting in Response to House Resolution No 73, Information Relating to the Seal Islands of Alaska.* 62d Cong., 1st sess., H. Doc. 93.

1914 *Minority Report, Fur-Seal Industry of Alaska* (July 27, 1914). 63rd Cong., 2d sess., H. Rep. 500, pt. 2, serial 6559.

U.S. Department of the Treasury, Special Agents Division

1898 *Seal and Salmon Fisheries and General Resources of Alaska.* 4 vols., serial 3576. Washington, DC: GPO.

Veniaminov, Ivan

1984 *Notes on the Islands of the Unalashka District.* Edited with an introduction by Richard A. Pierce. Translated by Lydia T. Black and R. H. Geoghegan. Fairbanks: The Elmer E. Rasmuson Library Translation Program, University of Alaska Fairbanks / Kingston, Ontario: Limestone Press (distributed by University of Alaska Press).

Index

Page numbers in **bold** refer to figures. Pages referencing endnotes include page, chapter, and note number (360n27:9 = page 360, note for chapter 27, endnote number 9.)

-Y-

-Z-